TREATING SEX OFFENDERS

Treating Sex Offenders

AN EVIDENCE-BASED MANUAL

Jill D. Stinson
Judith V. Becker

THE GUILFORD PRESS
New York   London

© 2013 The Guilford Press
A Division of Guilford Publications, Inc.
370 Seventh Avenue, Suite 1200, New York, NY 10001
www.guilford.com

Paperback edition 2018

Printed in the United States of America

This book is printed on acid-free paper.

Last digit is print number: 9 8 7 6 5 4 3

The authors have checked with sources believed to be reliable in their efforts to provide
information that is complete and generally in accord with the standards of practice
that are accepted at the time of publication. However, in view of the possibility of
human error or changes in behavioral, mental health, or medical sciences, neither the
authors, nor the editor and publisher, nor any other party who has been involved in the
preparation or publication of this work warrants that the information contained herein
is in every respect accurate or complete, and they are not responsible for any errors
or omissions or the results obtained from the use of such information. Readers are
encouraged to confirm the information contained in this book with other sources.

Library of Congress Cataloging-in-Publication Data

Stinson, Jill D.
  Treating sex offenders : an evidence-based manual / Jill D. Stinson,
Judith V. Becker.
    p. cm. Includes bibliographical references and index.
  ISBN 978-1-4625-0693-4 (hardback)
  ISBN 978-1-4625-3663-4 (paperback)
  1. Sex offenders—Rehabilitation. 2. Sex offenders—Psychology.
3. Sex offenders—Mental health. I. Becker, Judith V. II. Title.
  RC560.S47S76 2012
  365′.661—dc23
                                                          2012027423

About the Authors

Jill D. Stinson, PhD, is Assistant Professor in the Department of Psychology at East Tennessee State University. Dr. Stinson formerly served as the Sex Offender Treatment Coordinator at Fulton State Hospital with the Missouri Department of Mental Health. She has worked with sexual offenders with serious mental illness, intellectual/developmental disabilities, and personality disorders, as well as with sexually violent predators. Her research focuses broadly on psychopathology and sexual offending, self-regulatory processes in persons with a history of sexual offending and violent behavior, and specialized assessment and treatment needs of forensic populations. Dr. Stinson is a member of the Association for the Treatment of Sexual Abusers and the American Psychology–Law Society.

Judith V. Becker, PhD, is Professor in the Department of Psychology at the University of Arizona. Dr. Becker is a past president of the Association for the Treatment of Sexual Abusers and the International Academy of Sex Research, has served as editor of *Sexual Abuse: A Journal of Research and Treatment,* and continues to serve on a number of editorial boards. Her clinical research has focused on both adolescent and adult sex offenders as well as victims of sexual abuse and aggression. Dr. Becker is the author or coauthor of over 100 published journal articles and book chapters in the professional literature. She also consults on both criminal and civil forensic cases.

Preface

Why do people commit sex offenses, and what do we do with them? These questions continue to be of major concern to our society. We have viewed sexual offenders strictly as criminals—they commit sex offenses because of a personal choice, prompted by some combination of personal and situational variables—and unworthy of rehabilitation. At other times, sexual offenders have been viewed more sympathetically, through a lens of sexual and mental disorder, and attempts have been made to provide treatment and rehabilitation. At present, what we do with sex offenders seems driven primarily by social control policies that have been enacted in an effort to make society safer. Mandatory sentencing, sex offender registration and notification, indeterminate civil commitment, and other current practices emerge from this mindset. Yet the effectiveness of such policies in reducing the rate of sexual crime has not yet been empirically validated.

Although policies focused on control and safety have predominated over the years, there have also been attempts at treating sex offenders. Early treatment approaches utilized psychoanalysis, nonspecific group process therapy, and aversive conditioning (to decrease sexual arousal), among other models. During the 1970s and 1980s, a more comprehensive treatment approach was introduced, one based on principles of cognitive-behavioral therapy as well as relapse prevention, a treatment adapted from the substance abuse literature. The majority of such programs were designed as "one-size-fits-all" group therapies, seldom taking into account the heterogeneity of the population and specific needs an offender may have (e.g., intellectual or developmental disabilities, complex behavioral problems, serious mental illness). Disappointing results of outcome research from these models led to modifications in how offenders are classified. For example, the risk–needs–responsivity (RNR) model has gained in popularity partly because of its recognition of differing levels of risk, treatment need, and response to treatment among sex offenders. The more recent introduction of the positive psychology movement has led to the development of the good lives model and revisions to standard relapse prevention protocols.

In our previous book (Stinson, Sales, & Becker, 2008) we critically reviewed and evaluated existing etiological explanations for sexual offenses and developed one of our own based on the idea that self-regulation and self-regulatory deficits underlie sexual offending as well as other types of maladaptive or problematic behavior. This model—the multi-modal self-regulation theory—has undergone preliminary analysis and continues to demonstrate empirical validity. From this theory, we have developed a corresponding intervention approach, called safe offender strategies (SOS). This treatment has been in the pilot stages at three sites since the fall of 2007, with client populations consisting of forensic mental health inpatients, persons with intellectual and developmental disabilities, and high-risk sex offenders. For such challenging client cases, SOS has maintained a consistent theoretical framework while allowing for individualized differences in client need.

As treatment providers, we see ourselves as consultants to the patients; our role is to help motivate them, help them identify areas of potential change, and help them work through complex, interactive areas of need. Our basic philosophical premise is that people can change, and that our clients can reach the readiness to change in an environment of collaboration that will facilitate such a process.

Our treatment model consists of 10 modules, discussed in detail in this book. We provide not only the foundation for the approach we use but also the necessary tools and strategies to help clinicians with individualized treatment planning and the development of a productive and beneficial therapist–patient relationship. Key elements of this treatment include developing adaptive self-regulation skills, self-monitoring and self-management, forming healthy and normative interpersonal boundaries and social bonds, and addressing important life needs like emotional stability, balanced thinking, and a sense of self-control. Such needs cannot be met without compassionate and involved clinicians. Sex offender treatment is challenging for both clients and treatment providers. With this book we hope to help you with this task.

Acknowledgments

Writing this book involved the assistance and support of many people. Although we are unable to name all of them, we wish to gratefully acknowledge the contributions of the following individuals: Amanda Fanniff, Amy Hamel, Mary Jane Marcinkus, Tony Menditto, Lee Ann Morrison, Sharon Robbins, and Bruce Sales. We would also like to thank the faculty, staff, and clients of the Missouri Department of Mental Health, who assisted us in implementing and understanding this treatment.

Contents

CHAPTER 1

A New Approach to Treating Sex Offenders

Sex offender treatment is undoubtedly one of the more difficult and controversial areas of behavioral or mental health intervention. Treatment providers are faced with a number of challenges: sexual crimes that generate strong emotions and negative public sentiment, clients who are reluctant to participate in treatment and divulge deeply personal information about their sexual and violent behaviors, legislative policies that may stigmatize clients and detract from a focus on treatment, personal reactions and frustrations with the treatment process, ongoing concerns about victims and risk management, and questions regarding the effectiveness of available treatment approaches. Individually, any of these factors can make change more difficult. In combination, we face a daunting but not impossible task.

The field of sex offender treatment has evolved since its early days when psychoanalysis, aversive behavior conditioning, and a philosophy of containment prevailed. A number of services now exist for those in need of sex offender treatment. These draw from the broader mental health literature as well as from comparable literatures for addictions and criminology. Yet, as we discuss further below, existing treatment approaches have important limitations.

In this book, we introduce safe offender strategies (SOS), an innovative development in the evolution of sex offender treatment. SOS combines a skills-based curriculum with emerging research on the role of self-regulation in problematic sexual behaviors. This approach signifies a new direction in how we view our clients and the nature of their sexual offending. It builds upon a foundation of empirically supported etiological theory and psychotherapy to equip clinicians with new tools for sex

1

offender treatment. Unlike most other current approaches, SOS encourages treatment providers to foster a collaborative approach to treatment and elicit individualized change strategies that are consistent with the offender's stated goals and current treatment needs. In this book, we present the theoretical background, features of the client population, treatment techniques, and treatment intervention protocols that are integral to SOS. This text is intended for treatment providers who work with sexual offenders in a variety of settings, but particularly those who are interested in providing long-term or ongoing care for these challenging clients. Our main goals are to familiarize treatment providers with an evidence-based approach to sex offender treatment and to provide material that will be helpful in promoting treatment change across multiple domains.

In the remainder of this chapter, we discuss the current field of sex offender treatments, the limitations of each approach, and how SOS is designed to address these limitations. The chapter concludes with an overview of the rest of the book.

SEX OFFENDER TREATMENT: WHERE WE HAVE BEEN

Current forms of sex offender treatment include cognitive-behavioral approaches, relapse prevention, the good lives model, the risk–needs–responsivity model, sexual addictions, and pharmacological interventions. A brief review of these commonly used treatment interventions follows.

Cognitive-Behavioral Treatment

Recent surveys of North American sex offender treatment providers suggest that over half of all adult sex offender treatment programs use cognitive-behavioral treatment (CBT; McGrath, Cumming, Burchard, Zeoli, & Ellerby, 2010). This represents a wide range of possible interventions, given that there are few standardized or manualized CBT approaches for sex offender treatment. As with cognitive-behavioral treatments in general, the underlying theory is that people who commit sexual offenses do so because of offense-supportive beliefs and deviant sexual interests that have been reinforced and strengthened over time. Treatment is thus designed to alter these beliefs, expectations, and interests so that they are more normative and less supportive of offending behaviors. CBT also focuses on decreasing deviant sexual arousal and increasing or reinforcing normative sexual arousal. This is accomplished through a combination of cognitive restructuring, behavioral reconditioning of deviant sexual arousal, victim empathy training, and social skills training (e.g., Marshall, Anderson, & Fernandez, 1999).

A lack of standardization among different cognitive-behavioral sex offender treatment programs makes it difficult to compare outcomes, as there is much variability in which techniques are utilized, who is selected for treatment, and what outcomes or targets represent successful treatment completion (Rice & Harris, 2003). Though some studies evaluating the effectiveness of CBT for sex offenders have found positive treatment effects (e.g., Marshall, Jones, Ward, Johnston, & Barbaree, 1991; McGrath, Hoke, & Vojtisek, 1998), others have found no significant treatment effects or even found greater change effects in the control or comparison group than in the treatment group (e.g., Quinsey, Harris, Rice, & Lalumiere, 1993; Quinsey, Khanna, & Malcolm, 1998; Rice, Quinsey, & Harris, 1991). Although two recent meta-analyses of treatment effectiveness indicate success in reducing sexual recidivism among treated offenders overall (Hanson, Bourgon, Helmus, & Hodgson, 2009a; Lösel & Schmucker, 2005), Hanson et al. (2009a) caution that this effect is largely dependent on the design of the study rather than on any specific characteristics of the treatment itself. Stronger research designs have produced weak, mixed, or no results, whereas weaker research methodology has been more supportive of treatment effects (Hanson et al., 2009a). Further, few of the common targets of CBT, such as victim empathy, acknowledging the offense, or social skills training, have been significantly correlated with risk of future sexual behavior (Hanson & Morton-Bourgon, 2004, 2005). This finding suggests that targeting these and other related CBT goals may not result in the reduction of future sexual violence.

Relapse Prevention

The second most common approach reported by North American sex offender treatment providers (McGrath et al., 2010) is relapse prevention, a cognitively based therapy originally adapted from the substance abuse treatment literature (Laws, 1989; Laws, Hudson, & Ward, 2000; Pithers, Marques, Gibat, & Marlatt, 1983). Relapse prevention focuses on immediate risk factors that precipitate and perpetuate repeated sexual offending. But relapse prevention does not offer a specific explanation as to what initially prompts a sexual offense. Clients in treatment utilizing this approach are asked to recount their "cycle" of offending, describing environmental and internal factors associated with one or more of their offenses. The goal is to identify factors that present potential risk for future sexual offending and then to develop a concrete plan for avoiding or coping with these risks.

Critics have noted the inconsistency in clinical service across many programs labeling themselves as "relapse prevention," and marked differences in quality and duration of treatment services, research samples, and measures of treatment outcome (e.g., Hanson et al., 2009a). Much like CBT research, empirical evaluation of relapse prevention's effectiveness has been inconsistent and disappointing. The most prominent and well-designed study involving the use of relapse prevention with sexual offenders was the California Sex Offender Treatment and Evaluation Project (SOTEP). Initial findings suggested some positive trends (Miner, Marques, Day, & Nelson, 1990), but final project results confirmed that there were few, if any, significant differences between treatment and control subjects with regards to sexual recidivism during the posttreatment follow-up period (Marques, Wiederanders, Day, Nelson, & Van Ommeren, 2005).

Surveys have shown a steady decrease in the use of relapse prevention over time, particularly following the 2005 study cited above (e.g., McGrath et al., 2010). In addition to concerns regarding the lack of strong empirical support, other limitations include the adversarial approach and confrontational interpersonal style often associated with the delivery of relapse prevention (e.g., Mann, 2000; Serran, Fernandez, Marshall, & Mann, 2003), doubts about the effectiveness of avoidance as a viable strategy for lasting behavioral change (e.g., Mann, 2000; Mann, Webster, Schofield, & Marshall, 2004), and difficulties with implementing such a cognitively based treatment method with some populations of offenders (e.g., people with intellectual and developmental disabilities).

The Good Lives Model

A growing number of North American sex offender treatment practitioners are using the good lives model (McGrath et al., 2010), a strengths-based, positive psychology approach emphasizing client abilities and values (Ward & Brown, 2004; Ward & Mann, 2004; Ward, Mann, & Gannon, 2007; Ward & Stewart, 2003a, 2003b; Yates, Prescott, & Ward, 2010). The good lives model focuses on common goals and values, characteristics, or experiences associated with psychological well-being. These include concepts like healthy living, autonomy and self-directedness, inner peace, creativity, and social connectedness (Ward et al., 2007).

These values translate into treatment outcomes, so rather than targeting risk factors, practitioners help clients draw on these positive values to improve their circumstances and develop meaningful and satisfying lives. Conceptually, the basic principles of the good lives model harken back to CBT approaches, where beliefs, expectations, and behavioral contingencies interplay with values and goals to direct behavior. As a treatment approach, the good lives model could be described more accurately as a framework rather than a solidified treatment approach, though emerging work suggests that more specific methods of implementing the good lives model lie ahead (Yates et al., 2010).

Empirically, the good lives model has not yet been subjected to scientific study. Information available in the literature is mostly descriptive in nature. At present, no comparative or large-scale research has demonstrated the effectiveness of the good lives model in reducing sexual recidivism. In addition to limited empirical support and the lack of clear separation between the good lives model and the techniques of other treatments, this approach has also been criticized on the grounds of being paternalistic (Glaser, 2011).

The Risk–Needs–Responsivity Model

The risk–needs–responsivity (RNR) model (Andrews, Bonta, & Hoge, 1990; Bonta & Andrews, 2007) is a framework for treatment that is also commonly cited as an overarching treatment philosophy by many programs in North America (McGrath et al., 2010). The RNR model, in brief, posits that there are three crucial elements to be addressed during the course of offender treatment. First, the risk principle holds that we must tailor our interventions to the client's risk of future offending. Those at the highest level of risk should receive the most intensive and structured treatments, while those at the lowest levels of risk should receive less intensive and perhaps less restrictive or supervised forms of treatment and risk management. The needs principle examines the role of criminogenic needs, or targets associated with criminal and sexual offending like offense-supportive attitudes and sexual fantasies, poor social support networks, substance abuse, or other risky behaviors. And finally, the responsivity principle refers to factors that impact the individual's response to treatment, including motivation, engagement, cognitive or learning impairments, level of insight, and general progress in treatment.

These principles are applicable to sex offender treatment and risk management practices (e.g., Hanson, Bourgon, Helmus, & Hodgson,

2009b; Harkins & Beech, 2007; Becker & Stinson, 2011), though not directly prescriptive of treatment practices themselves. Treatment approaches already discussed that are consistent with this framework are CBT and relapse prevention, though it should be noted that because of the inherent focus on risk, the RNR model is generally incompatible with the good lives model (Ward et al., 2007; Ward & Stewart, 2003a, 2003b). Ample empirical evidence suggests that an RNR approach is useful and significant in reducing violent crime recidivism when working with correctional populations (e.g., Dvoskin, Skeem, Novaco, & Douglas, 2011), though this approach has not yet been thoroughly evaluated with sex offender treatment.

Sexual Addictions

Less frequently used but still noted among the literature and treatment provider surveys (e.g., McGrath et al., 2010) are approaches using an addictions model to address the problem of sexual offending. The sexual addiction treatment literature originates from the work of Carnes (1983) positing that sexual offending results from a sexual compulsion or addiction, comparable to alcoholism or substance dependence. The most common form of addictions treatment is a 12-step program promoting abstinence through faith-based support, disclosure, risk management and avoidance strategies, and the help of others undergoing similar problems. While these treatment programs are less often seen in Canadian or U.S. residential treatment programs, they are still prevalent in U.S. community-based treatment environments, where many choose to attend available support groups that use this philosophy (e.g., McGrath et al., 2010). There are virtually no controlled or descriptive empirical studies examining the effectiveness of such treatments (e.g., Gold & Heffner, 1998).

Pharmacological Interventions

Another intervention practice (often used in tandem with other approaches) involves using hormonal agents to reduce or alter sexual drive, more commonly known as "chemical castration." These hormonal agents, collectively known as antiandrogens (e.g., cyproterone acetate, gonadotropin-releasing hormone analogue, leuprolide acetate, and medroxyprogesterone acetate), work by either breaking down and eliminating testosterone, interfering with the production of testosterone by inhibiting leutinizing hormone, or increasing other hormones like estrogen and progesterone. Use of these agents may result in the reduction of sexual drive or physiological arousal, and the assumption is that this will produce a similar reduction in sex offending behavior. However, while some uncontrolled studies suggest that these agents do noticeably reduce sexual arousal (e.g., Maletzky, Tolan, & McFarland, 2006; see also Briken & Kafka, 2007), comparable reductions in sexual recidivism have not consistently accompanied such changes (e.g., Maletzky, 1991; McConaghy, Balszczynski, & Kidson, 1988). Furthermore, significant negative side effects (Giltay & Gooren, 2009), medical and legal ethical concerns, and compliance problems have plagued the use of such medications in many subsamples of men with histories of sexual offending.

A confusing picture emerges from this examination of current sex offender treatment practices. Though each approach has its strengths, notable limitations prevent us from knowing whether or not these interventions will promote change in persons with a history of sexual offending.

SAFE OFFENDER STRATEGIES

SOS offers a new, empirically based framework for treatment that is designed to address some of the problems of the other approaches described above.

Standardization

One of the most prominent criticisms for nearly all forms of sex offender treatment, including those most frequently used like CBT, relapse prevention, and the good lives model, is that there is little consistency across different sites and treatment providers. Each program calling itself "relapse prevention," for example, may look different. This is problematic from an empirical research perspective (e.g., Hanson et al., 2009a), and because one can never be sure that the treatment being claimed is in fact the treatment being implemented. Although these approaches have a common set of goals and treatment targets, there are no manualized protocols or structured texts readily available to assist treatment providers in consistently applying treatment principles. This is not so with SOS. This book presents a structured, manualized approach to treatment. It offers a common set of treatment principles, techniques, and protocols that are to remain consistent across sites and clinicians while allowing flexibility in individual treatment planning.

Multi-modal Self-Regulation Theory

Several of the treatments described above lack a strong, empirically based etiological foundation. This is especially true of relapse prevention, which does not address the development or cause of a client's sexual offense, but this is also true of other approaches that emphasize treatment targets not supported by the empirical literature as relevant factors in sexual offending (e.g., victim empathy, denial). Recent etiological research suggests that an important component in the development of many maladaptive behaviors, including sexual offending, is self-regulation and self-regulatory deficits (e.g., Stinson, Sales, & Becker, 2008; Ward & Gannon, 2006; Ward, Hudson, & Keenan, 1998). We have proposed a theoretical model focused on the role of self-regulation in the development and maintenance of maladaptive sexual behaviors. Called the multi-modal self-regulation theory, it explains these complex phenomena (Stinson, Sales, & Becker, 2008). Preliminary evaluations of the relationships between self-regulatory deficits and maladaptive outcomes have demonstrated significant correlations between these deficits and criminal behavior, substance use problems, suicidality or self-harm, and sexual behavior problems in selected samples of sexual offenders (i.e., sexually violent predators: Stinson, Becker, & Sales, 2008; seriously mentally ill sexual offenders: Stinson, Robbins, & Crow, 2011). We have incorporated these ideas into SOS so that the treatment identifies and targets offenders' self-regulatory deficits. Thus SOS not only addresses the immediate problem of sex offending but also improves the offender's ability to manage emotional, cognitive, and interpersonal distress that may lead to it.

Therapeutic Style and Clinical Strategies

Many approaches to sex offender treatment are characterized by detached and artificial therapeutic relationships, little attention to the client's goals in treatment, and client–therapist interactions that are harsh, confrontational, critical, and judgmental. Discussions of these problems have appeared in the sex offender treatment literature (e.g., Mann, 2000; Serran et al., 2003), and positive psychology approaches like the good lives model and individualized methods like the RNR model have sought to change how providers interact with clients and individualize their treatment. SOS also advocates a different philosophical and interactional style for effective intervention. It is based on the common elements that have been found to characterize effective psychotherapeutic treatment and includes the therapeutic alliance, therapeutic interpersonal style (e.g., warmth, empathy, and caring), therapist experience with a particular treatment, and client self-direction in treatment (e.g., Luborsky, Auerbach, Chandler, Cohen, & Bachrach, 1971; Messer & Wampold, 2002). These features have all been incorporated into SOS.

Empirical Support for Treatment Effectiveness

As noted, few current forms of sex offender treatment have generated strong empirical support. Research at best is mixed and at worst suggests no significant effect of sex offender treatment on sexual reoffending. The possible reasons range from inconsistent treatment implementation to weak research design to problems in the treatment itself. Also, some treatment-as-framework approaches do not readily lend themselves to rigorous empirical study. SOS has as yet only been subjected to pilot testing at three sites. Still, early findings (discussed in Chapter 2) suggest some support for the effectiveness of this treatment. Its standardization facilitates further research efforts.

SOS is also premised on a number of empirically based methods and therapeutic traditions, like the treatment targets and risk factors identified by the sex offender risk literature (e.g., the protective nature of social support, adaptive self-regulation, regulation of sexual urges and impulses, and prosocial beliefs and behaviors consistent with cognitive self-regulation; Hanson et al., 2009a) as well as the general criminology literature (e.g., the RNR model; Dvoskin et al., 2011; Hanson et al., 2009b). Furthermore, techniques like self-monitoring and skills-based therapy for the development of adaptive self-regulatory functioning are consistent with other empirically supported models like dialectical behavior therapy (DBT; Linehan, 1993), and other cognitively based approaches for mood and behavior management.

AN OVERVIEW OF THIS BOOK

In this chapter we have discussed the current approaches in the field of sex offender treatment and introduced some key features of SOS. Chapter 2 presents the theoretical basis of SOS, with a complete review of the multi-modal self-regulation theory and the empirical basis for this etiological framework. We also discuss how this theoretical viewpoint translates into a treatment approach. Some pilot data from early implementation using inpatient sexual offenders with serious mental illnesses and intellectual or developmental disabilities is also covered. SOS uses a modular treatment approach, with 10 distinct treatment modules, each spanning multiple sessions, that address clients' treatment targets and needs. Chapter 3 gives an overview of the 10 modules and their format along with a discussion of overall treatment length and structure. We additionally review other pragmatic considerations, such as therapist qualifications and target client population, as well as pretreatment tasks for the treatment provider and methods of measuring client progress. Chapter 4 emphasizes case conceptualization, individualized treatment planning, and fundamental conceptualizations of clients with the SOS frame. This chapter also includes discussion of building a therapeutic relationship with such challenging clients, and strategies for working with clients that will aid clinicians throughout the treatment process.

Subsequent chapters present the materials and protocols that are the fundamental components of SOS. Module 1 (Chapter 5) introduces the treatment. Treatment providers collaborate with clients to orient them to treatment and help them develop relevant treatment goals. In Module 2 (Chapter 6) clients are presented with a number of basic treatment concepts, including sexual health and education, the nature of sexual offenses, and the presentation of the theoretical causes of offending and the role of self-regulation for the clients. Module 3 (Chapter 7) is the first of three modules aimed at different domains of regulation. Here, we address emotional regulation, with a discussion of emotions, emotional distress, maladaptive behaviors, and emotion regulation skills. Sexual behaviors, including normative sexual interests, fantasies, masturbation, and pornography, are introduced in Module 4 (Chapter 8). Covering this material in therapy provides clients a basis for later discussions of sexual relationships and sex-related cognitions. Because personal commitment and individualized treatment goals are such a crucial component of this treatment, clients return to a review of their commitment to treatment, self-assessment of their readiness to change, and reevaluation of treatment goals in Module 5 (Chapter 9).

Module 6 (Chapter 10) turns to the cognitive domains of self-regulation, with a concentration on expectations and beliefs about interpersonal relationships and the ability to regulate thoughts and perceptions about others. This discussion examines important beliefs and expectations, how these may be linked to maladaptive sexual behaviors, and cognitive regulation skills. Interpersonal regulation is addressed in Module 7 (Chapter 11), reviewing the role of expectations and boundaries in relationships, conflict with others, problem solving, and interpersonal regulation strategies. The clients' own experiences of trauma or negative events as well as their reactions to their own harmful behaviors are included as the subject of Module 8 (Chapter 12). In this module, treatment providers cover key elements of the impact of trauma, acceptance versus forgiveness, and repairing damaged relationships with others. Finally, Modules 9 (Chapter 13) and 10 (Chapter 14) conclude the treatment with a review of self-management strategies, adaptive skills, and future treatment and aftercare needs, as well as a review of the client's commitment to ongoing treatment and progress made thus far. Tables and sample worksheets throughout these chapters will aid treatment providers in conceptualizing group discussion.

The book closes with a discussion of the role of families in treatment, aftercare, and community reintegration concerns, including the relationship between treatment progress and dynamic measures of risk (Chapter 15). Tables within this chapter provide additional materials and information to assist with aftercare planning.

Chapter 2 now details the theoretical and empirical basis for SOS. This foundation is important, as it facilitates our understanding of intricate relationships between the 10 modules of treatment and the therapeutic techniques designed to promote client growth and change. Learning these underlying principles will assist treatment providers in case conceptualization, the formation of therapeutic relationships, and ultimately the implementation of the therapy itself.

CHAPTER 2

Theoretical Foundation of Safe Offender Strategies

Sexual behavior is highly complex. Explaining "normal" sexual behavior is difficult enough, given great individual variability in sexual preferences, practices, and beliefs. But when trying to explain abnormal, deviant, or even harmful sexual behaviors, the complexity increases. People are not "born" as sexual offenders, nor do they awaken one morning to suddenly decide to commit a sexual offense. Thus, in order to understand the causes of sex offending behaviors, we should allow for some degree of complexity and specificity in our etiological explanations. Many etiological theories of sexual behavior problems have been proposed, but few of these are able to capture the multifaceted nature of this behavior. Hence, we have developed the multi-modal self-regulation theory (Stinson, Sales, & Becker, 2008), the theoretical foundation upon which SOS is based.

In this chapter, we describe the major tenets of the multi-modal self-regulation theory, relate these tenets to maladaptive patterns of behavior, including problematic or illegal sexual behaviors, and discuss the relationship between dysregulation and maladaptive behavior. These concepts arise from prior empirical work in this and other related fields. Also, because problematic sexual behaviors often co-occur with other maladaptive behaviors, signs of psychiatric illness, interpersonal difficulties, or other potential targets for intervention and treatment, we will highlight important relationships within a multidisciplinary literature that have contributed to our treatment conceptualizations.

MULTI-MODAL SELF-REGULATION THEORY

The multi-modal self-regulation theory was initially proposed by Stinson, Sales, and Becker (2008) in an effort to better understand the development of sex offending behaviors. This theory draws primarily from the clinical and developmental psychological literature, as well as from criminology and other domains of behavioral science. A fundamental premise of this theory is that individuals with deficits in self-regulation will engage in maladaptive behaviors—a premise that has already been evaluated in persons with self-injurious behavior (Linehan, 1993), aggression and criminality (Hirschi, 2004), alcohol or illicit substance abuse (e.g., Hull & Sloane, 2004), and difficulties with eating behaviors (e.g., Herman & Polivy, 2004). This can be extended to sexual offending as one form of maladaptive behavior from a similar source. The role of self-regulation—and the consequences of self-regulatory deficits—is paramount to our understanding of sexual offending.

Although many of the developmental antecedents described by the multi-modal self-regulation theory are common, we must remember that sexual offending is still relatively uncommon, even though increasing caseloads for treatment providers and enhanced media coverage of sexual violence (e.g., Anderson, 2008) suggest otherwise. Many individuals who struggle with self-regulation will engage in other maladaptive behaviors to the exclusion of sexual offending. However, a minority of persons with self-regulatory deficits will ultimately experience continuing problems with controlling their sexual urges, and these are the persons for whom SOS was developed.

This process includes a number of components: early biological predispositions, temperamental characteristics, learning and experiences from the early environment, perceptions of interactions with others, and changes in self-regulation ability over time. The development of maladaptive regulatory strategies is shaped by deficits in self-regulatory functioning, experience, opportunity, and reinforcement from varied and individual environmental contingencies. We examine each of these components in greater detail as we relate this process to sexual offending.

Biological and Temperamental Precursors

While we have already stated that people with sexual behavior problems are not simply born that way, initial biological factors and temperamental characteristics may still be relevant. These include genetic contributions, neurological development, and even prenatal development. If it is true that self-regulation plays a role in sex offending behavior, then we must consider how biological and temperamental precursors impact self-regulatory ability.

Areas of the brain most associated with self-regulatory processes include the amygdala and other components of the limbic system, which are responsible for processing emotional stimuli and learned reactions to fear, and some areas of the prefrontal cortex (e.g., anterior cingulate cortex, orbitofrontal cortex) that mediate behavioral response and impulse control (Davidson, Putnam, & Larson, 2000; Izard & Kobak, 1991; Linehan, 1993; Raver, 2004; Rothbart, Ziaie, & O'Boyle, 1992; Ryan, Kuhl, & Deci, 1997). These systems are often related, as areas of the prefrontal cortex are prompted to respond in association with emotional perception and memory. Research examining the role of these neurological regions in individuals with known self-regulatory deficits (e.g., individuals with borderline personality disorder, persistent substance abusers) have suggested overactivation of emotional response systems and corresponding underactivation of behavior control systems (Hazlett et al., 2005; Hill et al., 2009; Minzenberg, Fan, New, Tang, & Siever, 2007, 2008; Siegle, 2007). Thus, such persons may show early patterns of emotional reactivity and poor behavioral inhibition.

From a self-regulatory perspective, individuals have a homeostatic "set point" at which they are most comfortable—whether regarding emotions, perceptions, interactions, or physical and behavioral states. Disruption of this set point will result in discomfort, as well as a push to return to a baseline comfort level. This distress varies for each individual and is partly determined through genetics and biology. For example, from very early on, infants and young children show much individual variability in the ability to tolerate internal distress. This distress may be triggered by hunger, fear, sleepiness, or other physical discomforts. The ease with which the infant recognizes discomfort, becomes distressed, seeks aid from the environment, and remains distressed varies substantially. Behavioral manifestations of these processes are often described as individual temperament, or predictable ways of responding to environmental or internal cues. An infant who cries easily, loudly, and lengthily may be perceived as "fussy" compared to the infant who cries rarely, briefly, and less intensely. These early signs of temperamental differences may help us better understand the development of self-regulatory differences.

The developmental literature describes different presentations of temperament as early as infancy—while some appear to experience "normal" levels of distress or discomfort, others experience greater discomfort and reactivity. These differences are seen in four primary ways:

1. A low threshold for emotional stimulation (in comparison with other infants or children), where novel situations or environmental events will more easily elicit an emotional response (Davidson et al., 2000; Izard & Kobak, 1991; Malatesta-Magai, 1991; Scaramella & Leve, 2004).
2. A disproportionate emotional response, including heightened emotional arousal, emotional lability, irritability, and anxiety (Scaramella & Leve, 2004; Shaw, Owens, Giovannelli, & Winslow, 2001).
3. Difficulty returning to an emotional baseline (i.e., the set point described above) following an emotional reaction (Cole, Martin, & Dennis, 2004; Linehan, 1993; Malatesta-Magai, 1991; Scaramella & Leve, 2004).
4. A tendency toward negative emotionality, such as fear, sadness, or frustration (e.g., Hanish et al., 2004).

These factors in combination contribute to a temperament characterized by emotional sensitivity, reactivity, and intensity in response to interpersonal, environmental, and internal changes.

These processes have not been well studied in individuals with a history of problematic or illegal sexual behaviors. Research designed to describe neurological structures associated with emotionality and self-regulation using functional magnetic resonance imaging or other neurological imaging techniques has not yet included samples of sexual offenders. Similarly, little evidence exists regarding the early temperamental characteristics of sexual offenders, though some research has described problems with emotionality and emotional disorders in this population (Ahlmeyer, Kleinsasser, Stoner, & Retzlaff, 2003; Kafka & Hennen, 2002; Leue, Borchard, & Hoyer, 2004; Marshall, 1989, 1993; Seidman, Marshall, Hudson, & Robertson, 1994; Smallbone & Milne, 2000), as well as the potential role of negative affect in the offense process (e.g., Hall & Hirschman, 1991, 1992; Ward & Siegert, 2002).

Early Experiences and Socialization

Continuing development of temperament and self-regulatory processes occurs within the context of early experiences with family and peer socialization. The environment and those within it play a critical role in forming self-regulatory abilities and learning adaptive regulatory strategies.

Early interactions with others are important sources of learning and survival. Appropriate and beneficial caregiver responses to a child's distress or discomfort can help alleviate negative emotionality, provide reassurance and security, and increase adaptation to environmental change. These responses also serve as examples of helpful and effective regulatory strategies. The child is able to learn that his or her distress can be reduced, that others are willing to provide help and support, that environmental or internal cues can be tolerated, and that there are methods of regulating these experiences.

Experiences of distress or tension, including fear, hunger, or other salient needs, must be alleviated by caregivers in order for the child to survive and to facilitate the development of independent self-regulation (Cicchetti, Ganiban, & Barnett, 1991). However, not all caregivers are able or willing to satisfy these needs in an adaptive or healthy manner. Some are unequipped to adequately address the child's level of reactivity, sensitivity, or intensity of emotional experience. They may attempt to meet the needs of the child but are simply unable to do so. Some caregivers may not recognize the increased needs of these reactive or sensitive children. Others may respond inconsistently to the needs of the child, creating an unstable and unpredictable environment in which the child's distress is at times soothed and at other times unnoticed or ignored. Similarly, caregivers may completely ignore the child's needs, perhaps due to ignorance or preoccupation with their own distress, and never satisfy the child's needs for comfort. And finally, some caregivers may respond to the child's signs of distress in harsh, punitive, hostile, or abusive ways, which fail to address the problem and likely exacerbate it.

If caregiver interactions are insufficient, inconsistent, or hostile, they may inhibit critical learning processes. Research related to hostile or harsh parenting practices has supported this hypothesis, noting that children from abusive homes or who have experienced maltreatment show maladaptive emotional responding, hostile interpersonal interactions with others, ineffective strategies for coping with emotional distress, and other negative outcomes including aggression and psychopathology (Calkins, 2004; Cicchetti et al., 1991; Eisenberg, Fabes, Carlo, & Karbon, 1992; Eisenberg, Smith, Sadovsky, & Spinrad, 2004; Granic & Patterson, 2006; Maughan & Cicchetti, 2002; McCabe, Cunnington, & Brooks-Gunn, 2004; Moffitt, 1993; Scaramella & Leve, 2004).

A child who experiences a great deal of distress may, over time, elicit angry, critical, or hostile interactions with caregivers. These reactions may increase negative emotionality, potentially producing lasting deficits in self-regulatory functioning and inhibitory control (Eisenberg et al., 2004; Granic & Patterson, 2006; McCabe et al., 2004; Moffitt, 1993). In addition, some neurological evidence suggests that adverse or traumatic experiences in early childhood can in fact elicit change in areas of the brain responsible for the modulation of stress and cognitive and emotional regulation (Beers & DeBellis, 2002; Bremner, Elzinga, Schmahl, & Vermetten, 2007), further decreasing the child's capacity for self-regulation.

Another equally important influence on self-regulation is early experience with peers and others, including classmates, siblings, teachers, neighbors, or extended family members. Little research has examined the role of these important persons with regards to the development of self-regulatory functioning. Some empirical research explores peer relationships but focuses largely on peer interactions and social competence among children with early signs of temperamental or environmental distress. This research suggests that children who struggle with emotional and behavioral self-regulation, many of whom come from abusive homes (e.g., Maughan & Cichetti, 2002), are less socially competent and more isolated from their peers than other children (Eisenberg et al., 1992; Hanish et al., 2004; Maughan & Cichetti, 2002). They may also have greater difficulty self-regulating in the presence of peers, perhaps due to overwhelming anxiety or insecurity, intensifying their isolation and perceived social skills deficits (McCabe et al., 2004). Children who experience a great deal of negative emotionality and emotional reactivity may also be less likely to form friendships with their peers, and may in fact experience continued victimization (e.g., teasing, bullying, isolation, or criticism) by their peers as a result of their self-regulatory deficits (Hanish et al., 2004; Scaramella & Leve, 2004).

So why are these relationships important? Negative or abusive experiences within the home, followed in some cases by isolation, victimization, or limited peer relationships outside of the home, often predict negative psychological outcomes for these children as adolescents and adults (Hanish et al., 2004). Again, hostile, inconsistent, or insufficient responses to the child's distress in social situations will exacerbate this distress, and may even provide negative examples upon which to base regulatory learning (e.g., bullying behaviors). Children will fail to learn the diverse strategies used by others outside of their immediate family to regulate distress if the distress is in fact perpetuated by these individuals. In addition, some researchers have hypothesized that early failures in social competence in these peer relationships may interfere with the development of empathy, as highly dysregulated children are more likely to focus internally on themselves and their own distress than on the intentions, emotions, and motivations of others, all of which contribute to empathic understanding (Eisenberg et al., 1992; Leary, 2004; Vohs & Ciarocco, 2004).

The person's perceptions of events during critical periods of development and socialization are as important as the events themselves. Negative events are not the only factors to affect learning and self-regulatory functioning; how one perceives and interprets others' behaviors and intentions, and then subsequently develops explanations, beliefs, and expectations, also shape self-regulatory abilities or deficits. In other words, how the person learns to tolerate and manage distress also depends on his or her perceptions and understanding of these events.

People react to their environments and interactions with others, and these reactions may include changes in perceptions, beliefs, judgments, or expectations. If an individual struggling with emotional vulnerability or internal stress perceives that others are unhelpful, hostile, or critical, then he or she will react accordingly. If the individual adopts a view that the world, or even a particular person, is harsh and uncaring, genuine efforts to teach relevant and useful self-regulatory strategies will be met with suspicion, doubt, or fear. In a related vein, some may develop a strong sense of entitlement, where they feel that others owe them for the pain they have suffered, and their overwhelming sense of deservedness can interfere with attempts to teach them effective regulatory behaviors. Also, individuals may normalize their negative experiences, believing that harsh, hostile, or punishing behaviors are appropriate responses to internal or interpersonal distress. This may negatively impact the development of empathy for others when in a state of distress or tension, and could thus contribute to self-focused maladaptive behaviors.

Perceptions and socialization experiences may be particularly relevant during adolescence, as the individual enters puberty. During this critical stage, how the individual interprets sexual behaviors and views sexuality is impacted by perceptions of bodily changes and a shift from focusing on adult expectations to peer expectations. Additionally, adolescents are more likely to engage in risk-taking behaviors, particularly if those behaviors are endorsed by peers (e.g., DiClemente, Hansen, & Ponton, 1996), and interactions and everyday matters may become more sexualized due to hormonal and other developmental changes. The combination of peer-influenced behaviors, increased willingness to take risks, and sexualized perceptions and interactions play a crucial role in the development of relationships and beliefs about relationship behaviors (e.g., DiClemente et al., 1996; La Greca, Prinstein, & Fetter, 2001).

The available literature has not directly addressed how sex offenders' early socialization experiences and perceptions affect later outcomes. However, we do know, for example, that many individuals who have engaged in problematic sexual behaviors as adolescents and adults report serious histories of childhood maltreatment, including parental substance abuse and psychopathology (e.g., Becker, 1988; Briggs & Hawkins, 1996; Seghorn, Prentky, & Boucher, 1987, Stinson et al., 2011; Zgourides, Monto, & Harris, 1997), neglect, and various forms of emotional, physical, and sexual abuse (Briggs & Hawkins, 1996; Graham, 1996; Haapasalo & Kankkonen, 1997; Jonson-Reid & Way, 2001; Kobayashi, Sales, Becker, Figueredo, & Kaplan, 1995; Stinson, Becker, & Sales, 2008; Veneziano, Veneziano, & LeGrand, 2000; Worling, 1995; Zgourides et al., 1997). Less evidence regarding peer socialization among sexual offenders is available in the current literature. What is evident though is that these offenders were frequently victimized sexually, physically, or verbally by their peers (Hendriks & Bijleveld, 2004; Langevin, Wright, & Handy, 1989; Miner & Munns, 2005), often offended against their own peers, and affiliated themselves with other youths who engaged in illegal behavior (Blaske, Borduin, Henggeler, & Mann, 1989; Fehrenbach, Smith, Monastersky, & Deisher, 1986; La Greca et al., 2001). No studies have yet systematically evaluated the perceptions of childhood events among individuals who are known sexual offenders, though this topic offers a promising area for future study.

Self-Regulation and Self-Regulatory Deficits

We have already described self-regulation as the process through which a person modulates or controls various emotions, thoughts, interactions, behaviors, or even physiological states (i.e., biological urges like hunger or sexual drive) in order to maintain a comfortable, homeostatic balance of internal and interpersonal tensions. Each person is able to differentially tolerate experiences based on the biological and developmental precursors already described, establishing a unique homeostatic set point for the individual. Dysregulation occurs when there is imbalance or discomfort—when the set point is disrupted. Thus, the process of dysregulation is quite normal and happens to everyone, to a lesser or greater extent, with some regularity. When a person is dysregulated, he or she uses self-regulatory mechanisms to restore that homeostatic balance. We refer to someone as having a self-regulatory deficit when he or she is unable to adequately or adaptively deal with dysregulation (i.e., self-regulate). So though dysregulation itself is normative, the inability to effectively re-regulate once dysregulated is considered a functional deficit.

Discussions of self-regulation have centered primarily on four domains of regulation: emotional, cognitive, interpersonal, and behavioral. "Emotional regulation" is broadly defined as the ability to identify, monitor, and modulate emotional responses. "Cognitive regulation" refers to the individual's ability to modulate and regulate thoughts, expectations, and perceptions of others. "Interpersonal regulation" is the ability to monitor interactions with others, integrate feedback, and regulate interpersonal behaviors. And finally, "behavioral regulation" describes the ability to control, inhibit, and express behavior. These constructs have been seldom defined or empirically tested in sex offender populations, though we can gather evidence from the sex offender risk literature to inform our understanding of regulatory processes in sexual offenders.

Emotional Dysregulation

This is perhaps the most familiar form of dysregulation. Emotional dysregulation or distress is most readily addressed by many forms of mental health treatment, and also the type most often self-reported by clients when something is awry. It may be impossible to identify a specific point at which one becomes dysregulated, since each person copes with varying levels of emotion differently. However, an individual can often remember and describe the point at which he or she could no longer tolerate the experience of that emotion. This is when we would say that the person became emotionally dysregulated.

This may happen with virtually any emotion, whether positive or negative. They may reach an extreme point, which for negative emotional experiences may include anger, sadness, fear or paranoia, boredom, disgust, loneliness, or guilt; dysregulated experiences of positive emotion may include mania, excitement, infatuation, or overeagerness. Everyone experiences emotional dysregulation to some extent on a fairly consistent basis. Those with high thresholds for emotional experience, with greater emotional stability, or with highly efficient regulatory strategies may seldom notice strong emotional states. Others will struggle with understanding and regulating their emotional experiences. Much of this response depends on maturity, life experiences, personality and temperamental characteristics, available resources or opportunities, and self-regulation in other domains.

Sex offenders demonstrate some degree of emotional dysregulation, in that factors like feelings of rejection or loneliness (Hanson, Harris, Scott, & Helmus, 2007), anger or hostility (Hanson & Harris, 1998; Hanson & Morton-Bourgon, 2004), and generally negative affect (as measured in combination with other factors; Hanson et al., 2007) have been significantly linked to repeated sex offending behaviors. Though negative affect and low self-esteem are not always consistently linked with long-term sexual risk, it appears that more acute or immediate experiences of these emotional states contribute to risk in the moment (Hanson & Harris, 1998). Other research has described prominent mood symptomology (e.g., Ahlmeyer et al., 2003; Kafka & Hennen, 2002; Leue et al., 2004; Smallbone & Milne, 2000) and marked deficits in emotional regulation in relationship to frequency and severity of sex offending behaviors (e.g., Stinson, Becker, & Sales, 2008; Stinson et al., 2011).

Cognitive Dysregulation

Cognitive dysregulation may take several forms. The most obvious manifestation of cognitive dysregulation involves beliefs or expectations of others that may reflect judgment, blame, rationalization or justification, or all-or-nothing thinking. Examples of these thoughts may include "This is unfair," "He should / should not do _____," "It wasn't my fault that this happened, so I don't need to do anything about it," and so on. These types of thoughts have been traditionally labeled "thinking errors" or "cognitive distortions" in the classic cognitive-behavioral offender treatment literature (e.g., Beck, Rush, Shaw, & Emery, 1979; Blumenthal, Gudjonsson, & Burns, 1999; Bumby, 1996; Ward, Hudson, Johnston, & Marshall, 1997; Ward & Keenan, 1999; Yochelson & Samenow, 1976). However, while many conceptualize these thoughts as incorrect or distorted ways of viewing reality, these thoughts do reflect a very real manner of thinking that can characterize virtually anyone's cognitive experience. How much these thoughts impact other thoughts, emotions, and behaviors, and lead to discomfort or distress, varies by individual.

Delusional beliefs are also a type of cognitive dysregulation. Typically, these are strongly held beliefs that provoke significant distress and may change emotions, interactions, and behaviors. While the person may not have the insight to recognize the fallacy of such beliefs, he or she recognizes them as troubling or uncomfortable. As when under the influence of other dysregulated thoughts, an individual might utilize regulatory strategies to make the environment consistent with his or her delusional beliefs (e.g., avoidance and isolation for a paranoid individual), to reduce the strength of the delusions, or to distract from them. Delusions differ from other forms of cognitive dysregulation but may similarly contribute to problems with decision making, problem solving, and reality testing, though in perhaps a more persistent and pervasive way than other forms, like judgment or blame.

Another form of cognitive dysregulation involves how thoughts are processed or perceived, rather than problems with the specific content of the thoughts themselves. Racing thoughts, problems with abstract thinking, problem-solving deficits, or general cognitive disorganization also indicate deficits in monitoring and modulating cognitive processes. Regulatory strategies may be needed in order for effective information processing, attention maintenance, abstract reasoning, or learning to occur (e.g., Baumeister & Vohs, 2004, 2010).

Research on cognitive dysregulation among sex offender populations is limited to indirect empirical evidence of cognitive processes that support offense behaviors in sex offenders (e.g., Blumenthal et al., 1999; Ward, 2000; Ward, Fon, Hudson, & McCormack, 1998; Ward et al., 1997) and other criminal populations (e.g., Walters, 1995, 2002), problem-solving deficits and cognitive limitations in sex offender samples (e.g., Stinson et al., 2011), and risk predictors indicative of cognitive dysregulation like poor problem solving ability (Hanson et al., 2007), preoccupation with sexual thoughts (Hanson & Harris, 1998; Hanson et al., 2007), and deviant or offense-supportive attitudes and beliefs (Hanson & Morton-Bourgon, 2004), including sexual entitlement, justification of offending, blame toward others, and sexualization of victims (Hanson & Harris, 1998). Additionally, limited insight into risk (Hanson & Harris, 1998) is also predictive of problematic sexual behavior, so that offenders who minimize their potential risk (e.g., "I just know I won't do it again") demonstrate greater likelihood of continued sexual violence.

Interpersonal Dysregulation

How do interpersonal interactions become dysregulated? An interaction involves two or more people, perceiving and responding to one another, and modulating their behavior according to verbal and nonverbal feedback received from the other person or persons. Here, there are many opportunities for the interaction to become uncomfortable or unbalanced and to create distress in one or more parties. Distress may be prompted by arguing, making threats or issuing ultimatums, criticism, manipulation, deceitfulness, harassment, or avoidance behaviors such as ignoring or isolation. These are behaviors indicative of interpersonal dysregulation. They may be associated with strong emotions directed toward another person, such as anger, fear, or hurt, and thought processes reflecting negative judgments, blame, or specific expectations regarding what the other person should or should not do. Thus, interpersonal dysregulation is closely tied to the other forms of dysregulation described above. Note that some offenders, given their past experiences and reinforcement contingencies, may not feel particularly dysregulated by these interactions, but that the other person may experience discomfort or tension. Those who have become comfortable with lying or manipulation may make others with whom they interact dysregulated, and this is what counts.

Among sexual offenders (or any offenders, really), interpersonal dysregulation may be the construct most difficult to measure in an ad hoc fashion. Empirical research in this area is limited by perceptual and memory biases, as reporting interpersonal dysregulation is inherently colored by idiosyncratic perceptions of social and interpersonal cues. However, personality-disordered symptoms and problematic interpersonal interactions (Ahlmeyer et al., 2003; Davison & Taylor, 2001; Leue et al., 2004; Marshall, 1989, 1993; Segal & Marshall, 1985) have been recognized in samples of people with sexual behavior problems, and the presence of strong antisocial traits, including traits identified as diagnostic criteria for antisocial personality disorder in the DSM-IV-TR (American Psychiatric Association, 2000) or psychopathy as assessed by the PCL-R (Hare, 1991), are related to increased risk of sexual recidivism (Hanson & Harris, 1998; Hanson & Morton-Bourgon, 2004). The presence of any personality disorder has also been linked to greater risk (Hanson & Morton-Bourgon, 2004). Other sources of interpersonal dysregulation related to sexual offense risk include negative social influences, hostility toward women, relationship instability, and a lack of interest in or concern with other people (Hanson et al., 2007), as well as manipulativeness in treatment and supervision (Hanson & Harris, 1998). Also, traumatic interpersonal experiences in childhood or the formative years, including sexual and emotional abuse or neglect, are significant in identifying those at risk of repeated problems with sexual violence (Hanson & Harris, 1998), and abusive interactions are inherently dysregulated.

Behavioral Dysregulation

Though emotional dysregulation is more frequently discussed in general mental health treatment approaches, behavioral dysregulation is a common target of structured intervention. This is when behavior and behavioral urges are poorly monitored and poorly controlled. Behavioral dysregulation may have the most salient and immediate consequences for the individual. Evidence of more serious behavioral dysregulation includes criminal or aggressive behavior, illicit or problematic substance use, problematic sexual behaviors, suicidality and self-harm, disordered eating, or risky or reckless behaviors that could lead to harm. Evidence of less severe forms of dysregulated behavior may include procrastination, chronic lateness, irresponsibility or failure to follow through with commitments, or unhealthy habits. Behavioral dysregulation is sometimes seen as interrelated with other forms of dysregulation. For example, an individual who has engaged in some form of violent or aggressive behavior may later engage in self-harm or suicidal behavior in order to cope with emotional dysregulation following the aggression (e.g., guilt, shame, hopelessness). Similarly, those who use illicit substances may experience compromised cognitive functioning and decision-making capacity (i.e., cognitive dysregulation) and engage in further maladaptive behaviors. Therefore, one must consider the role of behavioral dysregulation as well when determining how dysregulation contributes to maladaptive outcomes.

We do know that these examples of behavioral dysregulation are common in a sex offender population. Sex offenders engage in frequent nonsexual criminal or aggressive behavior (e.g., Smallbone & Wortley, 2004; Weinrott & Saylor, 1991), problematic substance abuse (Abracen, Looman, & Anderson, 2000; Kafka & Hennen, 2002; Langevin & Lang, 1990; Langevin, Langevin, Curnoe, & Bain, 2006; Peugh & Belenko, 2001), and self-injurious behaviors (e.g., Pritchard & Bagley, 2001; Pritchard & King, 2005; Stinson & Gonsalves, 2011; Stinson et al., 2011). From a risk perspective, behavioral indicators of repeated sexual offending include the continued use of sex as a coping strategy, impulsivity, and a lack of cooperation with supervision (Hanson et al., 2007). Also relevant are irresponsibility, lifestyle instability, and the use of illicit substances (Hanson & Morton-Bourgon, 2004). Behavioral factors related to treatment include treatment dropout or refusal (Hanson & Harris, 1998; Hanson et al., 2007) and being uncooperative in treatment (Hanson & Harris, 1998). Again, these factors are all suggestive of behavioral dysregulation in the sex offender population.

Is Dysregulation Normal?

The view of dysregulation described in the multi-modal self-regulation theory posits that the process of dysregulation is a normal human experience. Feeling intense emotions, having distressing or unpleasant thoughts, or having uncomfortable or unhealthy interaction patterns with others are common and relatable experiences. Obviously, there is great individual variability. Some persons will feel emotions more intensely and negatively, will have highly problematic or uncomfortable thoughts, or will have perpetually negative or unhealthy social interactions. Others have these experiences more episodically or in a less intense way. But the process itself and the experience of being dysregulated is not necessarily pathological. Taken to extreme, it could be characterized as pathology (e.g., mood disorders, delusions, cognitive limitations, thought disorders, or personality disorders), but this is not the norm for most persons.

Where the pathology lies is in what people do when they are dysregulated. The multi-modal self-regulation theory holds that most individuals learn functional and adaptive ways of coping with dysregulation. Though these persons may engage in relatively low-level maladaptive strategies (e.g., procrastination, overeating, minor substance use), for the most part their selection of strategies reflects a healthy range of behavior. The fact that people select strategies to deal with dysregulation is also a normal part of this process. The problem—what isn't normal—is when people experience overwhelming dysregulation and are unprepared to cope with it, and when they select strategies that are harmful to others.

Thus far, we have described a process through which biological vulnerabilities—including natural individual variability in emotion processing, regulation of emotional response, and regulation of behavior during a state of emotional arousal—can create observable differences in the frequency, intensity, and lability of emotional responding. These characteristics may be demonstrated temperamentally, with increased sensitivity, reactivity, and duration of emotional responding as well. While some environments and caregivers are capable of managing or at least adapting to the individual's needs, other environments and caregivers are ill equipped to cope with an individual's high levels of distress. Insufficient, hostile or abusive, inconsistent, or indifferent responses can further exacerbate the distress and will fail to teach healthy regulatory practices. Similar reactions and isolation from peers and other important individuals outside of the primary familial relationship will have a comparable effect. Perceptions of these interactions during critical developmental periods will shape the person's view of others, impact his or her ability to learn from others, and further moderate his or her experiences of emotional distress, problematic beliefs and expectations, and unhealthy relationship behaviors.

This process leads to the ability to effectively monitor and manage a variety of internal states. Experiences of dysregulation create a drive to regulate, or restore a more comfortable balance. This drive is innate, and to a great degree involuntary. The desire to reduce discomfort is automatic and powerful. Throughout nearly every stage of life, we are constantly learning and practicing strategies by which to accomplish this goal. It is through these strategies that we regulate our internal states, and the strategies are either functional (i.e., they work) or not functional (i.e., they do not reduce distress), and adaptive (i.e., involve healthy, non-harmful behaviors) or maladaptive (i.e., cause or have the potential to cause harm to self or others).

Within the framework of the multi-modal self-regulation theory, those with the biological, temperamental, and experiential precursors described above will have significant difficulties with self-regulation. Given these circumstances, some individuals will turn to maladaptive strategies because (1) adaptive strategies are not functional, (2) adaptive strategies are functional but insufficient, (3) maladaptive strategies are more functional or readily available than adaptive ones, (4) maladaptive strategies have been modeled as functional by others, or (5) rarely, no strategies have been modeled as functional by others. A combination of adaptive and maladaptive strategies typically develops, each of which may be either functional or not depending on immediate circumstances, available opportunities, and the level of distress or dysregulation. Inability to self-regulate, or reliance on strategies that are insufficient, nonexistent, or involve maladaptive behaviors indicate a self-regulatory deficit—when an individual still must self-regulate but lacks the adaptive and functional skills by which to do it.

Many maladaptive strategies, whether they involve aggression, self-harm behaviors, sexual behaviors, overuse of substances, disordered eating, or other problematic behaviors, are seemingly impulsive and may be potentially harmful to self or others. They share some common features. First, they are frequently characterized by a need for immediate gratification, as an individual with limited ability to control or modulate distress is also unable to tolerate it for any great length of time. Because of this need for immediate relief, the strategies selected will be those that promise quick results. Second, these maladaptive behaviors involve little preparation or commitment and rely heavily on external influences for their effect. Maladaptive strategies can be relatively physical in nature, including aggression, self-harm, substance use, or oversleeping or over-eating. They may also include sexual behavior, in that the body can readily produce a strong physical response (i.e., sexual arousal or gratification). This does not mean these actions are always unplanned, as planning itself can also serve a regulatory function, but that they involve less internal effort than other, perhaps more adaptive strategies (e.g., deliberating pros and cons of a situation, using effective problem-solving techniques to resolve interpersonal conflict). For example, drinking alcohol can change one's mood, thoughts, and behaviors with little internal control over the effect or cognitive effort involved in the change.

The Role of Reinforcement

What ultimately determines the selection of self-regulatory strategies in any given situation depends on many factors. Behavioral reinforcement contingencies are an integral part of this process. Quite simply, behavior that does not achieve a desired outcome is unlikely to be repeated. How well a strategy reduces the dysregulation or distress will determine its likelihood of being used in the future. Again, behaviors must not always be adaptive or healthy in order to be functional. Obviously, this functionality will be mediated by other variables, but it is important to keep this in mind as we discuss behaviors that are, to many of us, simply untenable as reasonable strategies or solutions to everyday problems. Another important aspect of this is consistency—not only must the strategy be effective, but also consistent, in alleviating distress or dysregulation. And finally, the salience, impact, and consistency of negative consequences also matter. If these consequences are not perceived as negative, if they are less negative than tolerating or living with the dysregulation, if they are only inconsistently or occasionally relevant, and if they have little impact on the individual, then they will not deter maladaptive behavior.

Other relevant factors include the type and strength of the dysregulated state. If a strategy is not sufficiently successful due to particularly strong emotions or salient thoughts, or if the individual is habituated to that strategy due to repeated use, it may not be a viable solution. This may drive the person to seek stronger versions of the strategy or other strategies entirely when in a state of distress of this magnitude. Two other factors, closely related to one another, involve the perceptions of reinforcement versus negative consequences, as well as the weight given to the positive versus negative aspects of outcomes. There is a great deal of individual variability with regards to how people view consequences or outcomes. For example, many people, including treatment providers, would consider incarceration or hospitalization as a negative consequence, whereas some clients who come from particularly chaotic or stressful environments may benefit from the structure and support available in an institutional setting. Perceptions of what is reinforcing, what is a negative consequence, and the viability or likelihood of certain outcomes will all affect this process.

Sexual behavior, even maladaptive or risky sexual behavior, carries much potential for reinforcement. The most obvious form of reinforcement is, of course, the physiological experience of orgasm and the resulting sensation of sexual satisfaction or gratification. This is a powerful reinforcer that is typically consistent, relatively easily elicited in comparison with other potential sources of reinforcement, and often readily available when considering the accessibility of sexual fantasy and masturbatory practices (McGuire, Carlisle, & Young, 1964). Other kinds of reinforcement available from engaging in sexual activity include a feeling of intimacy or belongingness, a sense of being wanted or desired, increase in self-esteem or self-image, increase in confidence, increase in positive emotions, or a feeling of calmness or relaxation. Other research indicates that some individuals associate sexual offending with reinforcing experiences such as feeling powerful, dominant, or in control, a sense of superiority over others, or a sense of entitlement and self-justification (e.g., Baumeister, Catanese, & Wallace, 2002; Bouffard, 2010; Bushman, Bonacci, van Dijk, & Baumeister, 2003).

Personality and Cognitive Worldview

Within this context of self-regulatory development, beliefs about the self, the world, and interpersonal relationships are also developing. The developing personality and worldview shape behavioral choices and patterns of regulatory functioning. Certain personality traits or characteristics might be more associated with maladaptive strategy formation, particularly related to sexual violence or harm to others. An individual's beliefs can have a similar effect, mediating the relationship between dysregulation and self-regulatory deficits, and the selection of available and effective regulatory strategies. Several characteristics may be relevant, including egocentricity and limited empathy for others, resentment and entitlement, sadistic and psychopathic traits, sensation seeking, and offense-supportive beliefs (for further description, we refer the reader to Stinson, Sales, & Becker, 2008).

Research related to egocentricity and perspective taking has largely focused on the role of empathy, or the ability to consider the emotions and experiences of another person. An individual with limited empathy may be more likely to engage in behaviors with little regard for how they may impact another person, such as a potential victim (e.g., Caputo, Frick, & Brodsky, 1999; Porter, Campbell, Woodworth, & Birt, 2001). Also, limited empathy may be related to self-focused behavior, as the person concentrates almost exclusively on what must be done to meet his or her needs. Lack of empathy may be largely situational and can be driven by a state of dysregulation (e.g., Eisenberg et al., 1996). The empirical literature on sexual offenders and empathy notes that many offenders demonstrate selective empathy, meaning that they can identify the emotions or experiences of others in certain situations, but that they fail to do so reliably or meaningfully in relation to their own victims (e.g., Marshall & Moulden, 2001). Acutely dysregulated individuals often turn their focus inward on themselves, perhaps in a desperate attempt to identify the source of distress and search for strategies to cope with it. These two phenomena may be thus associated, in that offenders who are in a state of distress or dysregulation are more likely to focus on the self in an attempt to self-regulate and identify regulatory strategies, thus minimizing their likelihood of considering the needs, thoughts, or feelings of others in the process.

Resentment and entitlement, or thoughts and feelings of being "owed" or being "deserving" of something, are also associated with the selection of maladaptive regulatory strategies. Prior research has demonstrated a strong association between aggression and the perception that the world is a hostile and uncaring place (Lochman, 1987). This view could stem from early experiences or individual perceptions of important life events. Attributing hostility and apathy to others, along with a developing sense of "unfairness," fosters a strong sense of resentment and entitlement to have one's needs met. Sexual entitlement in particular may be a problem, as feeling deserving of sexual interactions and relationships or admiration from others could impact interactions and behavior.

A number of psychopathic and sadistic personality traits, including callousness, impulsivity, egocentricity, grandiosity, narcissism, and others (e.g., Hare, 1991, 1999), may also be a component of this process for some individuals. Those who enjoy hurting others, who have little regard for others' needs or emotions, and who act with little forethought or consideration of consequences, may be more likely to engage in these external forms of self-regulation, which require little effort and promise immediate gratification. These factors may also allow them to overcome social prohibitions more easily, to perceive opportunities in idiosyncratic ways, or to overlook the negative impact of their behavior on others (i.e., victims). While not all sexual offenders exhibit these traits, they exist on a continuum, and the presence of these characteristics may predispose some individuals to act in maladaptive ways in order to cope with their dysregulation. Empirical research has demonstrated a strong link between these characteristics and criminal and impulsive behavior (e.g., Hare, 1991; Millon, Simonsen, Birket-Smith, & Davis, 1998; Patrick, 2007), as well as maladaptive and violent sexual behaviors (e.g., Hart & Hare, 1997; Porter et al., 2001).

Sensation seeking has been consistently identified as a critical personality variable among individuals who engage in many risky behaviors (e.g., Hare, 1999; Millon & Davis, 1996). Those with a high threshold for excitement may seek behaviors that promise immediate thrills or excitement, are strongly reinforcing, and carry some potential risk. This need for greater stimulation may elicit boredom more readily, which is itself a dysregulated and uncomfortable state. This frequent need for stimulation and excitement can lead to habituation over time, thus reducing the effectiveness of any given strategy. This habituation may drive increasingly risky behaviors in order to achieve the same effect over time, or may push a move from fantasy to behavior for greater effect.

In addition to personality traits, the person's view of the world around him or her also factors into behavior and the selection of regulatory strategies. Offense-supportive beliefs, or a cognitive worldview consistent with sexual offending behavior, may take several forms, ranging from sexually entitled beliefs, beliefs related to victims, or attitudes and expectations related to the self and others. While research has not fully resolved whether or not many of these cognitive beliefs were present before the offenses occurred, or if they instead developed as postoffense justifications (see Stinson, Sales, & Becker, 2008), they may still provide a glimpse into the cognitive patterns that can lead to the individual's acceptance and normalization of some maladaptive behaviors. For example, negative views of women, including beliefs that women are inferior, that women should be controlled, or that men should make decisions regarding a woman's sexual behaviors, can facilitate an individual's willingness to engage in violent sexual behavior toward a woman. Similarly, sexual entitlement and sexual expectations of others may foster the use of sexual regulatory strategies in the absence of consent from another person. Those whose beliefs are consistent with maladaptive sexual behavior may be more likely to select these strategies and continue them over time.

To summarize, the multi-modal self-regulation theory describes a process through which developmental and experiential precursors impact the individual's ability to self-regulate moods, thoughts, inter-actions, and behaviors. For some, self-regulatory deficits will be mani-fested through a variety of maladaptive regulatory strategies, which may include maladaptive sexual behaviors. Reinforcement, personality characteristics, and cognitive beliefs may shape continued patterns of regulatory functioning and regulatory strategies over time. For sexual offenders, this carries important implications for prevention, research, and ultimately the treatment of problematic sexual behaviors.

TRANSLATING THEORY INTO TREATMENT

In Chapter 1, we described a number of current approaches to sex offender treatment and their limitations, as well as considerations from the broader treatment literature that could be incorporated into sex offender treatment practices. We propose that SOS is a viable alternative for treating sexual offenders. In order to translate the multi-modal self-regulation theory into a treatment approach (i.e., SOS), we must look at the core components of the theory that lend themselves to intervention and change. This includes identifying relevant treatment targets, factors related to the initiation as well as maintenance of problematic sexual behaviors, and expected outcomes.

With the multi-modal self-regulation theory as a guide, treatment providers and clients would target antecedent signs of dysregulation and self-regulatory deficits that prompted the use of maladaptive regulatory strategies like sexual offending behavior. Primary targets for treatment would be individual manifestations of emotional, cognitive, interper-sonal, and behavioral dysregulation. This would vary for each individual and would also necessitate a focus on other related behaviors—sexual offending is often not the only maladaptive strategy that may have devel-oped in response to dysregulation and self-regulatory deficits. Thus, treatment providers and clients may find themselves working together to identify not only sources of dysregulation but also a variety of maladap-tive behaviors resulting from it. An additional target or focus of treatment implied by this theory involves self-monitoring and self-management. Once sources or signs of dysregulation have been identified, it is crucial for clients to learn to self-monitor and self-manage these. Rather than emphasizing avoidance, SOS encourages a radical acceptance of dysregu-lation and the need to cope in a more appropriate and adaptive manner.

A second feature of SOS based on the multi-modal self-regulation the-ory involves the differentiation between causal and maintenance factors.

The initial causal factors here are assumed to be sources of dysregulation and self-regulatory deficits, including difficulties with managing anger, feelings of entitlement, thoughts of blame, negative or manipulative interpersonal interactions with others, or impulsivity or poor behavioral controls. These are different from maintenance factors, which may represent internal or environmental sources of reinforcement, such as temporary relief from negative emotional or interpersonal states, physiological or personal satisfaction, or feelings of belongingness or intimacy. SOS emphasizes both, as initial problems with dysregulation are still likely relevant issues, and the strength of maintenance factors may contribute to continued difficulties with adaptive self-regulatory skill development. Over time, some of the behaviors associated with maintaining the offending (e.g., planning of offenses, victim grooming) may also serve a similar regulatory purpose in that thinking about future relief of distress can itself be regulating.

The third major goal of SOS is the development of adaptive regulatory skills to aid in the regulation of uncomfortable or distressing states. As noted, the emphasis is not on avoidance of risk factors or dysregulation itself. These are considered normative, but they become pathological for some individuals who experience them to an extreme and who are unable to handle them in an adaptive manner. Negative emotions, strong urges, uncomfortable thoughts, or problematic interactions are addressed through the development of needed skills rather than avoidance strategies (e.g., learning to tolerate a specific urge rather than simply avoiding a source of it altogether). Replacement strategies are critical. Healthy relationships, boundaries, and skills are therefore needed to foster effective self-management of dysregulation and decrease continuing patterns of maladaptive behavior.

Finally, SOS assumes gradual or incremental progress in treatment, with a focus on harm reduction. Many treatments for sexual offenders aim to resolve these complex and serious behavioral problems within a relatively short period of time, often ranging from 6 to 12 months. Given the background factors described here and the widespread nature of self-regulatory deficits, we expect a gradual approach is best for learning and sustaining success. Behaviors and adaptive strategies must be shaped over the long term in order to be most effective and to provide opportunities for reinforcement. Initial efforts to develop and use new, unfamiliar strategies may lead to discomfort and frustration. This is expected, as more familiar strategies, though maladaptive, have been practiced and successful for a greater time. Treatment providers may also expect that other behaviors—some of which may be maladaptive—will emerge or increase during this process, as favored strategies are decreased or extinguished. Implementing new, adaptive strategies will take time and patience on the part of both treatment providers and clients.

PILOT PROJECT IMPLEMENTATION

In order to develop and test SOS with both clients and providers, this treatment was implemented at two inpatient mental health facilities (n = 220) and one facility for sexually violent predators (n = 50) in a midwestern U.S. state. These agencies had previously used relapse prevention as a primary sex offender treatment approach. Implementation efforts at these sites involved comprehensive and facility-wide training of professional and direct care staff members, as well as continued supervision, follow-up training, and monthly *in vivo* adherence monitoring to ensure continued fidelity to the philosophy and treatment materials of SOS. Pilot testing is ongoing at these three sites at the time of publication of this book. However, some early findings help us understand more about the treatment's effectiveness with these populations.

Clients at the two inpatient forensic mental health facilities present with a high degree of psychiatric impairment (see Stinson & Becker, 2010; Stinson, Robbins, & Crow, 2011), including rates of psychotic spectrum disorders at approximately 65%, intellectual and developmental disabilities at 40%, and substance abuse disorders at nearly 50%. Sex offenders in these studies often demonstrated histories of multiple arrests and psychiatric hospitalizations resulting from their sexual offending and other violent criminal behaviors, along with marked deficits in adaptive functioning (e.g., educational, relationship, and employment history) in comparison with standard correctional samples of sexual offenders (Stinson & Becker, 2011; Stinson et al., 2011). The pilot sample of civilly committed sexually violent predators is characterized by a lesser degree of serious psychiatric pathology and a higher degree of personality disorder and paraphilic sexual interests, as is comparable with other similar samples (Becker, Stinson, Tromp, & Messer, 2003; Vess, Murphy, & Arkowitz, 2004).

A number of outcomes have been tested as part of this pilot research. Behavioral outcomes, including verbal and physical aggression, contact and noncontact sexual offenses, suicidal and self-harm behaviors, and facility incidents of seclusion or restraint were coded for all participants for 1 year pretreatment as well as the first 2 years of treatment participation. Thus far, clients who have been in at least 2 years of treatment and who have attended at least 50% of offered SOS treatment groups (i.e., treatment participants) have shown significant reductions in incidents of verbal and physical aggression, noncontact sexual offending, and self-harm behaviors in comparison with those who had attended fewer than 50% of available SOS groups but who were participating in other empirically supported psychiatric programming (i.e., treatment nonparticipants; Stinson & Becker, 2010). Comparatively, measures of treatment progress using the Treatment Needs and Progress Scale (McGrath, 2005; McGrath & Cumming, 2003), such as self-management of sexual and aggressive behavior, treatment motivation and cooperation, and self-regulatory ability with regards to emotions, problem solving, and mental health stability, showed significant improvement for the treatment participants in comparison with no real change for nonparticipants (Stinson & Becker, 2010). Though these preliminary data were gathered and analyzed after only 2 years of treatment, it is expected that these trends will continue, demonstrating even greater client improvement in self-regulatory ability and adaptive behavior over time. Additional data continue to be collected with regards to posttreatment success in less restrictive settings, and the impact of this treatment with high-risk sex offenders in a civil commitment facility. These results are encouraging as we begin our discussion of SOS for sex offender treatment.

CHAPTER 3

Using Safe Offender Strategies
Pragmatic Considerations

Now that readers are familiar with the basic theoretical foundations of SOS, we will take a closer look at the treatment itself. In this chapter, we cover pragmatic issues to help treatment providers conceptualize treatment planning and implement SOS smoothly and effectively. Our coverage includes a brief outline of modules, treatment structure, therapist qualifications and client characteristics, pretreatment needs, compatibility with other programs or mental health care clients may be receiving, and measuring client progress. The primary goal of this chapter is to help treatment providers with the logistics and setup issues that are so important prior to beginning any new treatment. Questions like what treatment will cover, how long it may take, who it can help, how to ensure consistency, and how to measure outcomes are all important to consider in the early stages of treatment implementation. A secondary goal of this chapter is to facilitate treatment providers' understanding of the remainder of this text. By having a broad overview of the treatment itself, including main topic areas and features of treatment sessions, readers will be able to see how the 10 modules build upon one another, and how later concepts like treatment strategies (presented in Chapter 4) and measures of progress are interwoven throughout the use of this therapy.

MODULES OF TREATMENT

SOS is divided into 10 modules. Each module is distinct, yet all are important. The modules have been written and piloted as group therapy (typically with six to eight clients per group and two treatment providers) because the opportunity for clients to discuss their experiences and opinions as a group and to provide feedback about skills use offers a richness and diversity beyond that which can be provided in individual therapy. There is an assumption of two group facilitators are necessary for reasons of therapist safety and also so that treatment providers can use one another as examples and fodder for role-playing exercises.

Topics and Order of Modules

The 10 modules of SOS address several broad categories: motivation and commitment, different areas of dysregulation, and risk management and aftercare planning. (See Table 3.1 for a brief overview of these modules.) Treatment providers should not skip modules, nor should they introduce modules to clients in a different order than is presented here. The modules have been arranged to flow logically from one topic area to another; skipping any might result in the loss of important treatment information and difficulty with maintaining group cohesion and therapeutic alliance. If administered in an institution or other agency, clients may finish other treatment programming and prepare for transfer or release before the completion of all 10 modules. In such cases, treatment providers can recommend future treatment involvement in other settings emphasizing the concepts from any remaining modules that were not completed.

Early modules emphasize commitment to treatment and the client's own feelings about being involved in treatment. This emphasis facilitates several therapeutic processes. First, clients can explore and express their thoughts involving sex offender treatment. Treatment providers can thereby assess each client's level of willingness and troubleshoot early difficulties with treatment engagement or negative views of the treatment process. Second, engaging clients in discussions of commitment and barriers to treatment can increase group cohesion and set the stage for clients to better understand one another. Third, treatment providers can validate clients' fears, frustrations, and objectives to enhance the therapeutic alliance. Fourth, these early modules allow clients to develop the direction of their treatment through examining their strengths, treatment expectations, and goals for treatment change. Other activities in the early modules of treatment include understanding basic treatment concepts and discussions of clients' own sex offending behaviors, providing a foundation for later modules addressing dysregulation and adaptive skills building.

TABLE 3.1. Safe Offender Strategies Program Overview

The number of sessions shown following each topic point within the modules is an estimate. With more severely impaired clients, modules may require significantly more sessions than what we have suggested here.

Module 1—Why Am I in Treatment?

  Introduction and Orientation (Sessions 1–5)
  Stages of Change (Sessions 6–8)
  Identifying Treatment Goals and Expectations (Sessions 9–12)

Module 2—Basic Treatment Concepts

  Sexuality, in Brief (Sessions 1–8)
  Sexual Offending and Victimization (Sessions 9–14)
  Sexual Offending, Mental Illness, and Self-Regulation (Sessions 15–19)
  Behavioral Chain Analysis (Sessions 20–25)
  Self-Monitoring and Self-Management (Session 26)

Module 3—Emotions and Emotion Regulation

  Identifying and Understanding Emotions (Sessions 1–8)
  Origins of Our Emotions (Sessions 9–12)
  Experiencing Emotional Distress (Sessions 13–17)
  Emotional Dysregulation and Problematic Sexual Behavior (Sessions 18–22)
  Alternative Forms of Coping: Basic Techniques (Sessions 23–25)

Module 4—Sexuality and Sexual Behavior

  Sexuality and Relationships: A Review (Sessions 1–4)
  Human Sexuality (Sessions 5–10)
  Sexual Fantasies and Masturbation (Sessions 11–15)
  Pornography and Sexually Explicit Materials (Sessions 16–20)

Module 5—Review of Motivation, Commitment to Treatment, and Treatment Goals

  Being in Sex Offender Treatment (Sessions 1–5)
  Stages of Change (Sessions 6–8)
  Review of Treatment Goals (Sessions 9–12)
  Review of Expectations and Group Rules (Sessions 13–15)

(cont.)

TABLE 3.1. *(cont.)*

Module 6—Expectations and Beliefs about Interpersonal Relationships

Beliefs: How We View Ourselves, Others, and the World (Sessions 1–10)
Expectations (Sessions 11–15)
Cognitive Dysregulation: Getting Stuck (Sessions 16–20)
Thoughts, Cognitive Dysregulation, and Problematic Sexual Behaviors
    (Sessions 20–22)
Alternative Forms of Coping: Basic Techniques (Sessions 23–25)

Module 7—Dysregulation and Interpersonal Relationships

Expectations and Boundaries (Sessions 1–5)
Communicating in Interpersonal Relationships (Sessions 6–10)
Interpersonal Dysregulation (Sessions 11–15)
Working with Interpersonal Dysregulation (Sessions 16–22)
Alternative Forms of Coping: Basic Techniques (Sessions 23–24)

Module 8—Coping with the Past

Impact of Trauma (Sessions 1–10)
Thinking of Your Own Problematic Behavior (Sessions 11–17)
Repairing Relationships (Sessions 18–20)

Module 9—Making Good Choices: Managing Urges and Behavior in a Healthy
Way

Our Decisions, Our Behavior (Sessions 1–10)
Skills Building: Recognizing Adaptive versus Maladaptive Skills
    (Sessions 11–13)
Reviewing Skillful Behavior (Sessions 14–18)
Self-Management and Coping Ahead (Sessions 19–20)

Module 10—Motivation, Commitment, and Treatment Goals

Being in Treatment (Sessions 1–8)
Stages of Change (Sessions 9–10)
Committing to adaptive skills (Sessions 11–15)
Progress and Future Treatment (Sessions 16–20)
Challenges in Treatment and Aftercare (Sessions 21–23)
Termination (Sessions 24–25)

Subsequent modules emphasize emotional, cognitive, and interpersonal dysregulation.[1] Each of these follows a similar template, first focusing on general features of emotions, thoughts, or interpersonal relationships, followed by signs of dysregulation, discussion of how this dysregulation may relate to sexual offending, and ideas for the development and use of adaptive regulatory strategies. Interspersed in these discussions of dysregulation are materials related to sexuality and sexual development because clients need to explore these topics before they are fully able to describe relationships between dysregulation and their own maladaptive sexual behaviors.

Throughout the treatment, clients periodically review their motivation and commitment to treatment, as well as their progress toward achieving treatment goals and learning new adaptive regulatory skills and behaviors (see "My Treatment Progress" in Appendix B for a module review worksheet for clients). We encourage treatment providers to review key treatment concepts and progress toward goals following the completion of each module. The final components of treatment are designed to reinforce these points and develop a risk management and aftercare plan so that clients can continue learning adaptive skills and maintain the progress they have made thus far. These sections also review new strengths and healthy relationships and boundaries that clients have formed as part of the treatment process.

Duration of Modules

SOS conceptualizes sex offending behaviors as part of a larger problem: self-regulatory deficits. Treatment is broadly intended to improve self-regulatory functioning and to modify dysregulated patterns of behavior. Self-regulation is a major life function. Other behaviors that are considered major lifestyle changes, such as losing weight, improving physical health, quitting smoking or drinking, improving damaged or unhealthy relationships, or even getting out of debt, are presumed to take a significant amount of time to achieve and maintain. Brief episodes of treatment (e.g., less than 1 year) may be a good start, but may not lead to lasting

---

[1] Note that we have excluded a module devoted entirely to behavioral dysregulation or behavioral urges. This is because behavioral dysregulation—usually manifested as maladaptive strategies or behaviors—is the target of the treatment itself. Maladaptive or dysregulated urges and behaviors are often preceded by emotional, cognitive, or interpersonal dysregulation, each of which is dealt with more specifically within the treatment modules.

change. This is true of both low-level problematic behaviors and serious sexual offending and pervasive deficits in self-regulatory functioning. In addition, many clients participating in SOS also struggle with serious mental illness; cognitive, intellectual, or developmental disabilities; social skills deficits; and histories of trauma. These co-occurring problems only add to the complexity of the treatment experience. So the question remains: How long is treatment?

Within the chapters describing each module (i.e., Chapters 5–14) and in Table 3.1 we have provided guidelines as to how many sessions each section of treatment should take, assuming sessions of approximately 45–50 minutes in length. Generally speaking, most of the SOS modules (except for Module 1) require 20–25 weekly sessions. However, we caution readers and treatment providers that these are merely estimates, often assuming optimal group conditions and client responsivity.[2] While we have developed and implemented SOS as long-term treatment, just how long it may take depends on a variety of factors:

1. The number of clients involved in any given group.
2. The functional level of those clients.
3. The extent and seriousness of the sex offending behaviors to be addressed in treatment.
4. The clients' motivation and commitment to treatment.
5. The complexity of other client needs, including psychiatric symptoms, cognitive impairments, interpersonal deficits, and behavioral problems.
6. The pace at which group materials are covered.
7. Client retention of treatment concepts.
8. Whether sex offending behaviors continue during treatment (for institutionalized clients).
9. How frequently and how long clients meet for each treatment session.

Systemic variables may also have an impact on how long treatment takes. Treatment provider variability can be significant, with differences

---

[2]From our experiences with the pilot sites, involving 20–25 treatment groups and 150–200 clients, if you are treating a severely psychiatrically ill, behaviorally unstable, and largely intellectually and developmentally disabled population, the treatment will require more sessions per module. Pilot groups moved at an average pace of two to four modules per year.

in individual style, knowledge of the client, clinical experience, and personal expectations. Duration also depends on agency factors, such as the availability of trained treatment providers, the frequency with which groups are cancelled, structural changes that impact group composition, availability of other programming to supplement sex offender treatment, and the number of times that clients can meet per week for sex offender treatment.

The goal is for treatment providers to decide when clients have most benefitted from any given topic or group discussion, and then to move on. Managing the pace of treatment involves balancing the potential for missing important client revelations with the problem of staying so long on one area that clients lose interest.

Related to the length of treatment is the length of time before clients really begin discussing their sexual offenses. Clients do not discuss their sexual offenses in any great detail until the latter part of Module 2. This delay is deliberate. Skipping ahead to the referral offense or other past sexual offenses is not recommended. Doing so could compromise the effectiveness of treatment and the relationship-building components built into early modules. Additionally, while early in treatment, clients are often hesitant to discuss their offenses, either due to discomfort, hostility, shame, fear, or other reasons. This is a rational hesitation, as many of us would be loath to publicly admit shortcomings or socially unacceptable behaviors, all of which are likely much less harmful than what our clients have done. Clients are also not ready to discuss their offending within the context of dysregulation without first understanding what dysregulation is and how it affects behavior. Clients may be used to describing their offenses in a confession-like manner, describing blow-by-blow details of the offense itself. This does not accomplish SOS goals of identifying different areas of dysregulation and precipitating factors that may have led to an offense or the planning of an offense. An intricate description of the offense itself fails to include important emotional, cognitive, and interpersonal precursors that can aid clients in understanding future treatment and self-management needs. Before reviewing their offenses, clients must be committed, have goals, understand a common theoretical framework, and be prepared for the idea of self-monitoring and learning new skills. In SOS, clients discuss their offenses by using behavioral chain analysis, a technique that thoroughly elicits information regarding thoughts, emotions, and urges preceding a behavior. This technique is described in further detail in Chapter 6.

Balance of Process and Didactic Information

Group materials and concepts are covered through both didactic and process methods. A didactic approach allows clients to learn new concepts, whereas a process approach allows clients to discuss their experiences within the context of new information. The process portion of treatment is not a pure "process group," but instead involves guided discussion of clients' past experiences and examples relevant to the didactic portions of treatment. Other opportunities to focus on process include client discussions of goals, progress, and daily self-monitoring activities. With didactic information, it is best to avoid a lecturing style. Group leaders should instead incorporate concrete examples, role plays or pseudo-role plays (e.g., "Pretend that I've just embarrassed you in front of your friends. How might you respond?"), or even interactive or media examples to demonstrate treatment concepts. Clients' responsivity factors, including learning styles, are important influences on how one presents didactic information, as purely didactic sessions will often be too verbal, academic, or abstract for many clients.

Combining didactic and process learning, along with using concrete and specific experiential examples, fosters greater learning in lower functioning populations, whether clients struggle with verbal learning, abstract reasoning, attentional deficits, or interference from delusional beliefs or other psychiatric symptoms. Higher functioning clients can also benefit from such an approach, as they can have more complex and detailed discussions using the same basic set of concepts. This combination of techniques also facilitates the development of self-monitoring and self-management strategies, as clients can learn new strategies and then report their own experiences and give one another feedback throughout each module of treatment.

Worksheets and Homework Assignments

Within this text, we have described all treatment activities and discussions, with specific suggestions regarding the presentation and discussion of these concepts in a group or individual setting. We have also provided several figures throughout the text that represent sample client worksheets to visually represent some of the concepts. Treatment providers are free to copy these or develop their own such worksheets using the lists, exercises, and questions interspersed throughout the modules if they and their clients find them useful. However, given that many clients struggle with reading and writing, we have avoided too many written materials in order to avoid alienating clients who rely less on written learning.

Homework assignments are also a point of contention for many clients involved in sex offender treatment. Written homework, viewable by others, readily identifies them as sexual offenders. For some clients with reading or learning difficulties, it increases shame and limits their ability to fully participate in a group activity. At the pilot sites for SOS, we have discussed all topics and supplemental worksheets within session. Clients are thus able to ask questions, and treatment providers can examine client responses in the moment. Important beliefs or assumptions may be missed if clients complete assignments on their own, without the benefit of an open group discussion. Generally, the only outside assignments given include self-monitoring activities in Modules 3–10, when clients complete a daily self-monitoring sheet to demonstrate their growing capacity for self-monitoring and self-management. (Examples of such worksheets are provided in Chapter 6.)

TREATMENT STRUCTURE

How does one go about using SOS? Establishing effective treatment using SOS, whether in an institutional or an outpatient setting, requires certain early considerations on the part of administrators and treatment providers. While we cannot address all of the pragmatic details related to treatment implementation in this brief section, we will cover major concerns like group versus individual therapy, open versus closed groups, and length and duration of treatment sessions.

Group versus Individual Therapy

Traditionally, sex offender treatment has been provided in the context of group therapy. While many have suggested that clients make more progress when they can discuss and challenge one another's beliefs and behaviors in a peer group, the most likely reason for widespread use of group therapy is simply resource management. Many institutions and agencies lack the resources to provide individual therapy to all clients in need of sex offender treatment, and group therapy is a cost- and time-efficient alternative. While there have been no large-scale empirical studies evaluating the effectiveness of group versus individual sex offender treatment, there are advantages and disadvantages to both.

Group therapy is most cost-effective, requires fewer agency resources, decreases perceived pressure on any one client, broadens exposure to others' beliefs and experiences, and does provide clients with a similar peer group. Individual therapy, however, provides greater client privacy, limits negative peer influences (e.g., learning new offending strategies from sex offending peers), potentially increases honest responding in the absence of social pressure or social desirability effects, and allows for individualized treatment goals and intervention methods.

Choosing a treatment modality depends on individual client preferences and characteristics, interpersonal skills, availability and preferences of treatment providers, and other related variables. However, because most agencies and organizations are best equipped to provide group treatment, many of the lessons and activities in SOS are written in the form of group discussion. (Adaptations to individual therapy are described later in this section.) In an SOS group, clients can compare and contrast their opinions, behaviors, and regulatory strategies with those of others similar to themselves, leading them to critically evaluate their beliefs while exposing them to new ones. Group mix is important—clients should be matched in terms of cognitive, intellectual, or developmental level, and in some groups it may be preferred to match them on other characteristics (e.g., psychiatric symptoms, level of motivation or commitment to treatment) as well. Group facilitators can then ensure that clients share a similar understanding or similar expectations of treatment.

In an SOS group, the role of peer feedback varies. Unlike other forms of sex offender treatment, the role of peers in group is *not* to overtly challenge or confront denial, minimization, cognitive distortions, or treatment failure. These responses are invalidating and dysregulating, and will not create an atmosphere conducive to learning new skills. Instead, the role of peers is to educate, supply alternative viewpoints, provide encouragement or support, and reinforce treatment concepts or the application of new skills. It is acceptable for clients to challenge one another, though this should be done in a supportive and genuine manner.

The early treatment modules, particularly those emphasizing motivation, commitment, and basic treatment concepts, are designed to enhance group cohesion. In these modules, there are many opportunities for clients to share their views on sex offender treatment, commitment to change, goals in treatment, and the precipitants of sex offending behavior. Clients may also find that they share common goals, values, and strengths. This validates everyone in the group, not only in the initial stages of treatment but also throughout the treatment process.

Unfortunately, some of this validation and support is lost when SOS is applied as an individual therapy. Treatment providers must then work to maintain the usefulness of discussion topics, as these are opportunities for clients to reflect and learn from their past experiences. Some of these discussions can occur between client and treatment provider, but they will be less rich without the contributions of other clients who may have unique experiences to contribute. The treatment provider is also responsible for consistent encouragement, validation, and support, some of which may typically be provided by both treatment providers and peers. Individual therapy does, however, allow for more focused attention on one particular client's needs, so that therapeutic activities may be more detailed or in-depth related to one person's behaviors. For clients who are high risk or who have many areas to address in treatment, individual therapy may be a beneficial supplement to normal group processes, or could simply substitute as a far more individualized and intensive intervention. As an individual treatment, it could move faster, though this may not always be the case for high-risk persons, nor is faster treatment always desirable. It may be helpful to involve the individual therapy client in other forms of group treatment so that he or she will still have the opportunity to learn skills or strategies among peers. Thus, inclusion in other comparable skills groups (e.g., dialectical behavior therapy skills group, problem-solving or communication skills group, social skills group) is recommended.

Open versus Closed Groups

Assuming that treatment is to be provided in a group, we must then consider the use of open versus closed groups. We take the position that neither is significantly better than the other—each option has advantages and disadvantages. Treatment providers will make decisions that best fit the needs of their clients, their agencies, and themselves.

Closed groups, or those in which a set client group begins treatment together and no new clients are added until group is completed, are perhaps a luxury. The clear advantages of closed groups are that clients will know one another well, group process and cohesion will not be disrupted by the entering and exiting of group members, everyone in the group will receive the same components of treatment at the same time, and group leaders will know the clients, their interactions, and their needs and abilities well. Another potential advantage is that clients may be more open and trusting with peers with whom they have been in treatment for a long time. Some disadvantages of closed groups, however, are that they may limit the availability of treatment for new clients (e.g., they must wait for a new group to begin), groups may fall into maladaptive patterns together, group members may become so comfortable with group leaders and one another that they forget the seriousness involved, and they prevent the introduction of new group members who can sometimes provide fresh or unique perspectives. The reality too is that the duration of SOS may preclude the use of closed groups. If one group takes years to complete, it simply isn't feasible for clients to wait, and the clients who are new and waiting may not always fit as well with one another as they might with clients in already-established treatment groups.

Open groups, or those that allow new group members to join an already-established treatment process, are probably more common in institutions or agencies that admit new clients on a more frequent basis. In some cases, the frequency of new clients may allow for new groups to start. However, these new admissions are often sporadic and unpredictable enough that there are seldom enough new clients at one time who are similar enough to form an entirely new group. Thus, open groups allow for the rapid inclusion of new clients in treatment, introduce new ideas and perspectives in an already-existing group, and show new clients the commitment and progress of clients who have been in treatment for some time. For example, a new client who is hesitant or anxious about starting treatment may in fact be encouraged by entering a more established group with committed and more comfortable peers. Disadvantages of open groups, however, are frequent changes in group membership that can disrupt group cohesion, differences in the amount of treatment across individuals within the same group, missing or skipping vital components of treatment, and difficulties with maintaining openness when new clients are added. Open groups are also more challenging for treatment providers, who must constantly introduce new group members to the content in earlier modules while still keeping group concepts and topics fresh and relevant for all clients.

Ultimately, treatment providers and involved agencies will decide what is feasible given treatment demand, available resources, and best interests of the clients. Closed groups are fairly straightforward, but open groups are more complicated. How do we make open groups work? First, each new group member, regardless of point of entry, will still have to undergo the same pretreatment processes previously described. This will also include review of materials from Module 1 emphasizing motivation and commitment, positive and negative aspects of sex offender treatment, client reactions to treatment, and basic goals. Second, once the client has entered group, several group sessions can be dedicated to revisiting each client's goals in treatment, as well as his or her overall expectations and group "rules." Clients can then return to their normal topics of discussion. Third, at some point, each new client will have to complete a behavioral chain analysis of his or her offense, as described in Module 2. If a client enters significantly past that section of treatment, it may be helpful to have other group members briefly review important points of their own experiences with this process. Some clients may not be comfortable with doing this immediately, and this is okay. It should be done once new clients have somewhat acclimated to the group and its members. A final consideration is the discussion of dysregulation and self-monitoring. Again, new clients will be aided by more established group members who are able to identify their own areas of dysregulation or self-regulatory deficit that may have contributed to their offending and that they self-monitor daily. These procedures familiarize new clients with major treatment components and allow already-established group members a chance to review and reflect on these same concepts.

THERAPIST QUALIFICATIONS

If experience matters, then what kind of experience do clinicians need? The experience that is important in SOS is not specific to any mental health discipline or degree, but instead to the specialized interest, training, and style that support and facilitate client improvement. First, the treatment provider must be willing. It is difficult to expect willingness in our clients when we cannot find willingness in ourselves. And nothing can derail the development of a therapeutic relationship faster than a treatment provider who doesn't like the client, doesn't like the treatment, or who feels treatment cannot possibly work. Therefore the first qualification for treatment providers in SOS is that they have an interest in providing sex offender treatment, feel that SOS is a good match with their own style and beliefs, and believe that the treatment can help clients change.

Second, the treatment provider does need some experience in SOS, either through reading, studying, and preparing for treatment by using this text, or through additional supplemental training that can help troubleshoot and explain the implementation of treatment with more challenging client populations. Not everyone must have SOS experience, but training and familiarity are a necessity. Does this mean an SOS provider must have years of therapy experience otherwise? Not necessarily.

Though a completely inexperienced treatment provider may have difficulty navigating the therapeutic strategies described in Chapter 4 and elsewhere in the text, merely having more years of therapy experience does not equate to better therapy, particularly when someone does not have the requisite knowledge and understanding of the treatment itself.

A third qualification relates to the therapist's interpersonal style. Not all therapists must be the same—this is not only unrealistic but also undesirable. For clients to learn healthy boundaries and to see modeling of appropriate boundaries and adaptive skills, they must see the true variability of human nature. Each treatment provider brings something different to the therapy and the therapeutic relationship. Still, therapists with certain interpersonal characteristics or styles may be better matched with SOS and may be more successful in developing the type of therapeutic alliance that is needed to foster client commitment to change. Empathy, warmth, compassion, genuineness, caring—these are all characteristics of good therapists (e.g., Luborsky et al., 1971; Messer & Wampold, 2002). These characteristics also match the philosophical principles of SOS.

Finally, we must also consider the therapist's role. In traditional forms of sex offender treatment, the therapist may be viewed as a teacher, a lecturer, a judge, or an interrogator. In SOS, the role of the therapist is as a model of appropriate boundaries and relationships, a compassionate facilitator of client change, one who helps clients understand their needs, and a supporter as clients reveal their vulnerabilities and fears. Treatment providers are still in the position of eliciting information from clients, teaching them important concepts, and helping them describe areas of dysregulation that may have precipitated their offending. Thus, treatment providers are sometimes in the position of teaching or asking questions, but this is still done with the client's needs in mind and the ultimate goals of the therapy.

CLIENT SUITABILITY

Just as we must consider what makes a therapist or treatment provider suitable for SOS, we must address what makes a client suitable for this treatment. Merely having a history of sexual offending or otherwise problematic sexual behavior does not automatically dictate the most appropriate form of treatment. Sex offenders are a heterogeneous population, including contact and noncontact offenders, offenders with and without paraphilias, and persons with male or female victims, child or adult victims, or intrafamilial or extrafamilial victims. Some sexual offenders have mental illness, personality disorders, histories of trauma, or intellectual or developmental disabilities. Risk levels vary: low, medium, or high. This is only the beginning of the complex factors that differentiate and individualize people with histories of sexual offending.

When we look at the majority of sex offender research, including research into the implementation and effectiveness of sex offender treatment, it involves sexual offenders in correctional or community outpatient settings. This research is not fully representative of the sex offender population, as many sexual offenders reside in noncorrectional mental health or residential settings. Such clients may be significantly different from those in the correctional settings with regards to cognitive and educational level, mental health symptoms, personality pathology, level of risk, or range of adaptive functioning (e.g., Stinson & Becker, 2011). Therefore, we are treating specific facets of the sex offender population who may often be excluded from traditional sex offender treatment programs. These persons are certainly a challenge, even for the most experienced of clinicians, but because of risk and quality-of-life concerns, we cannot simply endorse large-scale exclusion of these groups. Few empirical studies have evaluated treatment effectiveness with seriously mentally ill and intellectually or developmentally disabled sexual offenders, though the need for treatment in these populations is significant (e.g., Lambrick & Glaser, 2004; Lindsay, 2002; Stinson & Becker, 2011). SOS was developed and piloted with these groups, with concrete and specific treatment content, goals of adaptive skill development, emphasis on therapeutic interaction strategies with challenging clients, and a long-term approach to treatment progress. While these methods can be tailored for other, perhaps higher functioning sex offender populations, those with special vulnerabilities need not be excluded from treatment. Treatment providers need not make deliberate changes to the materials presented here, other than to pay careful attention to manner of presentation (e.g., oral vs. visual for those with literacy or language limitations), level of comprehension, and repeated review of concepts. These materials were developed for seriously mentally ill or disabled clients, and pilot groups simply tailored the length, repetition, and review of concepts to the capacities of their clients.

We are also treating clients who are often less-than-enthusiastic about treatment. While some may embrace the opportunity to learn more about their offending and prevent such behavior from recurring in the future, the majority are mandated to treatment by the courts, probation or parole, or other comparable systems within mental health agencies.

We must thus acknowledge that we treat clients who may be resistant, frustrated, or afraid. Their negative attitudes will impact their progress, their interactions with treatment providers and other clients, their ability to learn, and ultimately their ability to effectively self-monitor and develop adaptive and functional self-regulatory strategies. SOS may be particularly successful with those clients who struggle with motivation, as this is a core element of the treatment itself.

PRETREATMENT

To set the stage for effective intervention, pretreatment tasks include assessment, describing treatment targets, identifying protective factors and client supports, and approaching the client. While many of these are important goals throughout the treatment process as well, they must also be addressed prior to treatment implementation. The RNR model (Andrews et al., 1990; Bonta & Andrews, 2007) is a guide for structuring and selecting clients for offender treatment programs. The premise of the RNR model is that treatment providers should tailor treatment interventions to the client's level of risk, address specific treatment needs, and consider responsivity factors such as the client's willingness and ability to engage in treatment. SOS should be implemented in a manner consistent with the RNR model, which is apparent in these pretreatment tasks.

Assessment

Decisions about treatment involvement should be made with some consideration of client risk. The most intensive interventions are applied to the highest risk offenders, with medium risk offenders receiving services at a moderate level of intensity, and the lowest risk offenders receiving not necessarily the least amount of treatment but treatment that is instead tailored to reflect their reduced risk. Some may interpret this as "more treatment vs. less treatment versus no treatment." This is not the case. Instead, intensity of treatment services can be determined by a variety of factors, including length and frequency of sessions, client-to-facilitator ratio in group treatments, overall duration of treatment, complexity of treatment targets, aftercare and supervision requirements, and depth of treatment discussions and assignments. In SOS, the treatment materials and procedures are fluid enough to allow for individualized client needs.

Treatment providers may find it helpful to consider available risk assessment instruments, including those that examine both static and dynamic risk factors, and ongoing research in the area of sex offender risk. A number of these instruments are available and likely familiar to readers, like the Static-99 and Static-99R (Babchishin, Hanson, & Helmus, 2011; Hanson & Thornton, 2000; Helmus, Thornton, Hanson, & Babchishin, 2011), the Static-2002 (Hanson & Thornton, 2003) the Rapid Risk Assessment for Sex Offense Recidivism (RRASOR; Hanson, 1997), the Minnesota Sex Offender Screening Tool, Revised (MnSOST-R; Epperson, Kaul, & Hesselton, 2005), the Sex Offender Risk Appraisal Guide (SORAG; Quinsey, Harris, Rice, & Cormier, 1998), the Sexual Violence Risk-20 (SVR-20; Boer, Hart, Kropp, & Webster, 1997), and the Stable-2000/Acute-2000 and Stable 2007/Acute 2007 (Hanson et al., 2007). While these may be more often used in release decisions or risk management planning, they can also assist in making more empirically or data-driven choices regarding appropriate treatment.

Pretreatment assessments must also focus on identifying the client's treatment needs. Sources of information may include the client's psychosocial and psychosexual history, criminal history, institutional behavior, medical and psychiatric evaluations, and client self-report. Research related to the RNR model notes a number of specific intervention needs for sex offenders, including offense-supportive beliefs and patterns of sexual arousal, offense precursors, emotional control, social skills and support, and risk management ability, as well as targets for general offender treatment (e.g., substance abuse, criminal lifestyle; e.g., Becker & Stinson, 2011; Hanson et al., 2009a, 2009b). We conceptualize these needs through the lens of the multi-modal self-regulation theory. These treatment targets are broadly divided into the domains of dysregulation: (1) *emotional,* including anger, hostility, and difficulty with emotional control; (2) *cognitive,* such as offense-supportive beliefs, perceptions, and attitudes; (3) *interpersonal,* capturing social and interpersonal skills deficits, manipulative interpersonal behaviors, and isolation or lack of social support; and (4) *behavioral,* which includes offense-supportive sexual fantasies and urges, aggressive or criminal behaviors, impulsivity, and substance use. Different clients will have different treatment needs, and these may not be readily apparent at the onset of treatment. Treatment providers will need to evaluate and prioritize referral issues and more salient pretreatment needs, continually assessing other potential needs throughout the treatment process.

Pretreatment assessment of responsivity factors will place clients in treatment according to their abilities and motivation. General responsivity factors to look for include motivation and commitment to treatment: any cognitive, intellectual, or developmental disabilities that may impact the clients' abilities to communicate and understand treatment materials; learning style and learning disabilities; level of supervision needed in order to conduct group safely; degree of psychiatric impairment; medical stability; or idiosyncratic variables like paranoia. Other specialized needs, such as deafness or linguistic limitations, may also drive decisions, in that treatment providers may need to ensure appropriate interpretive services. Though these are obviously not targets of treatment or factors immediately suggestive of increased risk, they will certainly impact client participation and progress in treatment. Responsivity factors can be gathered through a variety of means, including a review of history, client self-report, cognitive or achievement testing, or other psychological assessments. Assessment will be dependent on the client, the nature of the assessment or treatment services available at any given agency, and the time and resources available. It should be noted that the intention is not to require hours of assessment prior to treatment, but to gain enough information that treatment providers can best match clients with treatment programming and also have some awareness of potential areas of concern prior to the start of treatment.

Treatment Targets

As we have noted, treatment providers will need to conduct pretreatment assessment of potential treatment needs, including sex-offender-specific needs, as well as other generalized targets for intervention. In developing treatment targets, we must acknowledge multiple stakeholders in the treatment process. First, there is the client. He or she will have personal goals and preconceived ideas about what to do in sex offender treatment. This is a collaborative process, and clients may be more successful when they are allowed some degree of autonomy in focusing the direction of their treatment (e.g., Beech & Fordham, 1997; Marshall, 2005; Marshall, Ward, et al., 2005). Second, others may want a voice in client treatment, including supervision agents, the court, administrators at a treatment facility, victims, or the client's family. At times, we are mandated to abide by the goals of outside agents, particularly with regards to goals like "not reoffending." As a treatment provider, one can always exercise discretion in determining how successfully clients have met their goals and what other targets may be relevant on the way to addressing that ultimate goal. Third, treatment providers have their own goals and expectations to consider. These are determined by treatment approach, experience, and interactions with the clients on a day-to-day basis. We must strike a balance between these varying goals.

Identifying Protective Factors and Supports

Treatment is not all about risk. In SOS, it is also about developing and cultivating adaptive and healthy regulatory behaviors. Looking to clients for their strengths, supports, and protective factors can be a way of initiating and guiding this process. In the early stages of treatment (i.e., pretreatment assessment and Module 1) clients are encouraged to identify their strengths as well as support systems and other protective factors. These may include motivation, periods of stability or success, interpersonal strengths, past compliance with medications or treatment requirements, ability to ask for help, or even special abilities and talents that can serve as skills or adaptive strategies. A number of these protective factors, such as social support and prosocial (non-offense-supportive) beliefs and fantasies have also been empirically supported in relation to reduced risk of sexual recidivism (e.g., Hanson et al., 2009a).

This task also necessitates the assessment of realistically available supports, given applicable restrictions or situational factors. For example, if the client is in an institution, contact with family may be limited to certain times, or it may be solely dependent on administrative decisions. Clients in this situation who say that a primary support is family contact may find it useful instead to conceptualize this as "caring about others" or "being a supportive person," so that they see this as a strength available to them in their current setting. A focus on positive and supportive aspects of their abilities, relationships, and behaviors will also foster a positive therapeutic relationship from the outset of therapy.

Orienting the Client to New Treatment

We must also think about how to approach the client. While this pretreatment process implicitly assumes that the client is aware of pending intervention, it does not always mean that the client knows what to expect, the type of treatment being offered, or how to best interact with treatment providers. Typically, both clients who are new to sex offender treatment or who have participated in past forms of sex offender treatment are doing so as the result of either legal mandate or institutional policy. In other words, for many clients, treatment is not truly voluntary. Treatment providers are therefore tasked with the challenge of describing treatment in a way that generates client interest and hope. While we do not advocate for insincere or superficial treatment solicitations, clients may relate to the opportunity to focus on a variety of goals and to move at an individualized pace. Clients will also need to know the basic expectations of them in treatment, including attendance and participation in group discussions, commitment to treatment, and self-monitoring. Treatment providers must also acknowledge obligations to others, including the courts, institutions or agencies, or supervisory personnel. If agreements have been made with these agencies regarding regular reporting of treatment progress or activities, adherence to specific rules or policies, or meetings between treatment providers and other involved persons, then clients should be fully aware of these agreements at the outset in order to avoid any pretense of secrecy or deception, and so that the client will know the limits of confidentiality in treatment.

COMPATIBILITY WITH OTHER PROGRAMS

Some clients, particularly those who are in residential facilities or other forms of intensive treatment, may be receiving additional therapeutic services beyond sex offender treatment while they are also in SOS. SOS is compatible with other forms of psychosocial rehabilitation, provided that the philosophy and emphasis on self-regulation and development of adaptive skills remains intact.

Particularly compatible with SOS are programs utilizing dialectical behavior therapy (Dimeff & Koerner, 2007; Linehan, 1993), where the emphasis is on self-monitoring of dysregulated emotions and problematic urges and behaviors through the use of daily diary cards, skills groups to enhance adaptive functioning, and validation and skills coaching by treatment providers. Also compatible are programs for clients with intellectual and developmental disabilities that utilize positive behavior support (e.g., Carr et al., 2002), an approach emphasizing the function of client behavior and individualized treatment planning to enhance functional skills development and support networks. It also stresses the value of self-management of behavior, within the capabilities of that particular client.

Another possibility, however, is to modify SOS into a more comprehensive milieu program for exclusively treating individuals with sex offending behaviors, rather than just including it as one component of a larger treatment approach. This was the choice of our third pilot site, a civil commitment program for sexually violent predators. Given the broad and comprehensive nature of self-regulation, and the range of other maladaptive behaviors to address beyond just sexual offending (e.g., aggression, other criminal activity, substance use, self-harm or suicidal behaviors), SOS can be expanded into a series of groups and interventions such as groups addressing the various areas of dysregulation, more focused skills groups, behavioral chain analysis groups for continuing difficulties with sexual and other maladaptive behaviors, relationship effectiveness groups, and the like. The philosophy of SOS would also be expanded to broader programming efforts, and the activities described within this text can be applied in a more in-depth fashion for high-risk or long-term populations. (For example, SOS has been implemented as a milieu program at one of the three pilot sites.)

ASSESSING CLIENT PROGRESS

Traditional measures of treatment progress generally look for whether or not the client has improved since the initial treatment session. While behavioral and symptom improvements are certainly valid indicators of progress, there are many others that may be applicable in SOS. Progress is described differently by different persons—the client will have an internal measure of improvement, certain external agents (e.g., courts, administrators) may be mostly concerned with a reduction in sex offending behavior, and treatment providers will have a different and perhaps more in-depth view of the many factors that determine progress and treatment success. Progress falls on a continuum, and clients may vary throughout treatment in terms of how they demonstrate and maintain their progress. Below, we briefly describe several factors that incorporate dynamic risk and the clinical treatment literature to guide determinations of progress.

Measuring Progress

Improvement in Behavior from the Baseline

This is the most obvious and perhaps most traditional measure of progress in sex offender treatment. Put simply, has the client continued to commit sexual offenses? (This is most relevant for institutionalized clients.) If so, are they less frequent or less severe than they were in the past? People assume that fewer offenses means treatment success. This is true, to an extent. But when clients do not have access to preferred victims (e.g., pedophiles residing in an institution with adult peers), this is difficult to assess. It is also true though that sex offending behaviors do not occur that frequently, even for the most serious of offenders, so that any real reduction may take time to become evident. Also, sex offending behaviors are not the only relevant outcome, and other goals may still be salient even in the absence of clear sex offending behaviors.

Treatment Engagement and Willingness

By most standards, clients who are engaged and motivated are called successful treatment participants, whereas clients who are uncommitted, unmotivated, and disengaged are viewed as poor treatment participants. This is not the clear standard in SOS. It is possible for engaged and motivated clients to also continue having behavioral problems, struggle with applying treatment concepts, or show limited progress in other areas. Treatment providers must realize that commitment is a facet of progress that may operate somewhat independently of the others. Commitment and motivation should be fostered and reinforced, as this a first step toward more significant treatment changes. Keep in mind though that commitment varies according to the goal. Some clients may not be motivated to work on their maladaptive sexual behaviors, but they are committed to improve their relationships, control anger, or accept new beliefs.

Openness and Acceptance

Treatment providers who typically work with hostile, manipulative, or highly resistant clients can easily see the benefits of openness and acceptance in treatment. Being open and accepting of one's behaviors, limitations, or need for treatment are not the sole determinants of treatment progress, but when a client approaches treatment with an open mind and an accepting attitude, that person will gain more from treatment activities. With improvements in openness and acceptance come improvements in treatment performance. Acceptance, engagement, and willingness are all similar in that they do not always mean a "cure" for problematic thinking and behaviors, but they will facilitate learning and help clients remain in treatment for the duration.

Comprehension of Treatment Concepts

SOS consists of a variety of treatment discussions and activities, some of which focus on the client's behavior, and some of which more generally reflect principles of self-regulation and skills building. Clients may demonstrate a basic understanding of these concepts while still struggling with applying them to their own behaviors or even recognizing a need for treatment. This basic understanding is still important, because even as we see that a client does not understand his or her own offending, we can also see that he or she understands the general concepts associated with treatment and can apply them to relevant, though nonpersonal, examples. It illustrates where the need for continued treatment lies and guides future treatment planning.

Reality-Oriented Discussion of Concepts

Progress can also be measured by how well the client is able to relate treatment concepts to reality-based examples. This is more than just comprehension, as it reflects not only a basic understanding of terms and principles, but also the ability to think about them in context. For example, a client may be able to describe boundaries and give examples of what they are, but would he or she be able to recognize a boundary violation? And could the client verbalize why it's a boundary violation? In another case, a client may be able to identify characteristics of an unhealthy relationship, but would he or she be aware of being in an unhealthy relationship? Relating treatment topics to real examples in the moment gives us an idea as to how well the client will be able to apply these concepts in daily life.

Relating Treatment Concepts to Behavior

Does the client routinely apply treatment concepts to others' behaviors in group discussions or in situations outside of group? Can the client apply concepts to his or her own behaviors? If a sex offending behavior occurs during the course of treatment, for example, can the client recognize and describe important factors that precipitated this event? This measure of progress most certainly exists on a continuum; it is highly dependent on the behavior, its seriousness, its complexity, and other individualized factors. It is generally more difficult for clients to apply these strategies to their own behaviors than to others' behaviors, as they can observe others' actions more objectively. Treatment providers will be able to assess progress as clients move from (1) understanding concepts to (2) applying them in a reality-based way to (3) applying them to others' behaviors to finally (4) viewing them in the context of their own actions.

Self-Monitoring and Self-Awareness

A primary goal of SOS is to teach clients to self-monitor their dysregulation so that they can more easily interrupt dysfunctional or maladaptive regulatory behaviors and use adaptive strategies for modulating problematic emotions, thoughts, interpersonal interactions, urges, and behaviors. Seeing clients develop better self-monitoring abilities is therefore a key factor in describing client progress. Clients who maintain that they don't know when they are dysregulated, or that dysregulated states "just happen" without warning, clearly lack the ability to adequately self-monitor. This leaves them less able to use adaptive skills when they are needed most. Increased self-awareness and self-monitoring can also be used to measure client progress, dynamic risk, and needed supervision and supports as a client moves through treatment.

Responsibility and Insight

Responsibility and insight are very traditional measures of progress in sex offender treatment. Unfortunately, these measures are often simplified into their most basic forms: Does the client acknowledge culpability and harm? And does the client understand why he or she did it? These questions are not the only, nor even always the best, indicators of progress. There are many clients who fully acknowledge their behaviors and accept responsibility for them who are still very dangerous and who may have no real intention of changing. Sometimes those who minimize may in fact have a better understanding of the harm, social consequences, and judgments associated with their offending than those who openly acknowledge and even embrace their offending. More important though is balance. Clients may range on the continuum from hostile denial to almost prideful acknowledgment of offending. Somewhere in between are those who do understand and feel responsible for what they do. Insight into risk is also important. Clients who have progressed in other areas but who say that they are not concerned about risk because they simply *know* they will never do it again are those same clients who are unlikely to self-monitor or be self-aware of risk. Insight into one's own vulnerabilities, potential risks, or problems can be a powerful indicator of treatment progress, even in the absence of other signs of success.

Progress on a Continuum

As we have noted in the above discussion, client progress exists on a continuum, and when one considers the divergent but interconnected ways of measuring progress, progress in fact exists on multiple continuums. Clients, for example, may show improvement in behavior through the use of adaptive strategies but little insight into the seriousness of their behaviors or their need for risk management and self-monitoring. Such clients may be "going through the motions" without internalizing a need for doing so. Other clients may be strongly committed and motivated but show little improvement in self-management and use of adaptive skills. Still others may never show a commitment to change and begrudgingly attend treatment with no real goals for progress. Within this treatment frame, we meet clients where they are. (More is discussed about this topic in the following chapter.) Sometimes we have to face the reality that clients are not where we want them to be. There is little we can do to force change, but we simply note this lack of progress in any number of ways and continue working with the client to reinforce the progress or success he or she has had, and to illustrate other areas of potential treatment benefit.

CONCLUSIONS

In this chapter, we have reviewed many of the practical components of implementing SOS. We have introduced a summary of the 10 modules, considerations of treatment structure and startup, and suggestions for selecting clients and treatment providers. We have also discussed pre-treatment tasks like assessment and orienting the client to treatment, as well as ways to measure progress throughout the use of SOS. We now move from the practical to the philosophical as we look at overarching strategies to help put these ideas into practice.

CHAPTER 4

Case Conceptualization and Working with Clients

In Chapter 2, we described the underlying theoretical model from which we have derived SOS. In Chapter 3, we considered the practical elements of implementing SOS, including a brief description of the target population for whom SOS was primarily developed and piloted at three treatment sites. Now, we take a closer look at how we view clients within this frame. As readers are aware, not all sex offenders are the same. Each client has unique features that shape case conceptualization, development of treatment plans and treatment needs, building a therapeutic relationship, and using clinical strategies to facilitate treatment progress.

In this chapter we describe the philosophical elements of SOS. This includes how clients present with different features of dysregulation and self-regulatory deficits, how clinical case conceptualization will evolve over time, primary assumptions about clients, and important strategies to assist treatment providers in engaging clients in the therapeutic learning process. The primary goal of this chapter is to guide treatment providers through the clinical and philosophical aspects of understanding clients and their treatment needs in SOS. So while Chapter 2 focuses on *why* we have SOS (i.e., sex offenders have self-regulatory deficits), and Chapter 3 focuses on *what* you do in treatment, the goal of Chapter 4 is to learn *how* to do it.

A secondary but related goal is to ensure that treatment providers stay within the philosophical mind-set that is intended with SOS—a mind-set familiar to readers who have used other, compatible clinical techniques and approaches like those described in Chapter 3 (e.g., dialectical behavior therapy; Linehan, 1993) but perhaps unfamiliar to those who have exclusively practiced other forms of sex offender treatment. Adherence to a treatment model requires more than just doing the right worksheets or addressing topics in a certain order. In this case, it also necessitates thinking about and interacting with the client in specific, planned ways to enhance treatment effectiveness. The conceptualization of and interaction with the client in such ways also maintains the integrity of the etiological foundation upon which the therapy is based. The many elements of SOS as a treatment are tied together, and it is the view of the client that binds them.

WHO IS THE CLIENT?

In Chapter 3, we noted the heterogeneity of the sex offender population, and how SOS was developed to aid those clients who struggle with specialized treatment needs, including those with mental illness, personality disorders, or cognitive, intellectual, or developmental disabilities, as well as high-risk sex offenders with multiple offenses and a need for intensive therapy. Again, this is not to say that SOS will not work with other sex offender populations. On the contrary, it may be useful for other groups in need of more targeted intervention or who struggle with motivation to engage in treatment. However, for our purposes here, we assume the client to be a person with complex treatment needs who could benefit from a unique, integrated approach to treatment.

Case Conceptualization

Sex offenders enter treatment with vastly differing personalities, goals, and personal needs. Some have lengthy histories of formal arrest and conviction, whereas others do not. Some are contact offenders who have committed acts of sexual assault and child molestation, and some are noncontact offenders with histories of exhibitionism, voyeurism, and bestiality. Some offenders profess sexual interests in children or other nonnormative sexual stimuli, while others appear to have normative sexual interests and relationships apart from their offending behaviors. Is it possible for one treatment approach to satisfy the needs of such a diverse group?

When we treat sex offenders, we treat persons who exhibit deficits in their ability to self-regulate, and who have developed a series of maladaptive regulatory strategies over time. While the specifics of their dysregulation and the maladaptive behaviors they use are to some extent idiosyncratic—shaped by their experiences, reinforcement, and opportunity—dysregulation and self-regulatory deficits are a universal, shared occurrence that allows us a common theme to target in treatment. In other words, although each individual may struggle with his or her own form of dysregulation, the fact that it is dysregulation underlying the problem allows us to treat members of a heterogeneous group within the same general frame. Some examples of potential case conceptualizations utilizing this approach are provided below:

1. Rapist with hostile feelings toward women, psychopathic and sadistic traits
   a. Emotional—anger, entitlement, resentment, defiance
   b. Cognitive—judgment, blame, expectations of women, beliefs of sexual entitlement, egocentricity
   c. Interpersonal—hostility, manipulation, deceitfulness, dominance
2. Rapist with feelings of inadequacy and resentment
   a. Emotional—anxiety, resentment, hurt, loneliness
   b. Cognitive—self-criticism, self-judgment, all-or-nothing thinking, blame
   c. Interpersonal—isolation, sarcasm, intrusiveness, poor boundaries
3. Pedophile with depression and anxiety, poor relationships with adults
   a. Emotional—depression, anxiety, loneliness, helplessness
   b. Cognitive—beliefs about sexual interactions, problem-solving deficits, rationalization
   c. Interpersonal—isolation, poor social skills, manipulation
4. Noncontact offender (exhibitionist) with psychosis and poor social skills
   a. Emotional—paranoia, inhibited emotions, anger
   b. Cognitive—delusional beliefs, blame, cognitive disorganization, judgment
   c. Interpersonal—accusations, arguing, isolation, poor social skills
5. Opportunistic offender against adults and children, males and females, with personality pathology
   a. Emotional—entitlement, boredom, excitement, labile emotional experiences

    b. Cognitive—justification, sexual expectations and entitlement, perceptions of opportunity

    c. Interpersonal—hostility, manipulation, grooming behaviors, deceitfulness

Therefore, a client with a history of sexual perpetration against children, whose offenses are precipitated by loneliness, resentment, and social isolation, can be treated with the same basic approach as a client whose sexual assaults against adults are precipitated by his own anger, entitlement, and judgments about women. Teaching both clients to identify and self-monitor their dysregulated emotions, thoughts, and interactions, followed by teaching them learning strategies to help them cope more effectively, can address two very different illegal sexual behaviors. Working with both clients on their sexual boundaries, building healthy relationships, and other important needs they may share can also lead to positive therapeutic change.

Conceptualizing clients in this way allows for immense clinical flexibility. Each client has unique patterns of dysregulation and similarly unique or individualized difficulties with managing this dysregulation (i.e., self-regulatory deficits) and combinations of adaptive and maladaptive strategies used to partially or temporarily manage states of dysregulation. Therefore, the treatment landscape is constantly changing. Each client has his or her own set of self-regulatory needs, ways of managing self-regulatory processes, and evolution of these processes over time. As one area improves, deficits in another area may become more visible and present new challenges for clients and treatment providers. But again, the client's needs can be viewed through the same theoretical lens while still allowing for this flexibility. This is very important to remember as we move through all aspects of treatment.

Treatment Planning

Developing a plan for each client's treatment involves input from multiple sources, including the client, the treatment provider(s), and others who may be involved in the client's treatment referral (e.g., the court or some other facility administrative body). SOS is a manualized treatment. This means that the different components of treatment share an underlying theoretical and philosophical approach, common ideas about the conceptualization of the client, and a common view of client needs and treatment direction. However, treatment providers are encouraged to use flexibility in tailoring treatment concepts and materials to meet the educational, cognitive, and experiential needs of their particular clients. Providers can be creative in the way that they communicate treatment concepts to their clients, and the way in which they encourage clients to discuss and internalize important treatment components. Also, treatment providers have flexibility in determining the length of treatment, the depth and direction of group or therapeutic discussions, and specific examples or experiences described by the clients. Though different groups or clients may use the same basic materials to address the same ideas, the actual individual or group discussions will look very different depending on the examples and discussion points raised by each client.

Clients are also given much flexibility within this manualized framework in light of their individualized treatment needs and patterns of dysregulation and self-regulatory deficit. The discussions and activities are broad enough to allow for this individual variability. Discussing unhealthy relationships, for example, will allow each client to describe unhealthy relationships in his or her own way, drawing from individual experience. Individualized treatment planning also considers that some clients are more ready to work on specific parts of treatment than others, and some will primarily focus on enhancing their motivation and commitment, while others will demonstrate greater readiness to approach those issues more directly related to their offending behaviors.

Integration of Assessment Tools

In Chapter 3, we discussed pretreatment assessments that can aid in better understanding the client and his or her risk, needs, and treatment responsivity. Early on in the process of knowing the client and developing a treatment plan, we must integrate the information from the pretreatment assessment process. Clients' risk and protective factors, identified supports, and treatment targets will all be a part of the treatment. As clients move through early modules describing motivation and basic treatment concepts, these factors will play into client discussions. They will help determine client progress as well.

Important questions can be answered by integrating pretreatment information. Answers to these questions, in combination with the strategies described at the end of this chapter, will inform decisions about how to best interact with clients and present treatment information:

1. How do clients feel about treatment?
2. What is their risk level and how complex are their corresponding needs?

3. What other issues (psychiatric, behavior, interpersonal, etc.) may be relevant to treatment?
4. How can protective factors and supports be woven into treatment?
5. What are potential barriers or challenges that can impede treatment efforts?

By thinking about these questions and using the information garnered from pretreatment tasks, treatment providers can better plan and know their clients.

Evolving Conceptualization of the Client—Learning to Accept the Unknown

As with any complex situation, the rules are always changing. Sex offender treatment is no different, though the ultimate focus—managing sexual and other problem behaviors through adaptive self-regulation—remains the same. When clients improve and change in one area, other needs will arise and become more salient. Perhaps a client's vulnerabilities and intimacy deficits were hidden before by intense anger, hostility, and isolation from potential sources of support. Or maybe a client's symptoms of mental illness were masked by years of substance abuse and unhealthy relationship behaviors. Once such clients have made progress in treatment, other such issues become visible. Another possibility is that the client who has identified problems with dysregulation and is effectively using adaptive self-management is now faced with even greater challenges as he or she transitions into a different setting. Clients who move from residential to community treatment, for example, may be faced with many sudden changes in environmental structure, availability of treatment and support, expectations and responsibility, and the potential cost of failure. For such clients, the need for stability and self-management has just dramatically increased, as has the stress and potential dysregulation that they will face on a daily basis.

The challenge for treatment providers is to integrate the unknown into a client's treatment plan. Since the very nature of the unknown means that one cannot fully anticipate it, instead we encourage treatment providers to exercise flexibility in their treatment planning, and to prepare for natural evolutions in clients' treatment needs. This flexibility and preparation involves changing conceptualizations of motivation and willingness to engage in treatment, reformulations of primary goals and treatment targets, reconsideration of dynamic risk factors, and other recalibrations of a client's treatment plan according to natural changes that occur as treatment relationships become more knowing and complex.

HOW WE VIEW THE CLIENT

Sex offender treatment is a process of change. As treatment providers, we expect clients to make many changes concerning their beliefs, their attitudes, their interactions with others, their perceptions, their sexual arousal patterns, their everyday activities, and, most importantly, their behaviors. Realistically, these are high expectations, and we typically expect such change to occur quickly (over a few years) relative to the amount of time it took for these patterns to develop (a lifetime). We should be aware that our expectations shape how we view the client, which in turn shapes the client's attitude, engagement, and progress in treatment. To work effectively, we may need to examine our fundamental expectations regarding sex offenders in treatment.

• *First, the client is capable of change.* This is self-evident from a treatment perspective, but it is too easy to view sex offenders as hopeless or lost causes. The severity of their behaviors, stigma, obstacles to treatment, and extensiveness of their needs prevent us from seeing their capabilities for change. Remember though that change does not always have to be dramatic in order to be significant. A client who changes just a few small things is still demonstrating the capacity for success. These small changes may add up to more meaningful changes over time. But that the client is capable of changing something in treatment is a fundamental assumption of SOS. Remember too that because SOS allows for a variety of treatment targets, what the client wants to change may not always be directly sexual, but still represents treatment progress. Smaller goals, such as self-monitoring anger, practicing appropriate boundaries with females, or maintaining medication compliance, are all relevant indicators of change.

• *Second, the client is capable of making good choices.* Despite having made some poor choices in the past, clients are generally capable of learning new adaptive strategies and behaviors. They may need treatment in order to learn and use such strategies. The assumption, therefore, is not that clients will always make good choices, but that they can, given the right intervention, support, and opportunity. Relatedly, the client needs support to be successful. Unfortunately, sex offender treatment is one of the few areas of mental health intervention where being hostile toward and judgmental of the client is accepted or even encouraged. Methods of treatment that rely on shaming, confrontation, criticism, and judgment to "shock" or "break down" the offender are not a source of support and are not conducive to positive therapeutic change. Instead, treatment providers must facilitate success through support, genuineness (which may include honest but considerate feedback about progress and behavior), and respect for the individual.

• *Third, the client has been reinforced in the past for his or her maladaptive behaviors.* It is too simplistic to view sex offending as what the client just "likes to do." And it is not therapeutic to view the client as an evil or bad person, with sexual offending as evidence of his or her pervasively damaged character. All behaviors, especially within the context of self-regulatory development, are either effective or ineffective at modulating internal states and interpersonal interactions. Our value judgments about these behaviors can cause us to forget that they serve a purpose, and may have been reinforced in many ways. This does not mean that we no longer view the behaviors as harmful, dangerous, or unacceptable. But it does mean that we focus less on the intentionality of the client (i.e., he or she did it to hurt someone), and instead look to assist the client in learning new strategies to foster healthy self-regulatory ability and reduce harm to self and others.

• *Fourth, the client wants to change.* It can be hard to see client motivation through his or her defensiveness, resistance, shame, anxiety, and anger. Some struggle with these reactions so much that they say they are unwilling to change or simply do not need treatment. But generally, clients in sex offender treatment are rather unhappy with their current circumstances. They may feel guilt, shame, anger, or self-criticism. They may experience legal sanctions, restrictions on their freedom, loss of family or friends, and social isolation. Recognizing a problem, or at least being uncomfortable with the problem, lends itself to the possibility of change. We must not think of treatment motivation as an either-or condition. Instead, motivation exists on a continuum, and even those who appear to be the most unmotivated can identify something related to their sex offense that may lend itself to change. This may be as indirect as "I don't get along with everyone" (meaning perhaps the court, the victim, or even treatment providers) or "I don't want to be here anymore." SOS assumes that clients have some willingness to change, even though we may not always agree with what they think they should change.

Treatment providers must believe in that part of the client that wants change and foster it so that it may lead to greater treatment gains.

BUILDING A THERAPEUTIC RELATIONSHIP

In order to foster treatment motivation and treatment change, we must build therapeutic relationships with clients. The reason for this is clear: hostility does not beget meaningful change. There are always those who argue that "tough love" or harsh confrontation will expose clients to the rude realities of their behavior and shock them into taking a serious look at their actions. From that perspective, treatment providers help the client hit "rock bottom" so that he or she will have nowhere else to go but up, presumably toward the enlightenment of sex offender treatment. The reality, however, is that interpersonal conflict, confrontation, criticism, and hostility rarely evoke positive responses from clients. Instead, these interactions elicit strong dysregulation, thus minimizing the effectiveness of any effort to teach new information or strategies. Clients are experienced with harsh treatment and judgment from others. They do not learn from these persons willingly, nor do they view them as a source of support.

We must meet the client where he or she is at in the current moment. This involves the client's acceptance of his or her offending and the current situation, motivation to engage in treatment, and hope for future success. Treatment providers will find this easier with clients who are motivated, willing, and already making progress. But with clients who are not yet ready to engage, or who say they are willing but minimize or deny responsibility, treatment providers must accept this situation, for the moment, and help them develop a plan for making some positive gain from treatment. Clients will not always stay in that mind-set, and we can help them develop a more treatment-engaged mind-set through supportive guidance rather than judgmental confrontation. Treatment providers can still have their own internal expectations and plans, and we do not have to accept denial or minimization as truth. Clients do struggle with making a firm treatment commitment, and working with the client can build a relationship capable of supporting change.

A collaborative approach to treatment is central to SOS. An initial reaction may be "But I don't want to 'collaborate' with a sexual offender. That's not what therapy is." Some traditions in sex offender treatment view the treatment provider as a teacher, an interrogator, or a judge. Instead, we view the treatment provider as one who works with the client to learn about the client's behavior, to develop alternative strategies and plans, to continually assess client goals and progress, and to provide feedback related to ongoing treatment needs. This collaborative view aids the client in building a trusting relationship with the treatment provider so that he or she can express concerns, frustrations, and setbacks in an open way. It discourages secrecy and is accepting of flaws. This is therapeutic acceptance of the person rather than acceptance or justification of his or her harmful behaviors. The purpose of collaboration is to build a meaningful therapeutic alliance that facilitates change.

A more difficult point, however, is this: treatment providers must learn to cope with their own dysregulation. This is where we all fail at times, some more gloriously than others. It is easy to become hopeless and frustrated with a client's denial, lack of motivation, or failure to make progress in treatment. Clients who do not take treatment seriously, who are inconsistent in their approach, or who continue to engage in problematic behavior (seemingly on purpose) cause treatment providers to become detached, critical, and burnt-out. Frustration with clients causes tremendous damage to the therapeutic relationship, and as much as we would like to think it is the client's job to fix it, we must also accept some responsibility for our own dysregulation. So how do we do this? Consider the following:

1. *Clients have reasons for their behavior.* Denial, minimization, disinterest, or inconsistency all serve a purpose or could be related to other problems. Clients may deny or minimize because of their shame or resentment. They may engage inconsistently or not at all because, like many other people, they experience setbacks and give up during the change process. This is normal, though frustrating. Trying to understand the underlying reasons for client resistance can pull the treatment provider back into a therapeutic frame.

2. *We too must self-monitor our dysregulation.* Telling yourself that you do not become frustrated with clients, or that a "good therapist" does not judge, will only increase your dysregulation. Treatment providers must accept their own faults and frustrations and cope with them in order to provide effective treatment.

3. *Sometimes just being genuine with the clients can aid their progress.* This is a delicate maneuver. We do not advocate for treatment providers to share their own personal lives, struggles, or judgments and opinions with clients. Such sharing of personal information is potentially damaging to the client and his or her treatment, not to mention unethical. But

at times, expressing genuine emotion in a therapeutic way can help both providers and clients reach an understanding and strengthen their relationship. Saying, "I just don't understand why this is so difficult. Maybe I'm just thinking it's too easy. Help me see it," or "I know you don't want to be here. You've said that a lot. But hearing it over and over again when you're so angry makes it hard for me to be here too," can go a long way toward achieving this goal.

4. *Taking a break is allowed.* This doesn't mean quitting one's job, disbanding a group, or even going on an expensive vacation. These are not always realistic options, nor will they fix the problem. But talking with others about one's frustrations, seeking supervision from another professional, soliciting the help of other providers in leading a difficult group, or taking a "day off" by having group members do another, less intense activity, can help alleviate the pressure.

SPECIFIC STRATEGIES FOR THE TREATMENT PROVIDER

Each client has different needs, motivations, and goals. Struggles with denial, traumatic experiences, judgment and shame, and dysregulation in a variety of domains can all impact the client's progress in treatment. Specific techniques can facilitate client progress and bolster the therapeutic relationship. The core strategies discussed here include validation, dealing with denial, enhancing motivation and commitment, and skills building (see Table 4.1). Some of these strategies are associated with specific modules of treatment, whereas others may be used appropriately throughout the treatment program. Each of these stategies are introduced here and then discussed more specifically within the context of the group activities and discussions in Chapters 5–14.

Validation

The term "validation" is used rather broadly and inconsistently throughout the psychological literature. In some cases, it refers to empirical proof that a concept, technique, or tool bears scientific merit. For example, we refer to empirically "validated" treatments to communicate the belief that they have met specific criteria and have a discernable scientific basis. Other times, "validate" is used in a legal context to establish a standard of evidentiary proof or to substantiate a legal claim. One might think of

TABLE 4.1. Strategies for Enhancing Motivation and Commitment

Provider expectations of sex offenders in treatment
- Clients are capable of change.
- Client are capable of making good choices.
- Clients have been reinforced for their maladaptive behaviors.
- Clients want to change.

Validation (Linehan, 1993)
- Level 1—Listening and observing
- Level 2—Accurate reflection of what is stated
- Level 3—Articulating the unverbalized
- Level 4—Validating sufficient (not necessarily valid) causes
- Level 5—Validating as reasonable in the moment
- Level 6—Radical genuineness

Motivational interviewing (Miller & Rollnick, 2013)
- Exploring ambivalence
- Facilitating change talk
- Developing discrepancy
- Rolling with resistance
- Reflective listening
- Affirming positive aspects of clients' emotions and behavior
- Weighing costs versus benefits
- Accepting where the client is in the moment

the controversial "validation" studies undertaken to verify recovered or repressed memories of childhood sexual abuse.

Here, however, we define validation differently. Our view of validation originates from the work of Linehan (1993) in her discussion of core strategies of dialectical behavior therapy (DBT). The reason for this is twofold: First, DBT's psychosocial model of borderline personality disorder contains many common elements with the multi-modal self-regulation theory, including the belief that some problematic behaviors are maladaptive regulatory strategies, and that intense dysregulation in various aspects of a person's life may contribute to such behavioral difficulties. Second, sex offenders are often treated in a confrontational, invalidating, and at times openly hostile manner. Thus, the use of validation in this context provides a more accepting and motivating experience for these individuals, which is necessary to foster lasting therapeutic change.

But what is validation? Validation is a strategy to help clients understand themselves better by communicating to them that their responses are valid and understandable within the context of their environment (Linehan, 1993). Validation is the therapist's effort to have a meaningful and genuine relationship with the client, in which the therapist believes that the client is capable of change and that the client has real strengths and legitimate life goals. Validation is not simply making the client feel better or turning something into a positive statement; this may in fact trivialize the client's experience and be *invalidating*. In essence, validation allows the client to know that he or she has been understood and to help him or her make meaningful sense of current behaviors.

Why use validation in sex offender treatment? Validation builds rapport and a positive therapeutic relationship, increases the climate of acceptance and hope for the client, and assists the client in understanding his or her own behavior. While traditional delivery of sex offender treatment has not emphasized an inherent need to validate the client, it seems necessary in order to address difficult client behavior. Factors that influenced the client's decisions and behavior can be validated without excusing or minimizing his or her offense. Validation also "normalizes" the experience of dysregulation for the client, thus increasing the likelihood that a client will accurately self-monitor and report continuing struggles with self-regulation.

Therapeutic validation is best described on a continuum, with the *Levels of Validation* used in DBT (Dimeff, 2008). They progress from basic observation to more direct and genuine communication with the client.

Level 1 Validation: Listening and Observing

This involves careful, genuine, and mindful listening to the client's words and observing his or her behaviors. The therapist actively monitors verbal and nonverbal responses from the client. With regards to sex offender treatment, this monitoring includes listening to the client without making judgments or interpretations as to the meaning, intention, or legitimacy of what the client says.

> *Therapist validation*: "Tell me more." "What were you thinking when you just said that?" "Can you explain that to me?"

Level 2 Validation: Accurate Reflection of What Is Stated

This is accurately reflecting or summarizing what the client says. As with Level 1 Validation, the therapist avoids judgments or interpretations related to the client's responses. The goal is to communicate attentiveness and meaningful understanding. This does not mean that you have to agree with what the person has said, but only that you try to understand it.

> *Client example*: "I didn't tell her what was going on because she never listens to me anyway. Why bother?"

> *Therapist validation*: "So it seemed like it would have been pointless to tell her. She might not hear what you have to say."

Level 3 Validation: Articulating the Unverbalized

The therapist "reads" the client's behavior and imagines feelings, thoughts, or desires that the client might not have yet expressed. The therapist does not assume that a behavior was driven by its outcome, even if that outcome was reinforcing. This level of validation helps the client clarify his or her thoughts, feelings, and actions.

> *Therapist validation*: "It sounds like you were very upset/angry/hurt." "This must really be difficult for you." "Sometimes people are afraid to talk about these things in front of everybody, especially when you worry what other people might be thinking."

Level 4 Validation: Validating in Terms of Sufficient (but Not Necessarily Valid) Causes

The therapist validates the client's behavior given past experiences, perceptions (whether accurate or not), and biology. This means describing and reinforcing adaptive aspects of the client's behavior without emphasizing dysfunctional aspects of the behavior. The goal is for the client to make sense of the behavior in light of his or her life experience. Again, this does not mean that the therapist excuses or justifies the client's maladaptive behavior, but that the emotions, thoughts, or urges preceding the behavior were real.

> *Therapist validation:* "So when she turned you down, you were angry and embarrassed. You were thinking of every other woman who had ever rejected you. You were thinking of your friends, who saw this rejection and might have thought you were less of a man for just 'taking it' when she said no."

Level 5 Validation: Validating as Reasonable in the Moment

The therapist communicates that the person's behavior is reasonable, justifiable, meaningful, and effective in terms of current events, normative biological functioning, and the client's life goals. Unlike Level 4 Validation, where the therapist stops short of reinforcing the meaningfulness of a maladaptive behavior, this level of validation involves viewing the behavior, emotion, thought, or experience as reasonable and justified in the moment.

> *Therapist validation:* "You were really confused by that. I think most of us would have been confused at that moment. And so you got really angry and felt like you couldn't say anything about it." "I know you're having a hard time remembering what happened. It was a long time ago, and you weren't taking any medications then. You really want to work on this, but it's frustrating when your memory doesn't match the details of the police report. We'll do the best we can with what you do remember."

Level 6 Validation: Radical Genuineness

At this level, the client is treated as valid, that is, as a person of equal status to the therapist, due equal respect. The therapist recognizes the client as a genuine person with strengths and limitations, and believes in the client while seeing the client's struggles and pain. The therapist communicates without being patronizing or condescending.

> *Therapist validation:* "Being here is really difficult. I don't think I'd like to live here either. Sometimes I think about that, and I don't know how I would handle it." "What you did really scared people. I would have been scared too if I had been there." "No, I'm not angry with you because you're still having a hard time controlling your behavior. I guess I'm frustrated by the situation. I feel like we still haven't really figured things out just yet. And when we do, maybe it will be easier."

Using the levels of validation, treatment providers can emphasize and validate the *emotional* aspects of the client's response, such as letting the client describe his or her emotions, teaching how to monitor and label emotional experiences, recognizing nonverbal or indirect emotional cues from the client, and validating the inherent sense in the client's emotions (Linehan, 1993). Other strategies involve validating the *cognitive* components of the client's behavior, such as identifying and monitoring judgments, validating beliefs or expectations, helping the client learn differences between facts and judgments, and finding the truth in thoughts, emotions, or behaviors (Linehan, 1993). Finally, treatment providers should be prepared to provide validation in the form of support, encouragement, reinforcement, and realistic evaluation of the client's strengths and capabilities.

Validation is a challenging task. While most often the challenge is in deciding when and in what way to use validation, at times the challenge is to deliberately *not* use it. Validation should not be used for emotional catharsis (Linehan, 1993), nor should it be used immediately following a maladaptive behavior (e.g., sexual offending), as this kind of validation may only reinforce the behavior. And sometimes the challenge is how to validate something the therapist has judged to be problematic, distressing, or distasteful. In this instance, treatment providers will have an urge to challenge rather than to validate the client. One must remember that validation is not praise, nor approval, nor minimization of behavior. It is merely a tool to help the client learn from his or her own behavior, to increase the therapeutic understanding between client and treatment provider, and to feel understood, despite his or her flaws and problems. For example, a therapist is faced with a client who seems to be blaming the victim for a very violent, harmful offense. A therapist can still be validating by saying, "It seems like you're having a difficult time seeing why others held you responsible for that" or "It's sometimes hard to talk about the victim and what happened."

Denial

Those familiar with sex offender treatment—or any treatment aimed at correcting a problematic and stigmatizing behavior—are familiar with denial. Denial is a common response to any confrontation, challenge, or push for change. Denial results from perceived judgments; we may deny something to avoid others making judgments about us. Providers must be equipped to deal with offenders who deny all or parts of their offenses, as failure to prepare will lead to problems in treatment and strain the relationship between therapist and client.

Traditional sex offender treatments, including relapse prevention and cognitive-behavioral therapy, direct the treatment provider to confront and challenge the client's denial. An underlying theme of these treatments is that clients must admit their offending behaviors and the harm they have caused in order to make progress. Additionally, they must accept full responsibility for their behavior and not blame the victim or other external causes. Denial, minimization, and blame are confronted and immediately addressed. Treatment providers may respond to absolute denial by removing the client from treatment entirely. While many assume that this is an effective method for treating sexual offenders, most research indicates that confrontational methods damage therapeutic relationships, contribute to early treatment dropout, and inhibit client progress (e.g., Beech & Fordham, 1997; Marshall, Thornton, Marshall, Fernandez, & Mann, 2001; Marshall et al., 2005; Serran et al., 2003). It could also be argued that confrontation is more cathartic for the therapist than it is beneficial for the client.

SOS characterizes denial far differently. Denial is a mechanism through which the client presents him- or herself to the world in a more acceptable way—a way that is less subject to the negative judgments of others. Denial also serves to alleviate the client's guilt or shame. Thus, denial is perhaps a functional response to very real pressures. In order to better understand how denial is addressed in SOS, we will consider what it is in the context of the SOS philosophy, what treatment providers can do about it, and how clients in denial can still participate meaningfully in treatment.

What Is Denial?

Denial among sex offenders is fairly common; research suggests that a large number of sex offenders in treatment deny some, many, or all parts of their offense behaviors (e.g., Happel & Auffrey, 1995; Rogers & Dickey, 1991). Denial may be related only to parts of the offense (e.g., minimization of harm, denial of intent, denial of related fantasies), or it may be absolute and apply to the offense as a whole (e.g., "I didn't do it.") Both types of denial may prevent the client from engaging in and committing to treatment and could hinder the development of a positive relationship between client and treatment provider.

However, denial serves a function for the client. While denial of something as serious and harmful as a sexual offense may seem grossly maladaptive to us, we must step back for a moment and think about this process. First, what is more problematic? The offense or the denial? Most would agree that the sexual offense is the more serious problem. So what is the denial, if not the primary problem? Denial is the client's effort to counteract judgment, reduce stigma, and cope with shame and guilt. Denial occurs when we want to convince others of a different, albeit less reality-based, point of view. Denial, minimization, blame, and other derivations of this process are all-too-common human behaviors. While acceptance and openness are desired treatment characteristics, sometimes clients deny or minimize behavior because they *do* appreciate the seriousness of it and want to change how others view them.

For example, when we engage in some minor rule violation—whether it be a societal or a self-imposed rule—we often attempt to alleviate our own guilt or shame, or respond to others' judgments of that rule violation, by being deceptive in some way. When pulled over for speeding, most drivers do not say to the police officer, "Of course I know how fast I was going. Fifteen miles over the speed limit, to be exact. And I was talking on my cell phone and searching for my wallet at the same time." Most drivers say, "I had no idea, officer. Was I speeding?" Similarly, when one sets a goal to lose weight after holiday overindulgences, one does not say, "I ate that greasy cheeseburger and fries because I wanted them, and they tasted good, and I knew they contained more calories and fat than I'm supposed to eat in a whole day." After such a meal, most people might say, "I had a small burger and a few French fries. It wasn't too bad. After all, I had a reasonable breakfast and will exercise later today." Both of these examples illustrate denial, minimization, and justification of behavior. In the first example, denial is used to control self-presentation to an authority figure in the face of wrongdoing. In the second, minimization and justification serve to alleviate a sense of shame and disappointment with the self. Offenders are no different. They engage in these same processes, only the behaviors they deny are far more serious and have more negative effects on others. It is likely because the behaviors are so serious that we as treatment providers have such a strong reaction to denial in our clients. We must remind ourselves that the denial is not pathological. The *behavior* is pathological. We want to be cautious about reacting so strongly to the denial that we lose focus on what we are really treating.

What Do We Do about Denial?

From this perspective, we allow clients to be in denial without punishing them for it. Validation is a crucial part of this process. Validation communicates to the client that he or she is understood and helps the client view his or her own motivations and behaviors in a meaningful way. So how do you validate something as frustrating as denial? We must consider several questions. First, why might the client be denying, minimizing, justifying, and so on, his or her behavior? Is it because the client does not want others to believe he or she is capable of this type of behavior? Is it because this is difficult to discuss in front of others? Is it because the client fails to "take responsibility" in many areas of life and has difficulty accepting his or her own shortcomings and limitations? Or maybe the client truly believes someone else is responsible or should take some of the blame for his or her behavior? Treatment providers must understand the client's current position and his or her underlying motivations.

Second, what do we want to validate? The goal of SOS is to help the client identify areas of dysregulation that contributed to a sexual offense. The goal of validation is the same. Treatment providers can validate the client's dysregulation in the moment, rather than the actual denial or minimization itself. For example, when a client says that the victim wasn't seriously hurt, one could say, "It can be really hard to think about how we might have hurt someone else. No one likes to think of themselves as a person who hurts others." By avoiding the urge to confront, challenge, or correct the client, the treatment provider communicates the safety of the group environment, encourages the client to discuss his or her feelings about having potentially harmed someone, and allows the client to understand why he or she is having difficulty with the discussion.

Third, what effect might this denial have on the client? On other clients? On the group dynamic? A treatment provider saying "I understand" may lead to a rather hostile exchange in which the client says, "No, you don't understand. You're not a sex offender, and you're not in treatment." Other clients may view the therapist's validation as a hollow effort to empathize, feel that the client is "getting off easy," or believe that the treatment provider is justifying the client's failure to take responsibility. When selecting an appropriate validation, consider how it might impact all the clients. Be conscientious of others' feelings, the goals of using this strategy, and its impact on the group as a whole.

And finally, how do we deal with our own emotions and reactions when validating the client in denial? It is natural to confront deceptiveness or to become frustrated when someone blames others for their own problems. If we conceptualize denial as lying, as a pathological behavior, or as "wrong," then we will be unable to respond calmly and therapeutically. Being aware of your own reactions and dysregulation will assist in responding appropriately.

Can Clients in Denial Still Participate Meaningfully in Treatment?

In other forms of sex offender treatments, clients may be excluded from treatment until they can take full responsibility for their actions. This stance assumes that clients who openly acknowledge their offenses are more amenable to treatment, and that clients who deny or minimize will not make sufficient progress to justify the time and effort on the part of treatment providers. It has a somewhat punishing aspect as well, in that treatment providers can remove someone from treatment until he or she is ready to comply with the treatment providers' expectations. Exclusion does not work when the primary concern is providing beneficial therapeutic intervention to those who need it.

Admittedly, some clients are not ready to address their sex offenses at the start of treatment. This can be a frustrating experience for both providers and clients. We expect a lot when we want someone to talk about possibly the worst thing he or she has ever done to another human being, immediately upon starting treatment. Still, treatment providers can work with denial and minimization and still see treatment gains. Strategies for enhancing motivation (discussed later in this chapter) and pretreatment discussions of commitment can help clients navigate their own ambivalence or reluctance to openly discuss their sex offending behaviors (e.g., Garland & Dougher, 1992; Levenson, 2011; Marshall, Thornton, Marshall, Fernandez, & Mann, 2001). Those who refuse treatment and those who are typically removed from treatment because of denial and minimization may be two distinct groups of clients. Clients should therefore be given the opportunity to participate in treatment if they are willing to do so.

In the first treatment module of SOS, clients discuss their struggles with motivation and commitment. Additionally, clients are encouraged to establish their own treatment goals. In some cases, clients may need to work on their commitment and willingness for quite some time before setting higher level goals that are more directly related to their offenses. Treatment is a lengthy process, and it will ultimately be more effective for us to work *with* clients, encouraging and validating them as they struggle with their denial and commitment and emphasizing the value of voluntary change.

Enhancing Motivation and Commitment

"Treatment will not work for me, so why try?"

"Treatment is too hard. It's not worth the effort."

"I don't need it. This isn't a problem for me anymore. I can just stop anytime."

"My behavior doesn't really hurt anyone."

"I can do this on my own. I don't need a therapist or group."

"I can't talk about it. I don't want anyone to know."

"I'm comfortable with where I'm at."

As treatment providers, we have all heard these kinds of statements. The techniques from motivational interviewing (Miller & Rollnick, 2013; see also Miller & Rollnick, 1992, 2002) are very applicable to sex offender treatment. Understanding ambivalence and its impact on the client's efforts to change are integral to this approach. Ambivalence, or a sense of internal conflict regarding an important decision or anticipated change, is a common experience. When faced with two or more potential options, we naturally compare them and struggle with making a final choice. Ambivalence means that we hold multiple feelings or points of view at the same time, without knowing which of these is "wrong" or "right." Ambivalence is functional; it allows us to make informed and deliberate decisions. However, ambivalence becomes a problem when the person is "stuck" (Miller & Rollnick, 2013) and cannot settle on one option or point of view.

Many clients struggle with fully engaging with or participating in sex offender treatment. As treatment providers, we often attribute this situation to lack of motivation. And while it may be true that some clients are generally unmotivated, it may be the case that ambivalence has interfered with the client's commitment to change. In other words, part of the client may be motivated, but the other part is not, and this prevents the client from moving toward change.

In fact, we have to admit that there are many reasons why clients *should* be ambivalent about participating in sex offender treatment. Very few people are welcoming and enthusiastic regarding sex offenders. Clients are very aware of this negativity, given the attention given to sex offenders in the media and the political arena. They may also anticipate a negative reaction from treatment providers or others who know that they are in treatment, and they thus choose not to participate. Clients may experience a great deal of shame and self-judgment regarding their behaviors, and the thought of openly acknowledging and discussing these behaviors in front of others may be intimidating and emotionally distressing. These feelings of fear, anxiety, shame, or even anger can coexist with their desire to change. The primary goal is to resolve the underlying ambivalence and thereby motivate the client and enhance his or her commitment to treatment. This involves illustrating the ambivalence, exploring conflicting thoughts or emotions, and resolving them in a way that allows the client to make a decision.

Exploring Ambivalence

In order to understand ambivalence, one must talk about ambivalence. This involves describing positive and negative aspects of the current situation, identifying expectations of self and others, and voicing both positive and negative emotions regarding change. Other motivational interviewing strategies, including facilitating change talk and developing discrepancy between the two or more options (see Miller & Rollnick, 2013) can also assist in highlighting aspects of the client's ambivalence. Not all clients enter treatment at the same point of readiness, and movement through a change process is fluid (e.g., clients move through the stages of change, described further in Chapter 5; Prochaska & DiClemente, 1983; Prochaska, DiClemente, & Norcross, 1992). Attention to these and other aspects of the client's ambivalence may help him or her better conceptualize a direction in treatment, even if it may lead him or her away from change in the interim.

Validation

Again, validation is a very useful and broadly applicable therapeutic technique. The client expects specific and predictable reactions to acknowledgment of his or her offending and involvement in sex offender treatment. The client expects others to react in a negative and invalidating way, with little hope that someone will "understand" his or her feelings. Thus, validation can be quite helpful in building a supportive relationship. Giving voice to the client's fears, doubts, or frustrations can assist in describing the ambivalence. For example, simply saying, "Being involved in treatment can be very frightening. You feel like you don't know what people will think about you or what you did," can create an opportunity for open discussion and may eventually lead to a resolution of strong feelings. This strategy is also useful in maintaining motivation throughout the treatment process. Motivational interviewing techniques consistent with validation include rolling with resistance, reflective listening, and affirming positive or functional aspects of the client's emotions and behavior (Miller & Rollnick, 2013).

Weighing the Costs versus the Benefits of Treatment

As treatment providers, we are accustomed to focusing on why people *should* be in treatment and how treatment will help them. As a consequence of this attitude, we contradict or minimize why people *should not* be in treatment, or why they simply might not *want* to. This push from just one side results in strengthening the client's defensiveness and withdrawal from treatment, as we easily fall into a pattern of taking sides against one another. One strategy is to objectively examine both sides of the issue, without advocating for either. There are positive and negative aspects to engaging in treatment, as well as positive and negative aspects to withdrawing from treatment. Giving both sides full weight will help us understand the client's reasoning, assess realistic obstacles to treatment change, and aid the client in making a balanced and self-motivated choice regarding treatment involvement. Another related strategy is to take the opposite and unexpected side, and in fact lobby against change. This is commonly referred to as "playing the devil's advocate," and it often accomplishes the goal of making the client argue in favor of commitment. Discussing and validating real limitations, consequences, and obstacles and allowing the client to make a reasoned and voluntary decision leads to a more valued and lasting client commitment.

Emphasizing the Client's Goals, Values, and Strengths

Change interventions inherently assume that the client has done something wrong, and that it must be "fixed." This view reflects what others want the client to achieve, and obscures what the client him- or herself wants, as well as strengths that he or she may have. From the client's perspective, being told that what you are doing is wrong, and that someone else knows best how you should fix it, are probably not the most effective ways of eliciting motivation and commitment. Perhaps more effective are strategies that allow clients to select goals most relevant to them, find ways to meet these goals in a meaningful way, and stay true to their beliefs, values, and desires. Clients also enter treatment with strengths that can facilitate treatment participation and learning. Emphasizing these strengths and tying them to concrete outcomes may make the process seem less daunting and treatment success more attainable for hesitant, overwhelmed, or defensive clients.

Accepting Where the Client Is in the Moment

Change is a fluid process. "Meeting" the client in the moment in the context of his or her commitment can help facilitate commitment. This may be particularly important when the client's goals and the treatment provider's goals don't match. The key is to determine where the client is in terms of commitment, potential obstacles, and ultimate goals. This typically involves assessing ambivalence, emotions regarding the treatment experience, cognitive processes, available resources, and interactions with treatment providers and others involved in the process. Taking these into consideration can help us engage the client at a level where he or she is able and willing to participate. This may delay progress, perhaps lengthening the treatment process overall, but meeting clients at a place where they can and will commit, and can be successful, will enhance their motivation over time.

Building Skills

Effective treatment with SOS involves the development and use of adaptive regulatory strategies to replace strategies that are maladaptive, dysfunctional, or harmful to self and others. Replacement skills are necessary, as simply promoting the absence of a particular behavior is unlikely to be successful. In Chapter 2, we noted that individuals are innately driven to reduce dysregulation in some available and functional way, and we must present them with viable, healthy alternatives. In Modules 3, 6, 7, 9, and 10, clients will be asked to learn, practice, and review skills relevant to specific areas of dysregulation and maladaptive coping. Since each time clients will need to build skills, the process for facilitating this is skills building described here, rather than repeated within each module itself. Within the modules, the time frame given for learning new skills is generally two to three sessions. However, this time frame is not an accurate reflection of the actual time needed to learn, implement, and internalize new skills. That process continues throughout the treatment, as clients self-monitor their dysregulation and skills use daily, reviewed at the beginning of each session from Modules 3–10. Thus, setting aside two to three sessions at the end of the modules listed above is merely an opportunity to devote time for learning and discussion to specific skills, though it is expected that these skills training opportunities will permeate the remainder of SOS. Treatment providers may find it useful to refer back to this section for each of these modules to assist in planning group discussions and activities.

Identifying Skills

The first step is identifying new skills. Clients must know what a "skill" is. Many of them have an idea of "coping skills," but these are so vaguely and ubiquitously mentioned in various forms of CBT that few clients truly understand the meaning. For the purposes of this discussion, a "coping skill" is a strategy that allows one to deal with negative situations, emotions, thoughts, or interactions with other people. The skill doesn't necessarily change or fix the prompting event, but instead acts as a method for coping with it. When we say "strategy" or "skill," we refer to something used to modulate the individual's distress or discomfort.

Note, however, that this definition makes no assumptions regarding the skill's adaptiveness. A strategy or skill can be functional and effective (i.e., it works) while also being extremely maladaptive or unhealthy. Therefore, we should also help clients determine whether or not a skill is healthy. Unfortunately, this is fairly complex—the answer to "Is a skill adaptive?" is often "It depends." Treatment providers and clients will need to consider:

1. Does it hurt anyone, including the client?
2. What are the intended consequences of using this strategy?
3. What are the unintended consequences of using this strategy?
4. Are there long-term consequences that the client might not see now?
5. Are there other circumstances or vulnerabilities that this may exacerbate?
6. Is the client comfortable with this choice?
7. What will the client or others have to sacrifice in order to use this strategy?

Other concerns may be readily identifiable given the client's history and circumstances. These are important points to consider.

For example, clients often say that "walking away" or "sleeping" are viable alternative strategies for alleviating anger, anxiety, or sadness. There is truth in this, as momentary escape allows for "cooling off" time or an opportunity to think, and sleep can reduce vulnerabilities brought on by illness or sleep deprivation. However, these skills are not adaptive in all circumstances since avoidance can worsen the initial problem, or the person may be avoiding something important. The use of such avoidance skills prevents learning more direct and healthy problem-solving methods.

Identifying relevant skills also depends on opportunity. It does little good to rely on strategies that are not realistic or available. A client with diabetes who relies on chocolate or sugary candies as a coping strategy, an institutionalized client who expresses that "driving around by myself" is the only solution to dysregulated mood, or a socially isolated client who says that he will "talk to friends" to cope are examples of strategies that are not viable or realistic. We must encourage creativity in identifying and learning new skills, but we must also ensure that clients' attempts to develop adaptive regulatory strategies are grounded in the realities of their daily lives.

Practicing Skills

Once clients have identified potential skills or strategies, they must practice them. This part of the process is often overlooked and underutilized. Failure to practice new strategies leads to overconfidence, frustration, increased dysregulation and urgency, and ultimately skills failure. Practice provides opportunity for reinforcement, which will only further solidify clients' commitment to using new skills.

New strategies should be practiced repeatedly in the moment, not just in contrived therapeutic settings. These practice opportunities should include situations characterized by varying degrees of dysregulation or distress. The ability to recognize the need for a strategy, select a new adaptive strategy, use it in a state of dysregulation and vulnerability, and maintain that skill use despite potential failure, is very different from the guided skills coaching that occurs during a therapy session. Clients must practice not only with therapist guidance, but also in moments when the skill is most needed. Only through practice will the skill feel more comfortable and natural, thus ensuring a greater chance of success.

Modeling is also an effective component of skills teaching and practice. The client, other clients in group, and the treatment providers are all a part of this process. Modeling may involve simply describing one's own skills choices, such as "When I get angry, I like to. . . . " It may also involve more direct application of the skills in treatment, such as noting a client's (or treatment provider's) dysregulation and possibly relevant skills. For example, a treatment provider may report his or her own level of stress in the present moment, ask for feedback from the group about coping with stress, and then model some of those strategies as part of the session. Making this process more deliberate and conscious for the client in the beginning will help make their skills use more unconscious and automatic over time.

Challenges to New Skills

Clients and treatment providers will both experience challenges to using new skills. These challenges can cause frustration, impatience, or hopelessness about the effectiveness of alternative strategies. We therefore encourage both clients and providers to consider these challenges and discuss them at greater length in modules related to skills building.

First, new strategies simply may not work as well as the old ones. Old strategies, some of which were harmful or maladaptive, were comfortable and tested over time. At one point, these strategies were probably less effective too, but through repeated practice and reinforcement they became effective. The same process will occur with new ones. Also, the adaptive strategies may not promise the immediacy and ease of some of the maladaptive skills. It is true that they do not work in the same way, but they may have other benefits for the client. Validating the client's frustration or disappointment, problem solving if the skills fail to work, and encouraging and reinforcing use of adaptive skills are all tools for creating more effective skills use over time.

Second, the effectiveness of new strategies will vary. The skill's effectiveness depends on countless factors: the person's initial mood state; the strength of that mood state; whether or not other people are present; the person's thoughts, perceptions, and expectations; available time; situational demands; and so on. These variations impact the client's skill use, which in turn impacts the client's overall perception of whether or not the strategy will ever work. These factors cannot be controlled, nor should they be. They should most imitate the real-world, nontherapy environment in order to ensure generalization.

Third, clients may feel uncomfortable doing something new and unfamiliar. This can be overlooked, as clients feel compelled to say that a new strategy feels "good" or "better" than old strategies because of their own and providers' expectations. As with driving a rental vehicle, listening to a familiar song in a different language, or eating a favorite dish prepared in a different way, these changes may not be overtly negative or painful but are different enough to provoke discomfort. Clients will practice these new strategies while dysregulated or distressed, and adding discomfort will make it an even more unrewarding experience in the early stages of use. This discomfort will only lessen through repeated exposure and opportunities for the skill to be effective. Tolerating their discomfort will help clients move past this challenge.

Fourth, this learning process may actually increase the client's dysregulation in the moment. The client should be prepared for this eventuality. When a comfortable and familiar strategy is suddenly deemed "inappropriate" or "maladaptive" and denied to the individual, this leads to resentment, anxiety, and hopelessness. This, coupled with decreased immediate effectiveness of new skills, may make clients hesitant to rely on these new techniques. Open acknowledgment and carefully-timed extending interventions can be helpful. For example, treatment providers might say, "This is going to be really hard. You're probably going to have a lot of trouble, and you're even going to possibly feel worse. It just may be too difficult for you to change with all of that going on. In fact, I worry that you may just *have* to go back to what you did before." This strategy highlights dysregulation and challenges clients to practice new strategies regardless.

CONCLUSIONS

In this chapter, we have described the important philosophical underpinnings of SOS, highlighting core values and beliefs that should inform treatment and therapeutic relationships throughout this process. We have also provided treatment providers with tools and strategies to facilitate client progress. Now let us turn to the modules of treatment themselves.

CHAPTER 5

Why Am I in Treatment?

Each module of SOS focuses on specific treatment needs. Module 1 orients the client and introduces him or her to participating in sex offender treatment. Some clients will have already received sex offender treatment in prior settings, and some clients will be entirely new to sex offender treatment programming. Each client begins therapy with preconceived ideas, misperceptions, strong emotional reactions, and expectations of themselves and others. Module 1 helps orient the client to SOS and sex offender treatment. Concepts from this module will prepare them for important treatment changes ahead.

This module is meant to orient the clients and help them get ready for treatment. Clients need to understand the nature and purpose of treatment prior to making a commitment. In many cases, clients are court-ordered or otherwise mandated to participate in such treatment, but this does not mean that they shouldn't be involved in treatment-related decisions. Module 1 helps clients develop treatment goals that are meaningful, realistic, and achievable. Clients can also establish relationships with other group members and treatment providers. Another goal is to describe individual and group expectations to guide clients and providers throughout the treatment process.

Module 1 is also designed to aid treatment providers in assessing the client's level of motivation and commitment at the beginning of treatment and to determine potential obstacles or challenges to treatment, such as areas of resistance, emotional barriers to progress, conflicts or disagreements between group members, or assumptions and expectations that may be contrary to full treatment participation. Treatment providers can address these problems in a planned and therapeutic manner and develop an individualized approach to motivating and engaging clients in sex offender treatment. The concepts from Module 1 will be reviewed periodically throughout treatment (i.e., in Modules 5 and 10) in order to reassess willingness, motivation, and commitment as clients make progress.

INTRODUCTION AND ORIENTATION (SESSIONS 1–5)

Setting the Stage for Treatment

In a new group, it is important for group members and group leaders to introduce themselves and briefly note the reasons they are involved in sex offender treatment. This does not necessarily mean that group members must make a full confession of their offenses in the first session, though some may feel comfortable enough to explicitly state the offenses that led to their inclusion in sex offender treatment. These introductions may range from a client stating "I'm here to make some changes" to "I'm here because I was told I have to be" to "I committed a sexual offense and got arrested." Examples of provider responses that validate such sentiments include "It must be hard for you to do this then" or "I hope we can find a way to make this meaningful." As with all activities in this module, the client's responses allow treatment providers to gauge the client's level of willingness and commitment to treatment. Clients will also get some feel for each other, including similarities in referral issues, expected participation (e.g., probation requirement, court-mandated status), and level of commitment. (See Table 5.1 for an outline of these discussions.)

Treatment providers should also discuss the format of treatment. This includes the duration and frequency of group meetings; the anticipated length of treatment (if known); the type of homework or out-of-

---

TABLE 5.1. Introduction and Orientation (Sessions 1–5)

- Setting the stage for treatment.
  - Introduction of clients and group leaders; discussion of treatment format.
- Clients list and discuss reasons why people are included in sex offender treatment.
- Perceptions of sexual offenders and being in treatment.
  - Clients discuss how others (society) view sex offenders; compare and contrast this with how they themselves view sex offenders.
  - Clients discuss their emotional reactions to being in sex offender treatment.
  - Clients discuss their ambivalence—positive and negative aspects of being in sex offender treatment (pros and cons).

---

group assignments that clients are expected to complete; basic expectations regarding group confidentiality; limits of confidentiality or legal concerns; the structure of group sessions; other parties with whom information regarding treatment progress, participation, and risk will be shared (e.g., facility or agency treatment teams, probation or parole officers, or attorneys or officers of the court); and how individualized treatment planning will be used to enhance the client's progress and treatment experience. Prior to these discussions, treatment providers should clarify any expectations on the part of their own agencies or other interested parties to ensure that clients are fully informed regarding disclosure of offense-related information, contact with courts or other agencies, and how potential problems in treatment will be addressed. Then group leaders will be able to address questions in these initial treatment discussions and to provide the most accurate and up-to-date information possible.

Reasons for Sex Offender Treatment

The first group activity is a discussion of why people are placed in sex offender treatment. (For ease of discussion, group facilitators may find it helpful to list reasons on a board or other visual medium so that clients are able to follow along.) This does not have to be a list of specific reasons the clients themselves are in treatment, but instead a more general list of why sex offender treatment may be needed or recommended for some individuals. Some of these reasons may include the following:

1. *Legal problems.* Review a list of relevant sexual offenses and the legal consequences of such behaviors. Clients may even identify their own legal problems related to sex offending.
2. *Institutional problems.* Clients who reside in psychiatric, correctional, or other residential care facilities may be familiar with rules related to sexual behavior, as well as potential consequences and security restrictions that may result from engaging in rule-violating sexual behaviors.
3. *Victims.* Harmful or illegal sexual behaviors have an obvious impact on victims. Treatment may thus be recommended to prevent future victimization.
4. *Impact of sex offending behavior on family and important others.* Offenders, their families, and others in their lives are impacted when a sexual offense occurs. These others may view treatment as necessary to rehabilitate the offender and to restore a sense of trust and safety in these relationships.

5. *Societal expectations.* Members of society may want sex offending behaviors to stop, or at a minimum, they may want offenders to "learn right from wrong" and learn to control their behaviors.

6. *Personal reactions.* While not all clients may voice personal dissatisfaction with their behaviors, many do feel disappointed, ashamed, or self-critical following their behaviors. They may cite these personal reasons and a desire to change as motivators for treatment participation.

7. *Other treatment needs.* Offenders may want to address other concerns related to their maladaptive behaviors, including emotional and relationship problems, substance abuse, violence, and a history of trauma.

8. *Quality of life.* Some clients express a desire to achieve a more fulfilling and functional life, which may include developing healthy relationships with others, maintaining consistent employment and residence, or reducing other related problematic or maladaptive behaviors.

Perceptions of Sexual Offenders and Being in Treatment

Perceptions of Sexual Offenders

Clients are now prepared to discuss perceptions of sexual offending, as well as their own feelings about being in treatment. This builds group cohesion and provides group leaders with a measure of clients' reactions to treatment. The first discussion focuses on perceptions—clients are usually very aware of how others perceive sex offenders and deviant sexual behaviors. Clients can list these perceptions, which may include examples such as "They should be punished," "Sex offenders are sick," or "They should be locked up forever." This is an opportunity for group leaders to validate clients' reactions to such statements and consistently monitor their emotional states. While some of these perceptions may be justified (e.g., "Sex offenders need treatment"), group leaders can still be aware of clients' reactions and respond. For example, this may be an opportunity for treatment providers to note how feeling "trapped" into treatment by societal expectations can interfere with internal motivation.

This should then be juxtaposed with the second component of this discussion, when clients list their own perceptions of sex offenders and offending behavior. The side-by-side comparison of their own and others' perceptions can highlight similarities, such as "They need help" or differences like "They are bad people" versus "They did something harm-ful." Be cautious of certain reactions, as some clients might voice sui-cidal sentiments when discussing societal perceptions that sex offenders should be put to death or that they don't deserve to live.

Emotional Reactions to Treatment

Clients also have personal reactions and emotions related to being in sex offender treatment. Here, clients will review a number of common emotional reactions, including both positive and negative states that may result following the initiation of sex offender treatment. Some examples are anger, guilt or shame, fear, confusion, hopelessness, curiosity, relief, or interest. (See Form B2, "How Do I Feel about Being in Sex Offender Treatment?" in Appendix B, a client worksheet to facilitate this discus-sion.) Treatment providers should be sure to validate both positive and negative emotional reactions. This serves two purposes: (1) It allows cli-ents to feel understood and gives group facilitators the opportunity to read each client's motivation and notice potential barriers to treatment; (2) this demonstrates to clients that they can say things that would nor-mally elicit a negative and invalidating response (e.g., "But you shouldn't be angry about being here. We're trying to help you") and instead expe-rience validation and understanding (e.g., "It sounds like you're angry about it because you feel like you don't belong here. That must make it really hard to be here each week"). This sets the stage for later disclo-sures, when clients may reveal information related to their offenses, and lets the clients know that they will be safe in making such disclosures in treatment. Treatment providers who appear accepting of their nega-tive feelings toward treatment will also be presumably more accepting of some of the difficult revelations related to offending behaviors. Note, however, that this does not give clients permission for open hostility. Quick validation of negative emotions can diffuse strong emotions and negative attitudes so that the discussion does not become a venting ses-sion for client complaints. An additional benefit of this exercise is that clients can begin to see shared commonalities and build group cohesion as they review these issues.

Treatment Ambivalence

At this point, clients can also identify the pros and cons of being in sex offender treatment. This logically follows the previous discussion of how clients feel about being in treatment. Many of their negative emotional responses are related to the cons or disadvantages of treatment, whereas the positive emotions are related to pros or advantages of treatment. Common pros may be as broad as "getting help" or "learning," or even as specific as "learning to control urges" or "working on my problems with sexual relationships." Common cons or negative aspects of treatment may include being labeled, finding group discussions boring, feeling uncomfortable, or having to listen to others' problems. Again, it is important for group leaders to validate both positive and negative client responses in order to build therapeutic alliance and also to demonstrate that the group is a safe place for clients to appropriately reveal their true feelings regarding treatment and their behaviors.

During these early sessions, clients will reveal their own ambivalence about their sex offending behaviors, sex offender treatment, and efforts to change. This will lay the groundwork for a collaborative treatment process, so that group members can develop supportive relationships with the treatment providers and with one another. The use of validation techniques and motivational interviewing strategies can help illustrate this ambivalence and somewhat normalize the process for the clients. Clients' ambivalence is normal, even though the maladaptive nature of their behaviors is not. While some will loudly voice their resistance to treatment, others will be more reticent to openly express their reluctance to change, particularly if they have already acknowledged or disclosed their offending behaviors to others. They may feel that appearing resistant fundamentally conflicts with an admission of responsibility, and that it makes them appear callous or uncaring. In other words, if clients have already confessed to the police but then in treatment say that they don't need to change, a realistic fear is that others will think that they don't care, or that they don't appreciate the seriousness of their behaviors. In reality, it can be true that they acknowledge the wrongness of their behaviors but also have negative feelings about being in treatment. Thus, treatment providers may need to elicit this ambivalence and help them conceptualize their feelings to highlight the reality of where the client is at the beginning of treatment.

STAGES OF CHANGE (SESSIONS 6–8)

What Are the Stages of Change?

The five stages of change were introduced by Prochaska and DiClemente (1983; Prochaska et al., 1992) to describe how individuals approach the change process. These stages have been explored in multiple contexts, including general psychotherapy, addictions and substance abuse treatment, and weight management (e.g., Miller & Rollnick, 1992, 2002). The stages of change are also applicable to sex offender treatment. Clients should be introduced to these stages, with the discussion tailored to the client's comprehension abilities. To facilitate this discussion, we provide a brief description of each stage below. An overview of this section is provided in Table 5.2.

Precontemplation (or Prerecognition)

Sometimes people have substantial difficulty recognizing or acknowledging the need to change. They may be comfortable or satisfied with their behaviors, in spite of negative consequences or reactions from others. In many cases, they are unaware of a problem and may blame others for negative consequences that have occurred. Clients in this stage may say "I don't have a problem," blame their offense(s) on the victim(s) or others, or deny a need for treatment.

Contemplation (or Recognition)

Following a period during which clients are unable to see a need for change, they enter a stage of ambivalence, in which they view change as both desirable and at the same time unnecessary. This may be the point at which an individual first becomes uncomfortable with his or her behavior or problem. While the person sees that a problem exists, he or she has not yet made a decision regarding what to do about it. Clients in this stage may say, "I know what I did was wrong, but it will never happen again," fluctuate between denial and acknowledgment of offending, or express their belief that they can take care of the problem on their own.

TABLE 5.2. Stages of Change (Sessions 6–8)

- What are the stages of change?
  - Clients review the five stages of change, relating them first to neutral examples.
    - How do people think or feel about change in each of these stages?
- Stages of change and sex offender treatment.
  - Clients discuss how these different stages look during sex offender treatment.
    - How do they feel now? What stage are clients in?
    - How have they felt in the past? Have they been in other stages, at other times?

Preparation (or Planning)

At this point, the person has made a decision to change but has not yet taken any specific action, or has only made small, token efforts to modify behavior. Here, the intention is to change, and the individual is busy making plans and identifying goals related to what must he or she must do to make a change. Clients in this stage may recognize their need for treatment but are not sure where to start, say that they want to see what treatment is like, or start looking into different options for treatment.

Action

In this stage, individuals have made a strong commitment to change and are making important changes to their behaviors in order to reach their goals. Here, change may be apparent to others and results in noticeable differences in problematic behaviors. This stage may require more sustained commitment and energy than the previous stages. Clients in this stage are regularly attending treatment, aware of their behaviors and what precipitates them, and making concentrated effort to learn new skills and ways of interacting with others.

Maintenance

Following initial change efforts and behavioral improvements, a person enters the maintenance stage. This involves his or her ongoing efforts to maintain success and avoid or cope with pitfalls that could result in a return to old behaviors. There is no specific length of time for the maintenance stage, as some individuals may find themselves continually working to maintain progress over a lengthy period of time. Also, clients should also understand that maintenance is not always an "end point," as they can return to previous stages, or may move through them in a nonlinear fashion. Clients in this stage have already made significant changes to their behaviors and lifestyle and may be focusing on maintenance factors like improving social support, continuing to self-monitor, or working on other areas of companion treatment like substance abuse, mental health, or trauma interventions.

Stages of Change and Sex Offender Treatment

While these five stages were originally developed to describe the change process related to substance abuse treatment, they still apply to sex offending behaviors. Clients should first discuss each stage in a general way, unrelated to sex offending behaviors. This will help them learn the basic principles of these stages. Describing efforts to change health behaviors (e.g., dieting, exercise, smoking cessation) or improve day-to-day problems (e.g., procrastination, chronic lateness) can illustrate the stages and engage clients in the discussion without reference to their own behaviors, as their emotions or judgments related to their offenses can interfere with their learning at this point. After this, treatment providers can review the stages in the context of sex offender treatment, and have clients provide examples of what sex offenders might look like in each stage. For example, clients may point out that someone in the precontemplation stage may deny his or her offenses, blame the victim, or argue that his or her behavior was not wrong. Similarly, clients may note that persons in this stage may deny a need for treatment, saying that "I can just stop myself from doing it again."

Treatment providers can provide an open forum for discussion of these stages, allowing clients to describe thoughts or beliefs associated with each stage, using nondefensive and non-change-oriented validation. For example, while it may be tempting to challenge clients' statements involving denial, minimization, or treatment resistance, confrontation will prevent clients from learning about their own ambivalence and accepting treatment. When clients express the thought that being in precontemplation is fine for someone who was falsely accused, treatment providers can say, "Well, sometimes people feel that they have been unfairly labeled, or accused of something that they did not do. You're right—that would make it very hard for that person to want to be in treatment." This connects the person's ambivalence (i.e., "I didn't do anything wrong") with his or her reluctance to change behavior (i.e., "I don't need treatment").

Clients can then estimate their own willingness to change. The goal is for clients to acknowledge their actual stage of change. How accurately and objectively clients are able to describe their own stage of change depends on how much they were able to understand the stages in the context of impersonal or abstract examples. If clients were able to objectively identify thoughts or beliefs associated with decisions about health or lifestyle changes, for example, they will at least have a good foundation for understanding the components of each stage. Also, if treatment providers have sufficiently validated and normalized the ambivalence associated with each stage and the difficulties associated with the change process, clients may be better able to express their own struggles and ambivalence. Finally, avoiding judgments that certain stages are either "good" or "bad" makes a difference as well. Where clients are is simply where they are. The client's own estimate of change readiness demonstrates his or her willingness to engage in treatment, and the accuracy of his or her perceptions can inform progress even in this first module of treatment.

During this discussion, group members may feel comfortable providing one another with feedback. Feedback is intended to help develop group cohesion and support, not to encourage group members to openly confront or criticize one another. Clients may disagree with one another about the stages of change. Most often, a client who overestimates his or her stage (e.g., being in denial but stating that he or he is in the planning or action stage) will prompt others to comment. Clients can be steered toward supportive and helpful feedback, even when they may want to say something critical or negative by prompting clients to reflect back on times when they were in a different place with regards to willingness, or when they were not yet ready for change. This can establish an atmosphere of acceptance and help group members more supportively approach another client who overestimates his or her willingness and progress.

Clients will return to this discussion several times, most notably in Modules 5 and 10, to "check in" on changes in clients' willingness to change. These check-ins also allow treatment providers to identify other issues that have arisen in the meantime (e.g., new sexual offenses, emotional reactions to treatment activities) that may need to be addressed in treatment, or that may interfere with treatment progress. Those who use an open group format, or who notice changes in the goals and willingness of clients throughout treatment, may want to briefly discuss these concepts more frequently (e.g., at the end of each module).

IDENTIFYING TREATMENT GOALS AND EXPECTATIONS (SESSIONS 9–12)

Most forms of sex offender treatment or other interventions for problem behavior focus quite heavily on client deficits or problems, and they offer little opportunity for client input into the goal-setting process. In this section of Module 1, treatment providers and clients work together to understand protective factors, risks, and areas of treatment need (see Table 5.3).

TABLE 5.3. Identifying Treatment Goals and Expectations (Sessions 9–12)

- Client strengths and areas for improvement.
  - What are clients' strengths? How do these help them in treatment?
  - What kinds of things do others think they need to improve?
  - What do they think they need to improve?
- Long-term and short-term goals.
  - What is a long-term goal?
  - What is a short-term goal?
  - How do short-term goals lead to long-term outcomes?
  - Treatment providers assist clients in developing long-term and short-term goals for sex offender treatment. Try to discuss their goals in terms of behavior that can be easily identified or measured. Also, whenever possible, goals should be phrased in terms of things that they will *do*, not things that they will *not do*.
- Group expectations
  - Clients identify their expectations in treatment of:
    o Myself
    o My peers in group
    o My treatment providers/group facilitators
    o My case manager/treatment team
- Group rules
  - Clients develop group rules based on their expectations—a short (manageable) list of rules and consequences for persons who violate those rules.

Client Strengths and Areas for Improvement

While SOS does seek to improve problematic behaviors through self-management and skills building, it is important to first acknowledge the skills, strengths, and abilities that clients already possess. Clients and treatment providers will need to work together to identify these strengths and determine their role in treatment. These strengths may include motivation to change, consistent group attendance, verbal or written skills, maintaining supportive relationships with others, or being willing to ask for help. This initial discussion should be balanced with areas in which clients feel they need to improve, which can range from learning to be open, to very specific treatment needs related to their offending behaviors like controlling sexual urges or developing healthy relationships and boundaries. A helpful exercise could be to compare what clients identify as a treatment need, and what others have told them they should change about themselves. While there may be similarities, the differences in how they conceptualize treatment needs are telling. For example, clients will note that others expect them to "not do anything wrong," whereas their own goals may reflect desires to be in normative relationships or to control their urges. It is important for clients to describe their treatment needs in their own words, as this process informs subsequent discussions of treatment goals and expectations.

Long-Term and Short-Term Goals

Clients will now define their long- and short-term goals for sex offender treatment. First, it is important to clarify differences between long- and short-term goals. Many clients view their treatment goals in terms of long-term commitments: "I don't want to reoffend," "I want to get out of this hospital/prison/treatment facility," "I want to be back with my family." Less often do they think of their goals in terms of immediate, measurable outcomes that build toward long-term change.

In this section of Module 1, treatment providers must guide the discussion so that clients can readily identify realistic, attainable, and measurable goals related to sex offender treatment. Each client should first establish one long-term goal, while also identifying three or more short-term goals that will ultimately lead to the long-term goal. Clear and specific behaviors, tasks, or activities should be described for each of these goals. This will vary according to each client's needs, strengths, and level of commitment. It is expected that each client will have a unique or individualized set of short-term goals.

Below are two examples of different client goals. Treatment providers may find it helpful to write out such discussions on a board so that clients can more easily follow and conceptualize their goals. Note how each of them focus on areas of improvement that are unique to the individual:

Long-term goal: Graduate from sex offender treatment
1. Attend and participate in sex offender treatment group
   a. Go to group each week—work on willingness to go
   b. Try to say at least one thing in each group
   c. Pay attention to group discussion
2. Learn to control my anger
   a. Self-monitor and rate feelings of anger or other strong moods
   b. Learn new skills to help control anger
   c. Take care of myself better (take medications, eat and sleep regularly)

3. Get along better with other people
   a. Work on willingness and acceptance
   b. Self-monitor anger
   c. Learn and practice problem-solving skills

Long-term goal: Have a relationship with an adult partner
1. Build healthy relationships with others
   a. Be able to identify boundary violations
   b. Self-monitor interpersonal dysregulation
   c. Practice new social skills
2. Control sexual urges toward children
   a. Complete a behavioral chain analysis about sexual fantasies
   b. Self-monitor sexual urges toward children; self-monitor moods and thoughts that precede the urges
   c. Learn and practice skills to help cope with urges
3. Build self-esteem
   a. Build up my strengths—practice things that I am good at
   b. Listen to people who are positive and supportive
   c. Go to therapy and work on my self-image

These goals give the client a more specific idea of what is expected of him or her in treatment, and what he or she must work on in order to make significant progress. As you can see, these two clients have very different immediate goals, though the same treatment activities will help them build the necessary skills to achieve their goals.

Two problems generally arise. First, clients are used to describing their goals in terms of things that they will *not* do, rather than things that they *will* do. Learning new and more adaptive replacement behaviors is a more effective and concrete goal than the mere absence of a problem behavior. Thus, when clients say that the goal is to "not commit another sex offense," treatment providers must find ways to reframe this view of behavior into healthier behaviors that the client will do instead. Otherwise, clients won't have a clear idea of what they should do in treatment. This is comparable to other behavioral change goals. For example, nutritional experts caution against saying "I won't eat junk food" or "I won't eat as much," as these goals don't actually help dieters learn healthier eating habits. Instead, saying "I will eat more fruits and vegetables" or "I will eat 1,800 calories a day" are more measurable and realistic goals. As treatment providers, we are in a position to help clients learn what they should do instead of what they shouldn't do.

A second problem is that all clients are very different. One purpose of this module is to learn these differences and help clients adjust to treatment accordingly. Some clients will readily accept the idea that they need treatment and will be open to discussing goals related to their sexual urges, problematic relationships with others, or reliance on sexual behaviors as a coping strategy. However, some clients will be more resistant to treatment and unable to identify such goals. In the latter case, treatment goals should be consistent with the client's identified stage of change, approach to treatment, and level of motivation. Reasonable goals for such individuals are to attend group and listen attentively to treatment discussions. If the client says that he or she has no goals, then an appropriate goal is to figure out what the client can gain from treatment. This merely reflects the client's ambivalence but does not mean the client will not benefit from treatment. Clients who set low-level goals like "attending group" or "being more willing" have not successfully completed treatment once they have achieved these goals. For those who struggle with commitment, the client must achieve these simple motivational tasks before higher level goals can be set. It is also assumed that they will make some progress simply through exposure to treatment materials, as they may learn needed adaptive skills even when they have not expressly acknowledged their sex offending behaviors.

We expect clients' goals to evolve throughout treatment. Since SOS is longer term than other available sex offender treatment approaches, clients have ample opportunity to amend or change their goals as treatment progresses. As they meet their goals, or as the need for new goals arise, group facilitators may return to these discussions of long- and short-term goals. We encourage clients to briefly review their goals and progress at the end of each module of treatment to allow for needed adjustments.

Group Expectations

In order to more fully gauge willingness, commitment, and client needs, treatment providers need to understand what clients expect from treatment and those involved in the treatment process. Clients should discuss the following:

1. *Expectations of themselves.* What expectations do clients have of themselves in treatment? These may include externally observable goals

(e.g., attendance, completion of assignments, being polite) and internal or personal targets (e.g., honesty, seriousness, learning and change).

2. *Expectations of their peers in group.* What do they expect of each other? Often this issue will center on important concepts such as confidentiality, respect, open communication, or other elements of group cohesion. If clients are open about the newness of treatment, trust issues and unfamiliarity, and fear of judgment, this openness can prepare treatment providers for needed interventions should group members engage in harsh, critical, or dishonest behaviors with one another.

3. *Expectations of their group leaders.* What do clients expect of group leaders? The answers may often surprise you. At the pilot sites, the most frequent responses to this question were rather simple and straightforward: kindness, patience, respect, support, and honest feedback. (Helping clients recognize the importance of "honest feedback" may be needed, as some will expect direct and confrontational approaches, whereas others will say that they only want to hear the positives.) Clients will also expect to learn something from the group, and that treatment providers will take treatment as seriously as they do.

4. *Expectations of other supports (e.g., integrated treatment teams, probation or parole officers, friends and family).* Others are often involved in the treatment process. These others may include agency treatment teams, other therapists, or case managers; probation or parole officers or those related to the court to ensure that mandated treatment is being carried out as specified; or the client's own support group, consisting of family members and friends. So what do clients expect from these persons while they are in treatment? Some of these persons or agencies will receive feedback from treatment providers regarding treatment progress. Clarifying client expectations will aid treatment providers and clients in negotiating these relationships. (Note that we do not advocate for these support persons sitting in on treatment groups, merely that they are identified as supports.)

Role expectations are most salient during this discussion. Knowing, for example, that a particular client expects the treatment provider to be a source of support and strength can shape the direction of treatment for that client. This case is different than one in which the client expects treatment providers to help monitor and manage problematic behaviors. Also, recognizing a client's ambivalence or confusion regarding the role of outside supports can acclimate the client to the realities of communications between treatment providers and other agencies.

Group Rules

This discussion of expectations contributes to the development of standard group or therapy rules, emphasizing the importance of respectful communication, maintaining confidentiality, providing a supportive environment that is conducive to treatment, and the like. Clients will specify their own group rules, though these should be limited to a few overarching principles that will guide their treatment rather than a detailed list of many specific rules. They should then think about why these rules are important (e.g., "Why does confidentiality matter?") and what the ramifications and potential consequences are if these rules are violated. The consequences are not meant as punishments for those who violate the rules, but rather as a method for reestablishing trust and group cohesion. (It also gives treatment providers a glimpse of how well clients are able to understand the impact of their behaviors on others.) Temporarily removing someone from treatment for a period of several sessions, having that individual make repairs for the damage caused to the group (e.g., making an apology, completing an assignment about the importance of trust), or devising new methods of maintaining the group's cohesiveness may all be discussed.

MODULE 1 CONCLUDING SESSIONS

Module 1 involves orienting clients to treatment, exploring their feelings as they approach a new treatment group, and aiding group leaders in assessing client readiness to begin sex offender treatment. The module concludes with a collaborative effort to establish treatment goals that are realistic, measurable, and attainable. Treatment providers are encouraged to return to Module 1 concepts as often as is necessary, reviewing client emotions, pros and cons of treatment, commitment to change, and goals. From what they have learned, treatment providers can tailor their use of validation, motivational interviewing strategies, and teaching or discussion techniques to what will most benefit their clients. Client progress in this module is measured by simply assessing the client's openness, willingness, and the match between self-identified goals and the nature of their offenses. At this point, treatment providers can also recognize differences between true therapeutic alliance or willingness and a superficial (i.e., "I'm doing this because you expect me to") commitment from clients. It is possible to move forward, even with this latter form of client involvement. Clients can still benefit from some treatment activities, and treatment providers will merely recognize that such clients have additional work to do. In concluding sessions of this module, treatment providers can briefly list future treatment topics and concepts. This preview can alert clients to specific modules related to their treatment goals. At the end of this module, it is minimally expected that clients will have completed the following tasks: (1) described their emotional responses to being in treatment, including the pros and cons of treatment participation, (2) identified their current level or stage of commitment to treatment, (3) developed one or more short-term goals to address in treatment, and (4) discussed their expectations of themselves, group peers, treatment providers, and others involved in their care. Treatment providers should be sure to take into account the client's level of willingness and motivation, comprehension and retention of treatment concepts, and general level of participation. Once treatment providers feel that such concepts have been sufficiently addressed and understood by the majority of the clients, they will then be prepared to move on to the next module of treatment.

CHAPTER 6

MODULE 2

Basic Treatment Concepts

In Module 1 clients identified important treatment goals, discussed their ambivalence regarding behavioral change and treatment participation, and began forming a cohesive treatment group. Treatment providers have learned about clients' strengths and weaknesses, their readiness to change and expectations regarding treatment, and needed areas of treatment focus. During Module 2, clients will build on these ideas and begin discussion of basic treatment concepts to prepare them for the remaining modules of treatment. The primary goal of this module is to familiarize clients with the concepts and techniques that will be used throughout SOS, including terminology related to their sexual offending, principles of self-regulation, types of dysregulation they may experience, and how to differentiate behaviors, urges, emotions, thoughts, and interpersonal experiences. The chapter concludes with a discussion of behavioral chain analysis, a technique to aid clients and treatment providers alike in understanding the critical precursors to the clients' problematic or illegal sexual behaviors. These precursors will then be emphasized in remaining treatment modules.

Treatment providers must continually assess client motivation and willingness, highlight basic treatment components that are relevant to clients' individualized goals, and provide validation as clients struggle with exploring these concepts in greater depth. The materials presented in this module are a combination of discussion topics and more didactic lessons. Treatment providers should avoid a straightforward lecture style, even when materials may lend themselves more easily to that format (e.g., discussion of legal definitions of offending). For these sections, following a brief presentation of educational material, clients should be encouraged to share their own opinions, thoughts, and interpretations of these concepts, as well as relevant examples and experiences. Providers should also strive to use role plays or specific examples whenever possible to increase the realism of the concepts discussed. Some useful examples are provided throughout the text to facilitate this process.

SEXUALITY, IN BRIEF (SESSIONS 1–8)

Sex Education and Sexuality

To begin this module, treatment providers may remind clients that they will be discussing a number of fundamental concepts for sex offender treatment, including beliefs and knowledge about sexuality. While a later module of treatment is specifically devoted to sexuality and sexual expression (see Chapter 8, Module 4), early treatment discussions are informed by what clients have previously learned about sexuality, sexual behavior, and sexual relationships. Treatment providers should not assume that all clients have had sex education. A content overview of these sessions is given in Table 6.1.

Check Client Background on Sex Education

Some questions for clients may include "Why do we have sex education?," "What are your views on sex education?," "What should people gain from it?" Such questions will help treatment providers ascertain where clients are in terms of their understanding of sex education and a need to learn about sexual concepts. Emphasize the role of early sexual beliefs on the development of sexual behaviors and relationships—clients who have learned very little regarding their sexuality may also have corresponding deficits in their social and interpersonal knowledge related to the formation of intimate relationships. For clients with fairly limited histories of sexual education or limited sexual knowledge, treatment providers may choose to incorporate basic sex educational material, such as sexual anatomy, sexual development, or sexual practices according to the needs of the client. Others may elect to address these issues in Module 4, where there is a framework for further discussion that can be incorporated with other Module 4 concepts. If clients demonstrate prior knowledge of these concepts, then this education may be unnecessary.

Cultural Gender Roles

How much do clients understand differences between biological sex and cultural or societal gender roles? Clients with better abstract reasoning

TABLE 6.1. Sexuality, in Brief (Sessions 1–8)

- Sex education and sexuality
  - Check clients for past sex education
    - o Why is it important for people to have sex education?
    - o How many clients have had past sex education?
    - o What are your views on sex education (positive and negative)?
    - o What should people gain from having sex education?
- Gender and cultural gender roles
  - Do you know the difference between biological sex and gender (including gender identity, roles, and expectations; sexual orientation)?
  - What are some stereotypes of men and women (positive and negative)?
  - How do these stereotypes affect interactions and relationships?
- Sex and relationships
  - Public versus private behaviors
    - o What relationship/sexual behaviors do you think are okay in public? Only in private (e.g., hugging, kissing, touching, masturbation, intercourse)?
    - o Why do you think are there public prohibitions against certain behaviors?
  - Different types of relationships
    - o What are some different types of relationships (e.g., stranger, acquaintance, authority figure, enemy, friend, intimate partner, family member)?
    - o How do these relationships differ? (Draw out differences in how formed, level of trust, how one acts, expectations.)
  - Healthy and unhealthy relationships
    - o What makes a relationship healthy? Unhealthy?
    - o How do you know if you're involved in an unhealthy relationship (emotional reactions, expectations, physical feelings, etc.)?
    - o What are some of the negative consequences of being involved in an unhealthy relationship?
  - Boundaries
    - o What are boundaries?
    - o Can you describe one or more of your own personal boundaries in relationships (e.g., personal space, rules about privacy, how soon to reveal personal information)?

---

skills will be able to engage in more meaningful discussion regarding sexual orientation, gender identity, gender roles, physiological sexual characteristics, and body image. Clients who benefit more from specific and concrete concepts may focus primarily on gender roles and stereotypes. For all, a key discussion point involves gender role expectations and how these influence relationship behaviors. Put simply, clients should be able to identify a number of stereotypes about men and women. These may not necessarily reflect their own beliefs. Family beliefs or experiences;

inferences regarding gender roles obtained through television, movies, and other popular media; or even personal experiences in which others made assumptions about them can all be useful examples for group discussion. Using positive and negative gender stereotypes, clients can consider how these beliefs impact relationships or interactions with persons of both sexes and genders. For example, if clients say that women are more emotional than men or that men have different responsibilities in a relationship (e.g., traditional gender roles), they should also discuss how these kinds of stereotypical beliefs impact their own interactions with men and women, or how these beliefs may affect and shape important relationships. They may view women who are less openly emotional as "cold" or men who are emotional as "weak." Men who do not fulfill traditional relationship roles, or women who fill a more traditionally male role, may be viewed in a negative light or treated critically as the result of such beliefs. This discussion also provides treatment facilitators with groundwork for later discussions involving boundaries, interpersonal conflict, and cognitive dysregulation in interpersonal relationships.

Sex and Relationships

The concepts in this section, especially those addressing relationships and boundaries, provide an introduction that will inform discussions throughout the remainder of treatment.

Public and Private Relationship Behaviors

The first activity involves the identification of public and private relationship behaviors. For many of these behaviors, including hugging, kissing, and touching, their appropriateness in a public setting may be ambiguous or contingent on other factors. Clients may have strong opinions on these matters, or it may be something that they have never considered. Other types of behaviors, including masturbation, intercourse, and other explicitly sexual behaviors, will generate more definitive opinions among clients, even if they have engaged in these behaviors in public themselves. The point of this discussion is for clients to think critically about reasons for public prohibitions against certain behaviors (e.g., discomfort, values and norms associated with nudity and sexuality, gender differences). Examples that challenge clients with rigid beliefs are also useful discussion points. For example, when clients say public nudity is never permissible, clinicians can ask about gender differences (e.g., men vs. women going topless), situational factors (e.g., appropriate attire for beaches vs. church), or other specific scenarios (e.g., "You're camping in the woods and need to use the restroom. There are no restrooms. What do you do?").

Different Types of Relationships

This leads to more direct conversations about relationships. Many clients have a limited understanding of important differences in relationships. They confuse friendships with romantic partnerships, believe therapists are friends, or come from sexually abusive families. Clients will need to identify and describe different types of relationships (e.g., stranger, acquaintance, authority figure, enemy, friend, intimate partner, family member) and how they differ—how they are formed, level of trust, associated emotions, how one acts or behaves, or expectations. This clarifies boundaries between relationships and assists with subsequent discussions of boundaries, expectations, and healthy versus unhealthy relationship behaviors. Clients may also express a number of polarizing beliefs or expectations of others in this discussion, which will be fodder for further discussion in this section or later in Modules 6 and 7.

Healthy and Unhealthy Relationships

The next step is for clients to explore the characteristics of healthy and unhealthy relationships. Important questions to consider include the following:

1. What makes a relationship healthy?
2. What makes a relationship unhealthy?
3. How does a person know he or she is involved in an unhealthy relationship (e.g., emotional reactions, expectations, physical feelings, what others say, changes in the person's own behavior)?
4. What are some of the negative consequences of being involved in an unhealthy relationship?
5. What can a person do if he or she is in an unhealthy relationship?

These questions challenge clients to think about their interactions with others and whether or not they have engaged in or perpetuated unhealthy relationship behaviors. Validation is important—some clients may describe victimization, unhealthy behaviors in their families of origin, or shame regarding their own unhealthy interactions. This also calls attention to problematic beliefs about relationships to be targeted later in treatment. For example, clients may express that "being in love" is a characteristic of only healthy relationships. From pilot work, treatment providers heard with surprising frequency that one can "fix" an unhealthy relationship by getting married or having a child. (A common response was to solicit opinions of clients who had been married, or who did have children, to potentially refute such beliefs.) These may reflect experiences with healthy relationships or consistent maladaptive relationship patterns.

Boundaries

Boundaries are also first addressed at this point in treatment. Clients should discuss boundaries, including examples of what defines boundaries (e.g., personal space, revealing information, privacy, role expectations), how they are established, how they may vary according to situation or person, and how they may be violated. Role plays, demonstrations, or concrete and specific examples may illustrate these concepts and facilitate group discussion, particularly to those less tangible kinds of boundary violations. For example, treatment providers can plan ahead to demonstrate privacy by having one group leader pick up the other group leader's notebook or appointment calendar and begin reading it, ask a grossly personal question in front of other group members (e.g., "How much do you weigh?"), or take something that belongs to the other group leader like a pen or notepad and walk out with it. Clients who were unable to describe privacy boundaries or violations of privacy can quickly point out problems with these scenarios. This can also illustrate important differences between relationships: boundaries are different depending on your relationship with the person. Clients can include discussion of their emotional reactions to interpersonal boundary violations, how this impacts a relationship, and how this contributes to the overall health and functioning of a relationship with that person.

SEXUAL OFFENDING AND VICTIMIZATION (SESSIONS 9–14)

This topic requires preparation. Treatment providers will need to review relevant sex offending statutes in their state or jurisdiction so that discussion will be relevant to the group members. The goal is not to learn intricate legal complexities but instead to be able to familiarize clients with the types of offenses leading to arrest. Clients in sex offender treatment are heterogeneous. Some are referred for treatment as the result of an immediate arrest and conviction for a sexual offense. Others have both present and past sexual offenses that led to legal consequences. Still others engaged in harmful or problematic sexual behaviors that indicated a need for treatment but that were not formally sanctioned. Clients must therefore understand important distinctions between legal and illegal sexual behavior, as well as the role of consent in sexual interactions. Table 6.2 provides an overview of these sessions.

Sexual Offending

What Is a Sexual Offense?

Treatment providers can help clients understand where their behaviors "fit" in terms of legal responsibilities and explain concepts that are more legally ambiguous. Clients often struggle with legal definitions related to coercive sexual behaviors, sexual behaviors other than penile–vaginal intercourse (e.g., cunnilingus or fellatio, anal sodomy, or sexual touching

---

TABLE 6.2. Sexual Offending and Victimization (Sessions 9–14)

- Sexual offending
  - What is a sexual offense? Discuss your jurisdiction's statutory definitions of sexual offenses.
  - Discuss "violent" versus "nonviolent" offenses.
- Consent
  - What is consent? (Begin by defining in general terms, e.g., in medical decisions, financial contracts.)
  - What makes someone able to consent? What makes someone unable to consent? What does someone have to know in order to consent to sexual activity? What are examples of people who are unable to consent to sexual activity? Why?
  - Why is consent important?
  - Group leaders role-play situations involving sexual consent, while clients serve as "jurors."
- Sexual victimization of children and adults
  - What happens to someone after he or she has been sexually victimized?
  - Discuss with clients the physical, psychological, interpersonal, and functional effects of sexual offenses on victims and important others in the victim's life.
  - How does it impact people hearing a story about sexual violence on the news?
  - How does it shape society's views of sexual offenders? When people fear victimization, what do they think of offenders?

or fondling), and the statutory age criteria that define different classifications or categories of offending. A common question from clients is how
one sexual act or offense led to many charges, all of which may seem
similar (e.g., being charged with both forcible rape and sexual assault,
or child molestation and sexual assault of a minor). Knowing how these
charges are defined can help them better see the complexity of legal definitions of sexual offending.

"Violent" versus "Nonviolent" Offenses

Similarly, clients should discuss perceptions of "violent" versus "nonviolent" sexual offending. Traditional definitions of violent and nonviolent
sexual offending in the research literature have focused on the distinction between contact (e.g., rape, child molestation) and noncontact (e.g.,
exhibitionism, voyeurism) offenses, but clients may have their own perceptions. Clients may protest, for example, that their offenses were not
violent because they did not cause obvious physical harm to the victim,
or because it was "only" attempted rape instead of a completed rape. The
clients need to understand that "violence" is defined in terms of harm
and potential harm, which may include attempted contact offenses, use
of weapons, or explicit threats. This will be a difficult discussion for
the clients. Most clients do not view themselves as violent or dangerous
persons. They will struggle with the reality of these legal definitions and
descriptions of their own sexually violent behaviors. Highlighting the
nature of violent offenses, including the perceived threat of violence, use
of weapons, or physical contact with victims, in a matter-of-fact and nonjudgmental way helps clients understand how others view their offenses
without further increasing defensiveness or shame.

Consent

Consent is the ability of an individual to agree, comply, or approve of some
request. Following the discussion of legal definitions of sexual offending, treatment sessions should focus on consent. Early discussion should
focus on general consent (e.g., medical decisions, financial contracts)
and then move into the necessary components of consent in sexual relationships. Clients can provide their own definitions and examples when
discussing the following:

1. What is consent?
2. What makes someone able to consent (e.g., knowledge, experience,

understanding of consequences, capacity to make decisions, free will, voluntariness)?

3. What makes someone unable to consent (e.g., lack of knowledge or understanding, confusion or gross misunderstanding, poor decision-making ability, coercion or duress, incapacitation, manipulation)?

4. What does someone have to know in order to consent to sexual activity?

5. What are some examples of people who are unable to consent to sexual activity? Why can't they give their consent?

6. Why is consent important?

Role Plays

To ensure that clients understand these concepts and can apply them to a reality-based situation, a role-playing exercise can be useful. For example, one treatment provider could play the person seeking sexual activity, and the other provider could play a person who is unable to consent. The first provider can describe attempts to bribe, trick, or manipulate the other person, or efforts to coerce him or her into agreement. (Other examples may include instances where there is consent, but that it is ambiguous, as when one person voluntarily consumes alcohol to the point of intoxication.) Clients can serve as "jurors" or other decision makers to determine whether or not the situation was fair, if the person did or did not have the capacity to consent, what factors were involved that influence consent, whether or not the behavior is a problem, and what should be done about it. This role play could include elements of sexual behavior or nonsexual behaviors that would still capture the meaningful components of the consent process. The point is for clients to understand the complexity of giving consent, and for treatment providers to gain an appreciation of how well clients are individually able to understand and relate consent to sexual behaviors.

Sexual Victimization of Children and Adults

Clients will now build on their understanding of legal definitions of sexual offending and consent by describing the impact of these behaviors on victims. This should not be a discussion of clients' own personal experiences as victims of trauma, though many have had such experiences. Openly discussing their own experiences as victims at this point in treatment may be damaging or harmful to some clients, as they do not yet have the needed skills and abilities to cope with their reactions to trauma. (This issue will be addressed further in Module 8.) Here, we want clients to recognize the impact of sexual victimization in the abstract, without specific persons, situations, or experiences in mind. One could set this up by reminding clients that we will discuss their own victimization at some other point, or that we are not ready yet to discuss their own histories of abuse. The goal is for clients to understand what happens to someone after he or she has experienced sexual victimization.

Understanding victimization includes various facets of the victim's experience, including physical, psychological, interpersonal, and functional effects. These may impact the victim and important others in the victim's life, including family, friends, intimate partners, and others who are aware of the victimization. This affects persons in the offender's life as well, such as family members, friends, or employers. There are also effects for the legal and criminal justice systems, and support systems and treatment agencies for victims of sexual crime. Finally, sexual victimization also shapes the societal perceptions and beliefs that clients described in Module 1. For example, how does hearing a story on the news about an act of sexual violence impact those listening to it? When people fear victimization, what do they think of offenders?

During discussion of victimization, two opposing viewpoints will invariably arise: "They're fine" versus "They're irreparably damaged." The truth is likely somewhere in between these perspectives. Individual responses to sexual or other victimization vary on a continuum, and are highly dependent on idiosyncratic characteristics of the offense, the victim, and historical and situational variables. This individual and situational variability are hard to predict, though clients can at least generate a list of common responses. This will indicate how well they appreciate the seriousness and nature of sexual victimization, and how well they can verbalize its effect on others.

SEXUAL OFFENDING, MENTAL ILLNESS, AND SELF-REGULATION (SESSIONS 15–19)

Mental Illness and Sexual Offending

The research literature on sexual offenders provides wide-ranging estimates of the prevalence of mental illness and psychopathology in sex offender populations. Depending on the nature of the sex offender population studied, some research suggests relatively low rates of serious psychiatric illness among sex offender groups (e.g., Vess et al., 2004), while others indicate disproportionately high rates of personality pathology, paraphilias, and psychiatric problems among certain institutionalized samples (e.g., Stinson & Becker, 2011). Regardless of setting, it is probable that clients have struggled with symptoms of mental illness or personality disorders. This could also include cognitive deficits, as clients with such difficulties can identify how their problems have impacted relationships (e.g., being targets of bullying, problems with communication) and problem solving. These symptoms may play a role in clients' relationships, perceptions of self and others, behaviors, and problem-solving abilities. Clients can identify symptoms of mental illness, including delusions, hallucinations, impulsivity, shifts in mood or emotions, problematic emotional states, difficulties with thinking, and so on, that affect their thoughts, behaviors, and relationships. This should include sex offending behaviors as well. Simply having clients list symptoms of mental illness that might impact someone's thoughts, behaviors, emotions, or interactions can be a good start. Some clients may also have questions about paraphilias: what they are, what it means to be diagnosed with one, and what this means for changing patterns of sexual thought and behavior. The ultimate goal is educational. We want to help clients with psychiatric illnesses or diagnoses understand how these may contribute to behaviors or urges associated with their problematic sexual behavior. These discussions are therefore not meant for clients to challenge their diagnoses or to self-diagnose. An overview of these sessions can be seen in Table 6.3.

Self-Regulation and the Multi-modal Self-Regulation Theory

Clients in SOS need to appreciate the role of self-regulation and self-regulatory deficits in the offense process. Such appreciation gives them the necessary framework and tools that they will need to make progress in treatment. Clients need not understand all the nuances or facets of the theoretical approach in order to benefit from treatment, though it is important for them to learn those concepts most relevant to their own offending histories and areas of self-regulatory deficit. Overall the information can be broken down into several components, according to the needs and capabilities of the clients served.

Self-Regulation and Dysregulation

First, treatment providers should introduce the concept of self-regulation. This may be simplified into a discussion of regulation versus

TABLE 6.3. Sexual Offending, Mental Illness, and Self-Regulation (Sessions 15–19)

- Sexual offenses and mental illness
  - Clients describe relationship between symptoms of mental illness and sexual offenses. These may include paraphilias, if relevant.
    - o What are some symptoms of mental illness (like depressed mood, hearing voices, impulsivity, racing thoughts, paranoia, or unusual sexual desires)?
    - o How do these symptoms affect behavior?
    - o How do they affect sexual behavior?
- Self-regulation and the multi-modal self-regulation theory
  - Explain self-regulation and dysregulation.
  - Why do we self-regulate?
  - Describe the four domains of self-regulation—emotions, thoughts, interpersonal interactions, behaviors—and examples of dysregulation from each.
  - Encourage clients to identify domain(s)/area(s) they struggle with.
  - Discuss how these are related, and how maladaptive behaviors "help" with self-regulation.
  - Explain reinforcement and self-regulatory strategies.
    - o What is rewarding about sexual behaviors? Punishing? (Focus discussion more on positive reinforcement.)

dysregulation, perhaps using concrete examples that the clients can easily understand. For example, clients may relate to the idea of a see-saw, where too much weight on either end leads to imbalance. Other clients may relate to the idea of an engine, where routine maintenance, care, and attention (i.e., regulation) lead to a predictable and smoothly running vehicle, and erratic or inconsistent maintenance, excessive wear and tear, and harsh use (i.e., dysregulation) lead to an unpredictable, dysfunctional, and poorly running vehicle.

Why We Self-Regulate

This is also a discussion of why we self-regulate. When in a state of dysregulation, we are naturally driven to do something about it. A demonstration can be helpful in communicating with clients about differences in each individual's "setpoint" or point at which they are most comfortable. For example, clients can rate anger on a 1–10 scale, identifying urges, thoughts, and behaviors at each point. Then ask at what point they feel comfortable, uncomfortable, and out of control. A similar exercise with other emotions like sadness or fear will be further illustrative.

This will reveal wide variations among different members of the group and for different emotions. Some are better able to tolerate anger than sadness; some are more or less able to comfortably cope with fear. This is akin to someone stating that he or she "works well under pressure." For them, high levels of stress are not dysregulating. This naturally illustrates what it means to become "dysregulated." Treatment providers can provide their own ratings as well in order to be genuine with clients and demonstrate that these are normative feelings and experiences.

Domains of Dysregulation

The second major component of this discussion is describing the different domains of dysregulation. Clients and treatment providers can list examples of emotions, thoughts, interpersonal interactions, or behaviors indicative of dysregulation. An example of how these could be listed is provided in Table 6.4. Once clients are able to conceptualize imbalance, discomfort, or dysregulation in these domains, they will more easily be able to generate examples from their own experiences. Following this exercise, clients should also be able to identify important relationships between dysregulation in the different domains. For example, experiences of anger, blame, and judgment might manifest themselves through interpersonal difficulty (e.g., arguing, threatening) and behavioral dysregulation (e.g., aggression).

Ask clients which areas (domains) they struggle with most. For some, the primary area of dysregulation is emotional, whereas for others interpersonal and cognitive dysregulation in combination are more problematic. This is where clients' individual differences in self-regulatory functioning, maladaptive strategy formation, and ultimately behavior becomes most evident. This will allow treatment providers to

TABLE 6.4. Examples of Dysregulation in Four Domains

Emotional	Cognitive	Interpersonal	Behavioral
• Anger	• Blame	• Arguing	• Aggression
• Boredom	• Judgment	• Manipulation	• Substance use
• Fear	• Delusions	• Lying	• Sexual offending
• Loneliness	• "Blocked"	• Isolating yourself	• Overeating
• Sadness	thoughts	• Threatening	• Procrastination
• Mania	• Racing thoughts	• Issuing	• Self-harm
• Excitement	• Confusion	ultimatums	• Overspending
	• Worry	• Being selfish	

individualize and emphasize specific modules or discussions throughout the treatment to suit the needs of each client, still using the same basic theoretical and conceptual framework. Clients who understand these principles well may also benefit from knowing more about the development of self-regulation and self-regulatory strategies. Viewing maladaptive behaviors as a maladaptive strategy demonstrates important relationships between dysregulation, prior learning, and the reinforcement of behavioral patterns.

Reinforcement and Self-Regulatory Strategies

Finally, clients should discuss the role of reinforcement in the development of regulatory strategies, describing reinforcement versus punishment associated with sexual behavior. Treatment providers can ask clients to name different forms of reinforcement associated with both normative and nonnormative (i.e., maladaptive) sexual behaviors, including feeling wanted or included, sexual gratification, feelings of power or domination, or relief from strong sexual urges and impulses. Though they can generate a list of reinforcing or rewarding features of sexual behavior, they are perhaps more accustomed to describing negative consequences or sanctions. Negative consequences are important for brief review, but clients are already well aware of these.

BEHAVIORAL CHAIN ANALYSIS (SESSIONS 20–25)

The goal in this stage of treatment is to assess the client's understanding of internal states and sources of dysregulation, monitor willingness and commitment to treatment, and establish a sequence of internal events related to the offense process. Table 6.5 provides an overview of these sessions

Differentiating Thoughts, Urges, Emotions, and Behavior

Before beginning a process of exploring clients' thoughts, emotions, and urges precipitating their sexual offending, treatment providers need to ensure that they understand basic differences between these concepts. Have clients list examples of thoughts, emotions or feelings, behaviors, and urges for behavior to help clarify these differences. It may also be helpful for them to discuss how these are sometimes related, as clients

TABLE 6.5. Behavioral Chain Analysis (Sessions 20–25)

- Distinguishing thoughts, urges, and emotions
  - Make sure clients are able to differentiate between thoughts, emotions, urges, and behavior.
  - How can thoughts, urges, and emotions be related to behavior?
- Introduce behavioral chain analysis
  - Purpose: To change a behavior, clients must know the underlying factors that lead to it.
  - What is chain analysis?
    - It breaks down an event into its parts, examining in detail what preceded maladaptive sexual behaviors.
- Each client completes a behavioral chain analysis of one or more sexual offenses
  - Steps in doing a chain analysis
    - Identify one target behavior of one client.
    - Identify time frame for analysis.
    - Identify general situations and specific events that preceded the behavior.
    - Identify thoughts, emotions, and urges associated with each event.
    - Track client dysregulation through the sequence; have client rate intensity of emotions and urges.
  - Ask the group to reflect on the chain analysis.
  - What aspects of the analysis stand out?

may have difficulty separating emotions from urges, or thoughts from emotions.

Introduction to Behavioral Chain Analysis

For clients to change their behavior, they must know the underlying factors that contributed to it. We need to teach them to closely examine thoughts, emotions, urges, and events (as reported by the client) that preceded their maladaptive sexual behaviors. Describing and examining these precursors can reveal important areas of dysregulation to be targets for treatment intervention. As a technique, behavioral chain analysis has been applied to many behaviors, with the goal of learning what precipitates certain problem behaviors. This method may work particularly well with clients with intellectual and developmental disabilities, clients who are generally unaware of internal experiences, and clients who engage in seemingly impulsive behaviors with little forethought. Behavior chain analysis breaks down an event into simple yet specific components, so that clients can progressively and precisely identify relevant experiences, without having to independently generate a complex explanation for the offending behavior.

In this section of Module 2, the goal is for all clients in the group to complete a behavioral chain analysis of at least one of their sexual offenses. This may take several sessions per client, depending on the complexity of the behavior. This section overall may require several weeks or months of client time, and much of this should be done in a setting that allows all clients to comment and participate in the behavioral chain analysis for each person. The end result will be a detailed description of events preceding one specific incident of sexual offending, broken down into components that indicate areas of client dysregulation. We next describe the basic steps for completing a behavioral chain analysis and provide two examples of specific chain analyses of sexual offenses. Treatment providers will guide each client through this process in session, asking needed questions and eliciting responses for a coherent chain analysis.

Steps for Doing a Behavioral Chain Analysis

Identify the Target Behavior

The first step in behavioral chain analysis is to identify the target behavior. This may be the index or referral offense, a past sexual offense, or even an offense previously unknown to authorities or treatment providers. Treatment providers should simply ask the client what behavior he or she is going to discuss. It is important to identify a singular event, as trying to describe multiple offenses at once, or behaviors that were not specifically under the client's control (e.g., sexual victimization experiences), will not provide the same type of information or level of detail that is needed. At times, the client may not be fully ready to discuss his or her sexual offenses. While we do not want clients to avoid this altogether, if a client refuses to complete an analysis of a sexual incident, it may be helpful for the client to select another important maladaptive behavior, such as aggression or criminal behavior, instead. This will still provide some information regarding sources of dysregulation in the client's life.

Providers must first be familiar, as much as is possible, with the sexual offenses or other problematic sexual behaviors of the client, so as to make sense of the major events being described and to prompt the client's memory if necessary. Note, it is not always necessary that clients provide explicit details of the actual offense. Doing so may result in increased shame, embarrassment, fear, anger, or sexual arousal. Since the goal of behavioral chain analysis is to identify preceding events and internal experiences, a focus on specific and explicit details of the offense itself may not add additional beneficial information. Treatment providers must decide when to allow a client to discuss additional details related to offense behaviors. This may be appropriate when the behavior is part of a pattern, or to discuss reinforcers that perpetuated later sexual offenses.

Identify the Time Frame for Analysis

The second step is to identify the time frame of the offense for analysis. Some offenses appear relatively impulsive and may not entail lengthy periods of planning or forethought. Other offenses followed significant planning efforts or time spent with the victim(s). For the former, choosing incidents or events from the day of the offense or the hours immediately preceding the offense will suffice. For the latter, it is important to select relevant events spanning the days, weeks, or months before the offense.

Identify General and Specific Situations Preceding the Target Behavior

Within the selected time frame, treatment providers will help the client describe general features of his or her life at the time of the offense, such as problems in the immediate environment, relationships with others, work or financial status, emotional state and stress level, and the like. This is followed by identifying specific situations or events linked to the offense.

Identify Thoughts, Emotions, and Urges Associated with Each Event

The fourth step is to link thoughts, emotions, and urges to each of the events identified by the client in the latter part of step three. If clients have difficulty labeling these, treatment providers and other group members may make helpful suggestions based on other information the client has given. If the client has difficulty describing emotions, for example, treatment providers and other clients can review the thoughts already mentioned and ask what emotions were associated with each thought. Urges could be suggested based on what happened next in the chain of events (e.g., "You argued with her next. So at that point, did you have some urge to argue, or to tell her what you thought?").

Track Dysregulaton through the Sequence

Rating the intensity of emotions and urges helps track clients' level of dysregulation throughout the sequence. The most important part of this step is to elicit signs of dysregulation that led up to the offending behavior. Again, it is not always necessary that clients provide explicit details of the actual offense.

The Clients Reflect on the Chain Analysis

Finally, once the chain analysis has been completed, the client and other group members can reflect upon the discussion. Notice aspects of the chain analysis that stand out, whether it is the intensity of urges and emotional experiences, the content of the thoughts described, the self-reported internal states, or any other information that may be relevant. A nonjudgmental approach best helps clients learn from their experiences. This information can later be used to aid clients in self-monitoring relevant types of dysregulation.

Example 1

A 45-year-old male has been convicted of attempted rape of a female case manager in a community home. This is the target behavior for the chain analysis. He has a lengthy history of psychiatric hospitalization and incarceration for aggressive behavior in the community, though his history of sexual offending is limited. Initial discussion between the client and treatment provider (i.e., "What was going on in your life at the time this happened?") reveals that the client had been residing in the community home for approximately 6 months before the offense, that he had lost contact with his family in a nearby city, and that he was feeling "stressed out" by his job at a grocery store and the demands of paying bills for his rent and transportation services. In this case, however, when asked about the time frame of the event, the client identified relatively immediate precursors from his interactions with the victim that day. The treatment provider elicited specific emotions, thoughts, and urges associated with these immediate events and asked the client to rate their intensity during this progression of events.

In this example, a progression of events, both internal and external, shown in Figure 6.1 is clear. External stressors contributed to feelings of disappointment, frustration, fear, and resentment, thoughts of "unfairness" and specific expectations about himself and how he should

Events	Thoughts	Emotions	Urges
Had a meeting with my case manager	I don't like it here. I can't pay all my bills. She's a nice lady.	Sad—6 Disappointed in myself—5 Frustrated—7	Give up—8 Talk with her—10
Talked about feeling stressed; I asked if she could come meet with me more often so I would feel better	Nobody talks to me. I miss my family. She wants me to get better.	Sad—8 Appreciative—4 Resentful—5	Cry—5 Hug her—10
She said she can't, and that I can make it on my own	That's not fair. I thought she liked me. Nobody likes me.	Angry—8 Sad—5 Hurt—8 Disappointed—10	Cry—8 Yell at her—4 Hug her—5
She said it was time for her to go	She can't leave. Why did she say no? Doesn't she like me? I'll show her.	Angry—10 Hurt—10 Sad—6	Yell at her—7 Grab her—5 Run away—5
I grabbed her, hugged her, and told her how pretty she is	Now she'll understand. I deserve this.	Scared—7 Lonely—4 Happy—5	Hold her—10 Sexual urges—7
She pulled away and told me to "back off" and leave her alone	That's not fair. I didn't do anything wrong. How dare she say that to me?	Scared—10 Angry—8	Run away—4 Hit her—7 Sexual urges—7
Pushed her to the floor; she was screaming for help	I'll show her. She can't treat me that way.	Angry—10 Hurt—10	Hit her—9 Sexual urges—9 Pull off her clothes—8
Tried to pull off her pants; other clients intervened and called police	I'll show her. This will be easy.	Angry—10	Sexual urges—10

FIGURE 6.1. Behavioral chain analysis for Example 1.

be functioning, as well as expectations of his case manager and what she should be able to do for him. These thoughts, emotions, and interactions facilitated several urges, some of which the individual acted on in the moment. For the purpose of treatment, the client has now identified a number of areas for potential intervention, including sources of emotional, cognitive, and interpersonal dysregulation. These areas of dysregulation, rather than a lengthy description of actual sexual behaviors involved in the offense itself, are the most important components of the behavioral chain analysis. Because of the richness of the information provided by the client in this exercise, treatment providers may be able to overlook minor discrepancies in the client's self-report of events in comparison with the victim's or witnesses'.

Example 2

A 22-year-old male was convicted of child molestation following several incidents of fondling and sexual touching of a 5-year-old niece, who his mother was babysitting at the time the offenses occurred. This was identified by the client as his target incident for the chain analysis. This client has no prior legal history of sexual offending, but interviews with family members revealed additional suspected incidents of child molestation since his adolescence. All of the known victims were young females, including both family members and other young children from his neighborhood. At the time the most recent incidents of sexual offending began, the client was reportedly unemployed and living at home, abusing alcohol and marijuana on a daily basis, and often arguing with his mother regarding his lack of income and substance use. The client has previously received disability services due to cognitive impairments but was not in any form of treatment at the time of the offense.

As shown in Figure 6.2 we can see a progression of events leading to a sexual offense. Again, this client has selected a relatively concise series of events that occurred on the day of one incident of sexual abuse. The client's reported thoughts, emotions, and urges provide us with an idea of what occurred immediately before the offense. In this case, negative interactions with his mother, a buildup of frustration and anger resulting from his current life circumstances, and other negative interactions, boredom, and a history of sexual behavior and urges involving children are all relevant targets for treatment intervention. The treatment provider is able to identify not only the sources of dysregulation but also implied difficulties with accepting responsibility, expectations and

Events	Thoughts	Emotions	Urges
Woke up late; in a bad mood from the night before	I hate being here. I'm tired of people telling me what to do. I wish I could just stay in bed.	Irritated/ annoyed—6	Go back to bed—8 Yell at someone—5
Ate breakfast; mom griped at me because I got up so late	Leave me alone. She's so stupid. I hate putting up with this.	Irritated/ annoyed—8 Angry—5	Leave—5 Yell at my mom—8
Mom said I had to help out with chores while she babysits	I don't need this. Why do I have to do this?	Angry—5 Frustrated—6	Leave—7 Drink—4
Mom had to go to the store; told me I had to watch my niece while she was gone	Why couldn't she do this? This isn't my job. This is boring	Irritated/ annoyed—4 Frustrated—4 Bored—7	Call my friends—4 Watch TV—5 Shut myself in my room—8
Niece kept bugging me to play with her	I just want to watch TV. This is boring. Where's mom? I just want something to do.	Irritated/ annoyed—5 Bored—8	Watch TV—6 Leave—5
Niece started poking at me and I started tickling her	She needs to quit it. I need to find something to do. She'll like this.	Irritated/ annoyed—3 Bored—6 Excited—4 Hyper—6	Tell her to quit—5 Sexual urges—3 Touch her—7
Kept tickling her and touching her everywhere	This is fun. She thinks this is fun.	Excited—8 Hyper—8 Happy—5	Sexual urges—6 Touch her—10
Started touching her sexually	This feels good. She likes this.	Excited—10 Happy—8	Sexual urges—10

FIGURE 6.2. Behavioral Chain Analysis for Example 2.

blame of others, and limited ability to self-monitor potential risk. Note that the client indicates that his niece began touching or poking him first (blaming the victim) and he further implies that his mother should not have left him with his niece (minimizing personal responsibility). Some of the frustrations this client mentions are not simply his own perceptions (though perceptions are still important), but recognizing the role of his cognitive deficits in low frustration tolerance, his difficulty with managing boredom and unstructured time, and his sense of resentment over his family's expectations will help us understand this client's dysregulation.

Troubleshooting

Sometimes treatment providers may become frustrated with a client's participation in the process of behavioral chain analysis. A number of questions may arise. Several common concerns are addressed below, and we then provide several sample chain analyses.

• *"What if the client says he or she can't remember, or gives conflicting information for the chain analysis?"* This is a difficult process for the client. He or she is being asked to describe the offense in a level of detail that may not have been expected or required by other forms of treatment. In other models, describing grooming behaviors, thoughts about the victim, or decision-making processes may be the extent to which clients have been asked to explore inner experiences related to the offense. Here, you are additionally asking him or her to reveal important emotions and urges that occurred at each step of the offense process. This may be far more personal and uncomfortable than simply describing observable behavior. The client may report difficulty remembering or give differing accounts of events, and treatment providers should validate or at least acknowledge the normality of his or her hesitation, resistance, or difficulty in describing such personal events.

Also, the client may be engaged in treatment at a time long after the offense actually occurred. This passage of time may realistically interfere with memory, as can other potential factors, such as cognitive deficits, psychiatric medications, or emphasis on other information since the time of the offense (e.g., other treatment approaches that focus on different features of the offense, like situational risk factors). When clients report memory failures or give contradictory information, treatment providers must gently elicit what seems most important in relation to the event. Asking other group members for general input about what may have logically happened next (e.g., "It seems like he was pretty angry, and had strong urges to 'make her pay.' What might have come after that, if you were in this situation?") may also help alleviate client concerns about others' judgments and also reinforce other clients for participating in the process.

• *"The client is giving me a lot of irrelevant information. How do I know what to focus on?"* Sometimes clients want to describe minute or irrelevant details that they consider crucial to the offense. Treatment providers will guide and shape the information that is used in the chain analysis. Providers must first be familiar, as much as is possible, with the sexual offenses or other problematic sexual behaviors of the client, so as to make sense of the major events being described. For example, if the client gives a confusing and nonsequential account of a known offense—perhaps describing things that happened after the offense while at the same time talking about what the victim said or did prior to the incident—a treatment provider may say, "Oh, so that's what happened afterward. That's when she talked to the police. I want to go back up here though where you had just gone into the room and saw her there. We'll get to that other part in a minute."

Providers can also emphasize certain parts of the client's experience and reinforce those, while at the same time deemphasizing or moving away from seemingly irrelevant details or off-topic elements. Reminding clients of the importance of each of these events can guide this process as well (e.g., "So what really seems to be the next major part is what you said here, about what the victim said when you showed up. That's when things really starting changing."). Clients will become more familiar with behavioral chain analysis as they observe others complete this process. In this part of Module 2, it is expected that earlier chain analyses may require more shaping than later ones.

• *"What the client says doesn't match the police report. Is this a problem? Should I say anything about it?"* It depends. How much of a discrepancy is there? Is the rest of the discussion consistent with known offense information? Again, the primary goal of behavioral chain analysis is to elicit information related to dysregulation that may have preceded the sexual offense. Clients may not always provide completely accurate and factual information about the events, but still give enough information about their own thoughts, emotions, and urges to allow treatment providers to identify dysregulation.

Efforts to alter, deny, or minimize situational events are therefore less problematic, provided that the reported internal experiences seem genuine. Also, this type of information may be more difficult to deliberately fabricate—attempts to do so will appear illogical in the overall sequence of events. When reported emotions, for example, suddenly and inexplicably change in a manner that is inconsistent with reported events or thoughts, it is noticeable. A client who reports being uncontrollably angry, judgmental, and wanting to harm someone who then reports that his or her next emotion was "happy" will stand out. This provides material for discussion, as treatment providers can express confusion or misunderstanding of this sequence of internal events. These types of inconsistencies are more problematic than those regarding time of day of the offense, the client's age at the time of the offense, or even the exact age or identity of the victim.

• *"What if the client denies the offense altogether?"* This is certainly more challenging. In this instance, the client may need to delay the chain analysis until a later (more willing) point in treatment. He or she could select several areas of dysregulation to monitor, or could monitor willingness and commitment, until such time as the client is ready to attempt a chain analysis on the offense. An alternative would be for the client to complete a chain analysis on another type of maladaptive behavior (e.g., aggression, substance abuse, a different arrest), as this may elicit signs of dysregulation similar to those precipitating the sexual offense.

SELF-MONITORING AND SELF-MANAGEMENT (SESSION 26)

As clients complete their behavioral chain analyses of sexual offending behaviors, they should become more familiar with the areas of dysregulation that precipitated their offenses. Once all clients have had an opportunity to complete a chain analysis, treatment providers next introduce self-monitoring. Treatment providers may find it helpful to explain the purpose of self-monitoring in other contexts, such as monitoring food intake, exercise, and daily or weekly weight in a nutritional program, or keeping track of time spent doing normal daily activities in order to improve time management. Self-monitoring is simply a process that increases awareness, and this increase in awareness is needed to precipitate change. Clients may already be familiar with self-monitoring in some respect, as it is central to many anger management programs (i.e., monitor your anger so that you can address it) or substance abuse treatment approaches (i.e., monitor factors that increase your risk of substance use).

Providers and clients should then discuss what areas may lend themselves to continuing self-monitoring; some of these areas of dysregulation are probably still present, even if they do not result in repeated or frequent sexual offending. Table 6.6 provides a quick reference for this session's content. Some clients may focus on emotions related to the offense (e.g., anger, resentment, loneliness), whereas others may note greater difficulties with thoughts, interpersonal interactions, or urges (e.g., blame, judgment, self-criticism, sexual urges, hostility toward others). Each client should identify four or five areas to be monitored and rated on a daily basis for discussion at the beginning of each session in the remaining treatment modules. Some examples are provided in Figure 6.3, using the chain analyses from our two sample clients described above. Treatment providers will need to collaborate with clients to develop individualized self-monitoring logs such as these based on what clients identify during behavioral chain analysis. Typically, clients will discuss daily self-monitoring activities in their weekly treatment group, though clients with very complex self-monitoring needs and a high degree of risk may need a separate individual or group session each week so that they are able to more fully process and discuss dysregulation and skills use.

Some clients may be unable or will have difficulty identifying areas of needed self-monitoring on their own. Treatment providers and other clients may be able to suggest important components from their chain analyses and try to elicit agreement. For those clients whose treatment goals are unrelated to their offense (i.e., clients who deny their offenses or who refuse to talk about their offending), they may need to self-monitor emotions, thoughts, or urges related to their continued struggles with commitment to change. For example, some clients may need to rate their commitment or willingness on a daily basis. Others may need to rate

---

TABLE 6.6. Self-Monitoring and Self-Management (Session 26)

- Introduce self-monitoring
  - Purpose: Self-monitoring helps clients increase their awareness of dysregulation in their daily lives and alerts them to opportunities for skills use. It also makes them more aware of vulnerabilities and situations in which they are more vulnerable to strong urges.
  - Clients will now develop a self-monitoring log (see Figure 6.3) using sources of dysregulation from the behavioral chain analysis. Clients select their own self-monitoring targets and share them at the beginning of each group from this point forward.

Behavioral Chain Analysis for Example 1

	Sadness (1–10)	Loneliness (1–10)	Anger (1–10)	Judgment (name who)	Sexual urges (1–10)	Skills used
Monday						
Tuesday						
Wednesday						
Thursday						
Friday						
Saturday						
Sunday						

Behavioral Chain Analysis for Example 2

	Boredom (1–10)	Resentment (1–10)	Expectations (name who and what)	Sexual urges (1–10)	Blaming others (yes/no)	Skills used
Monday						
Tuesday						
Wednesday						
Thursday						
Friday						
Saturday						
Sunday						

FIGURE 6.3. Sample self-monitoring logs.

their anger or resentment regarding being involved in treatment. Though these do not directly relate to sex offending behavior or its precursors, they are still legitimate areas of treatment emphasis and may actually aid in improving client motivation and engagement.

At this point, the structure of treatment sessions will change. Following the development of a self-monitoring worksheet for each client, sessions from this point forward will begin with a brief discussion of major points during the week—times when the client was highly dysregulated, or successes in using adaptive skills to cope with dysregulation (to be discussed at greater length in each module). Treatment providers can use these discussions to monitor and track client progress, given that clients are monitoring, reporting, and describing their experiences in a genuine manner. Each module of treatment henceforward will address specific areas related to sexual offending or different domains of dysregulation, thus building on the basic concepts covered in Module 2.

MODULE 2 CONCLUDING SESSIONS

In modules like this one that present new concepts or didactic information, treatment providers should be sure to review the major topic points discussed before moving on to other areas. For Module 2, these points include relationships and boundaries, sexual health, consent, how victims feel, and dysregulation and its role in sex offending behaviors. Treatment providers may wish to use Form B1, "My Treatment Progress," in Appendix B to generate summary discussion of how these topics relate to their own treatment goals, progress thus far, and future treatment needs.

CHAPTER 7

MODULE 3

Emotions and Emotion Regulation

Clients are now ready to begin working on specific forms of dysregulation. This dysregulation may have preceded their offenses, and could continue to cause them distress and functional impairment in their current lives. In this module, we start with emotions—something often overlooked in sex offender treatment but crucial for understanding the basic motivation behind human thought, learning, and behavior. Emotions drive our decisions, shape our interactions with others, and often influence our sense of self and general well-being. In terms of self-regulation, emotions are often the first and most easily described form of distress. They may also be the most uncomfortable, leading to maladaptive behavioral strategies for some individuals. People can generally list maladaptive or unhealthy behaviors that are linked to emotional dysregulation, including problematic eating, relationship stress, aggression, problems with drinking or drug use, and many others.

The primary goal of this module is to help clients better understand their own emotional experience. This larger goal consists of a series of smaller goals, including recognizing the complexity of emotional states, how they interplay with thought and behavior, the origin of emotions and how we learn emotion-related behaviors, qualitative features of emotional experience, and the relationship between emotions and maladaptive behavior. Clients will also explore the role of risky emotional states (i.e., those that are commonly linked to dysregulation and sexual offending) in their own sex offending behaviors. This module concludes with a discussion of adaptive regulatory strategies that may be useful in more effectively modulating emotional experience. Clients should now be completing a daily self-monitoring sheet, in which they describe important emotions and other experiences identified either during discussions of self-regulation versus dysregulation, or during behavioral chain analyses. Group sessions hereafter will begin with a discussion of these self-monitoring sheets, with clients identifying important events, emotions, urges, or other relevant factors from the week. This may include some discussion of self-regulatory successes or failures as well. While this should only absorb a brief period of each session, it is still a crucial part of treatment. This is the opportunity for clients to work toward more effective self-monitoring and self-management, and to also engage them in ongoing learning about their patterns of behavior.

As in prior modules, the materials presented combine teaching and discussion, perhaps leaning more heavily toward client discussion of concepts. Several completed sample worksheets are provided within the text to give providers additional ideas about communicating these concepts. Such activities can primarily be done in session to aid clients with reading or other cognitive deficits that preclude routine homework assignments. Early sections of this module focus on general issues related to emotions, later moving into specific emotions that may have been related to clients' sexual offending behaviors, and then adaptive skill development. Examples and troubleshooting tips are also provided to aid with facilitating such discussions throughout the module.

IDENTIFYING AND UNDERSTANDING EMOTIONS (SESSIONS 1–8)

Basic and Complex Emotional States

Before focusing on emotions and emotion regulation, we must focus on some basic principles of emotional experience: What are emotions, how do we experience them, and how do we track them over time? These questions may be all the more important for clients with impairments,

---

TABLE 7.1. Identifying and Understanding Emotions (Sessions 1–8)

- Basic and complex emotional states
  - Eight basic emotions
  - Thoughts, other emotions, physiological sensations, and urges/behaviors related to these basic states
  - Relationship between basic and more complex emotional states
- Describing emotional states
  - Intensity and duration of emotions
  - Why and how we self-monitor emotional states

emotional disorders, or limited experience with feeling and describing emotional states. This focus will prepare them for later discussions of dysregulation, when emotions feel uncomfortable or "unbalanced." We refer readers to Table 7.1 for an outline of this section.

Basic Emotions and Their Impact on Other Internal States

Clients with a history of dysregulation and maladaptive behaviors have a rather limited understanding of their own and others' emotional experiences. For clients to effectively manage their emotions (dysregulated and otherwise) and related behaviors, they must first gain a better understanding of what emotions are, where they come from, and how they impact interactions and behavior. The first sessions of this module are devoted to a discussion of basic and complex emotional states. The most basic of emotional states—those that are largely innate and consistent across cultures and generations—are the foundation for understanding more about emotional experience. As a group, clients will discuss each of these basic states: (1) happiness, (2) sadness/anguish, (3) anger, (4) fear, (5) surprise, (6) disgust, (7) shame/guilt, and (8) love/interest (e.g., Tomkins, 1962, 1963, 1991). Clients should identify thoughts, physiological sensations, other emotions, and urges or behaviors associated with each of these states. For example, when discussing fear, clients can identify physiological reactions associated with the sympathetic nervous system (e.g., fast heartbeat, sweating, feeling hot, muscle tension), other emotions that are more complex variations along a continuum of fear (e.g., anxiety, panic, apprehension, discomfort), specific thoughts or general characteristics of their fearful thinking (e.g., judgments, worry, racing thoughts, inability to think), and urges or behaviors prompted by fear (e.g., run away, fight back, hide). Treatment providers should challenge clients to think about these emotions in depth and compare them to one another. Many will find it easier perhaps to describe negative emotions, as they are often less accustomed to thinking about positive emotions. They may also notice important similarities and differences in these experiences, along with complexities or facets of emotional responding that they had not before recognized.

Basic versus Complex Emotions

This should lead into discussing the development of more complex emotional states. These are emotions that are often secondary to the more primary or basic emotion, such as resentment leading from anger, hopelessness leading from sadness or fear, or embarrassment leading from guilt or shame. Alternatively, some conceptualize complex emotional states as manifestations of the basic emotion at varying levels of intensity. For example, happiness exists on a continuum with elation, euphoria, contentment, and satisfaction. Clients already identified or considered many of these more complex emotions in the preceding discussion of emotions related to the eight basic emotional states. Clients may find it useful to start thinking about their self-monitoring experiences, and the types of emotions that they've been reporting in group. Are they basic or complex? How are they related to one another? How do the complex emotions develop (i.e., what sequence of emotions, thoughts, and urges can lead to a more complex emotional state?). How do they experience these emotions in comparison with the more basic ones? For example, is resentment different than anger? Are hopelessness and loneliness different than sadness? These types of questions will help clients with recognizing, understanding, and describing their emotional experiences, and will ultimately improve their abilities to regulate these states.

Describing Emotional States

How do we describe strong emotions? Clients often describe their emotions in terms of extremes—they either feel a particular emotion quite strongly or they don't feel it at all. This doesn't mean that the moderate or less intense emotional experiences aren't there, but that people may not think about them or label them unless they are noticeably felt. Most people experience emotions in multifaceted ways—one emotion is mixed with another, and emotions can be experienced at different levels of intensity throughout even a single event or interaction. Furthermore, emotions are not experienced in the same way by each person, so describing emotional experiences is highly idiosyncratic and depends on historical and personal factors. Because of these individualized differences, clients will need to learn how to label, describe, and communicate their feelings more effectively.

Clients will discuss the *intensity* and *duration* of emotions, using specific examples from the previous section on basic and complex emotions. Some questions to consider:

Intensity

"How strong is it?"

"How do you feel the same emotion 'differently'?"

"How does this compare with others' experiences?"

"Do you think you experience emotions more or less intensely (or the same) as others?"

"How do you know when it's too intense?"

"At what point do you feel like you're not in control of your behavior?"

Duration

"How long does it last?"

"How long does it take for you to return to 'normal'?"

"How do you know it's over?"

"What makes it last longer?"

As a group, clients should create a rating scale for a few selected emotions. Since there are differences between individual clients, have them describe what the emotion "looks like" at each point on a 1–10 scale. This description can include bodily sensations, thoughts, or behaviors. Also discuss when the emotion changes, and at what point clients return to their "normal" emotional baseline. Note that for some individuals, the baseline may be a 3 or a 4 on the scale, whereas for others it is higher or lower. Point out differences for negative versus positive emotions. This is helpful for later discussions involving dysregulation, as some clients become more easily dysregulated at lower levels of emotion than others, and for some the dysregulation may be more intense and of greater duration. This series of points allows for participation from each client. Their differences will show not only individualized needs but also illustrate the importance of self-monitoring—no one else can describe their emotional experiences as well as they can themselves.

Self-Monitoring Emotional States

Clients are now ready to list reasons why we should rate and monitor our emotional states. Again, self-monitoring of emotions and emotional dysregulation is an important step toward learning effective strategies for modulating emotional experiences. Being able to recognize emotions; understand their impact on the body, mind, and interactions with others; and discern changes in one's emotional state will all build toward more adaptive strategy formation. As clients monitor their emotions, discuss how this self-monitoring has changed or altered their view of emotional experience, whether they are now more aware of their emotions, or if they have begun to think differently about the way that they describe and rate their emotions. As a practice in DBT (Linehan, 1993), members of a DBT consultation team also self-monitor important emotions, urges, or behaviors. This helps them keep themselves balanced and also heightens their own awareness of client experience. The therapist engages in the same types of therapeutic assignment that the client is asked to. For new treatment providers with SOS who are unfamiliar with self-monitoring as a therapeutic technique, it may also be useful to practice self-monitoring emotional states for a brief time. These do not need to be reported in group, but the experience can offer insights into what the clients are learning as they learn to self-monitor.

ORIGINS OF OUR EMOTIONS (SESSIONS 9–12)

Treatment providers will now prepare to help clients understand where emotions come from. Even clients who are aware of emotional experience may lack a basic appreciation of how their emotional responses have developed over time. We have provided an outline of this section in Table 7.2 and several examples of completed client worksheets in this section for further assistance.

Why Do We Have Emotions?

Emotions are a natural part of being human. Unfortunately for those who struggle with strong emotions, they may be a very unpleasant or

TABLE 7.2. Origins of Our Emotions (Sessions 9–12)

- Why do we have emotions?
  - Biological and learned emotional responding
  - Adaptive nature of emotions
  - Pros and cons of emotional experience
- What causes my emotions?
  - Clients list examples of four precursors/triggers for their emotions
    - Situational factors
    - Cognitive factors
    - Interpersonal factors
    - Emotional factors

unwanted part of the human experience. Some view emotions as purely biological, unpredictable reactions within the brain. Others view them as learned responses to our cognitive interpretations of events. In reality, emotions are a bit of both. As a teaching point, group facilitators should describe for clients how biology and the environment work together to produce emotions and related behaviors.

Biological and Learned Emotional Responding

Clients might begin to see that some of our emotions, such as fear, anger, sadness, or happiness, are present at birth (e.g., Izard, 1991). Even babies and small children are able to experience and express these emotional states, so our reactions to these emotions are somewhat automatic. However, we also learn about emotions from those around us, including family members, friends, cultural or societal practices, and popular media (e.g., television, video games, or music). Each of these sources communicates something about emotions: whether a particular emotion is good or bad, what causes the emotion, how one should or should not express the emotion, or what results from having that emotion.

Clients should now be able to identify some of their learned experiences related to emotions. (See Figure 7.1 as an example of how to present this step, and refer to Form 7.1 at the end of the chapter for a client handout.) For example, a client may state that his father often yelled or cursed when angry, teaching him that anger is expressed in loud or threatening tones. Another client may say that as a child, he was punished for crying or expressing sadness, teaching him that sadness is an emotion to be hidden or ashamed of. Treatment providers should also prompt clients to think about how emotional responses are portrayed in movies or other media (e.g., if you're angry, you shoot someone; if you like someone, you have sex with them). Also be sure to emphasize how emotions may be reinforced or punished, as this is also a basic form of learning. Clients will recognize that some emotions are considered "bad," while others are labeled "good." Client responses will vary according to their experiences and environments. In the two examples used above, anger may have been perceived as more acceptable or good, whereas sadness was punished or ridiculed. This reinforcement versus punishment reaction was likely dependent on individualized factors, like familial or cultural beliefs, gender role expectations, observed behaviors, and even deliberate education.

Really spending some time on this can help illustrate for clients where their emotional responses originated. Recognizing, for example,

Many of our feelings are things we are born with. They come hard-wired into our brains.

This includes emotions like anger, fear, sadness, or happiness. Even babies are able to feel these emotions. The body may react to one of these emotions automatically. For example, think about what your body does when you are very scared . . . or angry . . . or happy.

We also learn about emotions from the environment we live in. How we act when feeling some emotions is mostly learned. We learn from:

1. How others act when they feel that way.
   Family, friends, or others who are important to us. (Ask clients how their family and friends act when angry, sad, or hurt.)
2. Messages from our culture about that emotion.
   Television, movies, video games, and traditions. (Ask clients what people in movies or video games do when they're angry, sad, or alone. What role does culture play?)
3. How we are reinforced or rewarded in some way for our own emotional behavior.
   (Ask clients how others have reacted when they are upset, afraid, or happy. How do others react to what they do when they're emotional?)

What have you learned about each of these types of emotions?

Emotion	What I learned	How I learned it
Anger	That it's okay to yell or throw things when you're mad	My dad
Happiness	To buy whatever you want	My mother
	Be nice to everybody	My minister
Sadness	That you shouldn't cry	My dad and movies
	Drinking will make you feel better	TV ads and family
Fear	You can't ever show fear, or some-one will take advantage of you	My dad and brothers
Loneliness	Having sex will make you feel loved	Movies and friends
Love	You show your love through sex	Movies & music videos
	People who love you will hurt you	Parents

FIGURE 7.1. Sample client worksheet—"Emotions: Biology and Learning."

that one's family members handled anger through violence, drinking, or arguing, and also seeing similar patterns in one's own behavior, can help make sense of how maladaptive strategies developed. This insight "normalizes" the clients to the extent that they can see how they learned such behaviors and that it's not simply because they're bad people (as they might have been told). This recognition can depersonalize or detach them enough from how they respond that they are more amenable to changing emotion-based behavior.

Adaptive Nature of Emotions

Clients should also consider the adaptive nature of emotions—if emotions are "hard-wired" into our brains, why? They are not random, though clients with negative emotional experiences may view them as useless, unnecessary, or punishing. Emotions, even the negative ones, still serve some adaptive function (Izard, 1991). Being able to recognize this reality may help clients understand and accept their own emotions better. Some examples to discuss with clients include the following: (1) Fear may help you avoid harm; (2) anger may alert you to problems or potential threats in your environment; (3) love may prompt you to protect others or stay with others who will protect you; and (4) disgust may help you avoid something negative or harmful. There are many other examples of the function of emotions, though treatment providers and clients may have to think creatively. Thinking about what life would be like without emotions, emotional learning (e.g., fear responses), and emotion as a motivator may help.

Pros and Cons of Emotional Experience

This discussion topic naturally leads to a consideration of the pros and cons of emotions. Some clients experience many negative or intense emotions or have been punished as a result of having strong emotions or acting problematically because of them. Such individuals may argue that emotions are "all bad" or that they would be better off without them. However, there are positive aspects of having emotions, including the adaptive functions reviewed above, as well as the role of positive emotions in developing healthy relationships, positive self-esteem or self-image, and a more productive and satisfying life. Although some clients struggle with identifying these goals for themselves, the purpose of such a discussion is to introduce balance into their beliefs about the way that they feel. They can have both positive and negative emotional experiences, and their responses to emotions can become more balanced. This may take work, which is the purpose of this module and this treatment.

What Causes My Emotions?

Beyond broad explanations of biology versus learning, clients may have a difficult time understanding why they feel the way that they do. For many of them, emotions seem to occur "all of a sudden," or may rapidly shift from one mood state to another. While some truly do experience emotional lability in a more pathological sense, it is more common that clients are simply unaware of their emotions until they become very strong, or do not recognize what prompts their emotions to change.

Here, clients will discuss four types of precursors, or triggers, that can elicit an emotional response. Clients should provide their own examples from recent experiences.

1. *Situational factors*—notable events or environmental stressors. These may include major life events, such as loss of a job, recent success, relocating or changing residence, or loss of a friend or family member, as well as minor or temporary situational circumstances, such as drug or alcohol use, being in a crowded place, hearing your favorite song, or being late for an appointment. Challenge clients to think how these and other examples affect their emotional state.

2. *Cognitive factors*—thoughts or beliefs. Specific kinds of thoughts may change one's mood state. For example, self-critical thoughts may elicit sadness, guilt, or self-directed anger. Judgmental thoughts (toward others) may prompt feelings of disgust, anger, or resentment. Beliefs may have a similar effect. Believing that things are going well and that people are generally fair, for example, may lead to feelings of happiness and hope. Again, have clients generate examples of how their thoughts or beliefs influenced their moods.

3. *Interpersonal factors*—specific interactions or types of people. Interpersonal interactions are very likely to elicit emotions, whether they are positive emotions like happiness, love, or appreciation, or negative emotions like hurt, fear, or rage. Similarly, some types of people (or our perceptions of these people) may trigger our emotions. We may feel frustrated or defiant toward those who are bossy or demanding. We may feel ashamed around someone who is highly critical. Our clients, like

everyone else, interact with others on a daily basis and should be able to provide ample evidence of how their emotions change in these interactions.

4. *Emotional factors*—other emotions that precede the current mood state. Sometimes emotions lead to other emotions. Feeling hurt, for example, can provoke anger toward the one who caused the hurt. Being disgusted or angry can cause feelings of guilt or shame. This connection between emotions should remind clients of the prior discussion related to basic and complex emotions.

How we act in response to these triggers is a combination of biology and learning. Certain triggers may lead to an emotion, but how we act, think, and feel is dependent on experience. Our decisions and actions are what we can change—not the emotion. For clients, how they respond to emotions and what they do following one of these triggers is one of the major targets of treatment.

EXPERIENCING EMOTIONAL DISTRESS (SESSIONS 13–17)

Emotional Distress and Dysregulation

Emotional distress and dysregulation are relative. (It may be helpful for clients to briefly review types of emotional dysregulation from Module 2. Also, see Table 7.3 for the sequence of discussion in this section.) Certain elements of emotional experience help define distress and dysregulation. The first of these has already been discussed in this module, but bears repeating: *intensity*. Clients and treatment providers are typically able

---

TABLE 7.3. Experiencing Emotional Distress (Sessions 13–17)

- Emotional distress and emotional dysregulation
  - Facets of emotional distress and dysregulation—emotional and physical responses
    - Intensity—how strong is it?
    - Sensitivity—how much does it affect you?
- Relationship between emotions and maladaptive behavior
  - Reacting to extreme emotions
  - How are reactions maladaptive?
  - How are maladaptive behaviors or reactions to extreme emotions reinforced?
  - Emotional coping—adaptive and maladaptive

---

to identify the point at which an emotion becomes so intense as to be uncomfortable. Knowing an emotional threshold enables clients to better utilize their self-monitoring sheets and preventatively use adaptive skills to cope with increasing emotional intensity. Again, clients can use a rating scale to help them identify dysregulation for a variety of emotions. Clients should also describe things that cue them to increasingly intense or dysregulated emotions, like physiological sensations or urges.

Intensity

Here is a key question for clients: What happens when your emotions are very intense? Their answers could include both positive and negative emotions, as even positive emotions can be uncomfortable or distressing in the extreme. To help illustrate this point, treatment providers can consider questions like: What happens when you're too excited? Have you ever felt uncontrollably angry? Can sadness or loneliness be too much to handle? What happens when you're too angry, too sad, or too afraid? Clients may want to revisit their comments and examples from Module 2 discussions of emotional dysregulation in thinking about these questions. Remember that dysregulation is a variable threshold, reached when the emotional intensity becomes uncomfortable.

Sensitivity

A second component is *sensitivity*. Different from intensity, sensitivity is best described as how easily an emotion is elicited and also how it affects the person. Those with increased sensitivity to emotions are perhaps more reactive, feel emotions more easily, or are more affected by their emotions. Those with less sensitivity or who experience little emotional valence may underreact to emotional stimuli, feel emotions in a superficial way, or think and behave largely independent of emotional feeling. Sitting too much on either extreme—being overly sensitive or being callous and insensitive—are both indicators of emotional regulation problems. However, even normal emotional sensitivity can lend itself to experiences of dysregulation, given individual and experiential variability.

For clients, their sensitivity to emotions influences the intensity of the emotion as well as the experience of distress or dysregulation. Consider the following questions in relation to sensitivity: How easily do you feel that way? What else may affect your sensitivity to a certain emotion (e.g., preceding mood state, relationship factors, past experiences, or physiological states like hunger, pain, or tiredness)? How much control do you have over these factors? In answering these questions, concrete illustrations, role plays, or recent examples from group may be useful. Treatment providers could, for example, create a hypothetical situation in which the individual's sensitivity to emotion does change the outcome. Different physiological precursors (e.g., "You didn't slept well the night before" or "This incident happens in a bar, when both individuals are quite intoxicated"), relationship factors (e.g., "You feel like he never listens to you" or "Talking with her always ends in an argument"), or preceding mood states (e.g., "You woke up in a bad mood" or "He comes into this situation having just lost his mother and feeling very sad and lonely") could be substituted within the example to highlight real differences in one's sensitivity to emotion.

Emotions and Maladaptive Behavior

Reacting to Extreme Emotions

Giving in to emotional dysregulation impacts behavior, relationships, decision making, self-esteem, and the intensity and nature of one's urges. Therefore, dysregulation can be not only uncomfortable, but can lead to extreme and damaging outcomes. Many examples from clients' own experiences readily illustrate these points. (See Figure 7.2 for a sample client worksheet for discussion, and Form 7.2 at the end of the chapter for a client version of this handout.) Still, being emotionally dysregulated and acting accordingly is also a natural human experience. Many people have acted rashly or impulsively "in the moment" of intense emotion. It may be important to normalize this experience in order for clients to feel more comfortable discussing it. We want them to be able to talk about their maladaptive and harmful behaviors within the context of emotional responding. Sometimes clients are hesitant to talk about the emotional aspect of these behaviors, as they have been punished or discouraged from doing so in the past. For example, describing their anger or loneliness within the context of a violent sexual offense would typically cause the listener to criticize them, accuse them of minimizing the behavior, or say that they're trying to deflect responsibility. Anger and loneliness may be legitimately related to some of their behaviors. This relationship does not lessen the seriousness or wrongfulness of the offense. The problem lies with the behavior or action, not the actual emotion that preceded it. Learning to accept some degree of emotional distress and dysregulation

Think about specific examples from your past of how emotions led to impulsive behaviors, poor decisions, or behaviors that may have harmed you or other people.

Emotions	Behavior	Harm caused
1. Anger	Yelled at family members	Hurt others' feelings
	Later felt guilty	Hurt self
2. Anxiety	Felt like people were judging me	Irresponsibility
	and didn't go to group	Missed treatment
3. Excited	Felt like nothing could go wrong	Impulsivity
	and acted on my emotions	
	without thinking	
4. Paranoia	Isolated myself and got high	Hurt self and family

FIGURE 7.2. Sample client worksheet—"Extreme Emotions and My Behavior."

while separating it from value judgment will help clients more effectively monitor and manage their strong emotions.

Reinforcement of Maladaptive Behavior

Many people—not just those who commit sexual offenses—act on strong emotions. But some individuals act in maladaptive ways. By now, clients are probably able to recognize some relationship between their emotional state and the offending process. Emotions they have mentioned in prior discussions, behavioral chain analyses, and self-monitoring activities are related to their sexual offenses and other maladaptive behaviors, including substance use, aggression, self-harm or suicidality, criminal behaviors, or lying, arguing, and other problematic relationship behaviors.

If extreme or dysregulated emotions can lead to impulsive, harmful, or maladaptive behaviors, what happens to the emotion in the end?

The goal of self-regulation (and the use of a self-regulatory strategy) is to reduce or change emotional intensity or dysregulation. This change occurs when a strategy works, regardless of whether it is adaptive or maladaptive. This change –alleviation of dysregulated emotion—is reinforcing. Admittedly, it is hard to conceptualize maladaptive behavior as reinforcing. So many negative consequences or societal beliefs get in the way. But it's not the behavior that's reinforcing. Rather, the reinforcing part of it is the relief it provides from an intense, uncomfortable, or unbalanced emotional state. In the end, the relief from dysregulation may soon be overshadowed by other consequences, such as guilt, self-criticism or judgment, and disappointment, all of which are additional forms of dysregulation. Maladaptive strategies for strong emotions are not long-term solutions for dysregulation, but they certainly produce an effect and are self-perpetuating.

Clients understand this process, though it is a concept fraught with difficulty. Knowing that a maladaptive strategy "works" to reduce strong emotionality does not justify or excuse the behavior, nor does it mean that the client intentionally sought such an effect. We simply want them to understand the process so that they can substitute more adaptive strategies at the needed time. Clients can give examples of this process using a number of maladaptive behaviors with which they are familiar, including substance use (with the most obvious impact on mood), verbal and physical aggression, or other disordered behavioral patterns. A next step is for clients to identify other behavioral "strategies" that they have used to cope. They should think about whether or not these strategies worked, what happened when they did not work, and what influenced their decision to engage in a maladaptive behavior. Important factors to consider may be available opportunity, strength of the emotional state, or the ease of using said strategy in a given moment or circumstance.

EMOTIONAL DYSREGULATION AND PROBLEMATIC SEXUAL BEHAVIOR (SESSIONS 18–22)

We now turn to how emotional dysregulation and how maladaptive behaviors or regulatory strategies may precipitate sex offending behavior. While not all clients will have strong emotions related to their offending, many will. These emotions and other factors may have already been identified through the process of behavioral chain analysis, and may be better understood through further discussion in this section of the module. See Table 7.4 for a summary of these discussions.

TABLE 7.4. Emotional Dysregulation and Problematic Sexual Behavior (Sessions 18–22)

- Specific emotional states related to sexual offending
  - Clients define and identify how these states are related to their own and others' sexual offending behaviors
    - Entitlement
    - Anger
    - Resentment
    - Defiance
    - Boredom
    - Excitement
    - Sadness
    - Loneliness
    - Disappointment
    - Anxiety or fear
- Precursors to risky emotional states
  - Review of situational, cognitive, interpersonal, and emotional triggers for these specific states

Specific Emotional States Related to Sexual Offending

Some emotional states are more significantly related to sex offending behaviors, including anger, entitlement, loneliness, boredom, and others. Clients may have already mentioned these in their behavioral chain analyses, and some of the same emotions have been recurrent topics in this module as clients describe their own examples of emotional dysregulation and maladaptive behaviors. There are certain risky emotional states that clients can discuss within the context of their everyday experience, sexual behavior, and their own sexual offending.

- *Entitlement.* This can be both a mood state and a way of thinking. In this discussion, we want to emphasize that feeling of deservedness, self-justification, and pride or envy that defines entitlement as an emotional state. Clients may identify with the egocentricity or "rush" of power that accompanies entitlement. Related to sexual offending, some experience feelings of sexual entitlement, when they feel justified or deserving of sexual contact (perhaps regardless of another's refusal). Others may describe feelings of hurt or anger toward a specific person (i.e., victim), and that sexual offending humiliates the other person so that he or she knows how important and powerful the offender is (e.g., Baumeister et al., 2002; Bouffard, 2010; Bushman et al., 2003; Hanson, Gizzarelli, & Scott, 1994).

- *Anger.* Anger is commonly associated with violent sexual behavior (e.g., Smallbone & Milne, 2000). Some offenders report being angry at their specific victims, while others report being angry at a larger group, of which the victim was a member (e.g., women, persons of authority). Sometimes this anger results from feeling rejected or ridiculed by the victim, feeling mistreated by others (thus also prompting entitlement), or simply wanting to take one's anger out on another person in a humiliating or degrading way.

• *Resentment.* Resentment includes elements of both entitlement and anger and is also sometimes related to violent behavior (Baumeister et al., 2002; Bushman et al., 2003). Clients may recognize resentment as the feeling of bitterness that accompanies jealousy, or the feeling that they didn't get something they "deserved." Angry resentment can exacerbate feelings of vengeance or entitlement, also leading to offending. For example, clients who know the victim may resent that person (e.g., "She had no right to treat me that way, and she does that all the time") and feel that mistreating him or her is justly deserved. Some offenders may also report feelings of resentment that precede sexual entitlement.

• *Defiance.* For many offenders, defiance may be strongly linked to a victim's rejection, refusal of sexual advances, or negative interpersonal interactions (e.g., Baumeister et al., 2002; Bushman et al., 2003). Defiance and thoughts of "I can do whatever I want" could lead to impulsive sexual acting-out, or going through with a sexual act even after the victim has refused to participate or comply.

• *Boredom.* Boredom is often overlooked as an emotional precursor to sex offending and impulsive sexual behaviors. A bored person will seek excitement or novelty in order to alleviate boredom (Hare, 1999; Millon & Davis, 1996). In the absence of adaptive means, this seeking may be something risky or impulsive. For those with prior sexual offenses or a history of offense-supportive fantasy, the promise of sexual gratification or other reinforcement may be a viable strategy for relieving boredom. Boredom can then perpetuate future sex offending. For those without such a history but who have poor sexual or interpersonal boundaries, the possibility of sexual excitement can modulate boredom.

• *Excitement.* Excitement is typically viewed as a positive, desirable emotional state, but can lead to a dysregulated state (e.g., feeling "hyper," giddy, or overly emotionally aroused; for some may be associated with mania). Excitement in the extreme may set the stage for a sense of urgency, impulsivity, poor decision making, or desperate attempts to prolong the positive mood state (e.g., Anestis, Selby, & Joiner, 2007; Nezu, Nezu, Dudek, Peacock, & Stoll, 2005; Whiteside & Lynum, 2001). Feeling overly excited in interpersonal interactions could facilitate sexual arousal or efforts to solicit sexual interactions.

• *Sadness.* Some clients report feelings of sadness or depression preceding their sex offending behaviors. This sadness may stem from personal loss, interpersonal failures, or self-criticism, among other sources. It can lead to attempts to regain personal or interpersonal satisfaction through external means. Some clients may expect a sexual interaction to make them "feel better" about themselves or a relationship, or to in fact strengthen a failing or unhealthy relationship (Marshall, 1989, 1993).

• *Loneliness.* Many offenders may struggle with both loneliness and sadness (e.g., Cortoni & Marshall, 2001; Marshall, 1989, 1993). They may solicit sexual interactions or sexual relationships with others to alleviate loneliness. Sometimes loneliness may also be related to resentment or entitlement, as some clients feel that they deserve sexual contact or relationships with others, and that they perceive their loneliness as "unfair."

• *Disappointment.* People experience disappointment every day. But for some, disappointment is overwhelming. Interpersonal rejection, failure, loss, or self-criticism—all are potential sources of disappointment. Some react with sadness, while others may react with anger. Either way, those who experience intense disappointment may act in impulsive, vengeful, or desperate ways (e.g., Marshall, 1993; Marshall, Anderson, & Champagne, 1997). This may include sexual acting out or efforts to initiate sexual interactions with others.

• *Anxiety or fear.* Anxiety or fear may not often directly precipitate sexual offending, but they are related to other emotional states or situations that could precede an offense. Anxiety in an interpersonal interaction, coupled with anger and disappointment following another's rejection, could create enough dysregulation to trigger maladaptive behavior (e.g., Marshall 1989, 1993; Marshall et al., 1997). Some clients may report paranoia associated with their offending, which is an exaggerated or extreme form of fear (e.g., Guidry & Saleh, 2004; Stinson & Becker, 2011). Coupled with anger or entitlement, paranoia may exacerbate existing aggressive or sexually aggressive impulses and weaken behavioral controls.

Virtually any emotion can create the right circumstances for maladaptive or harmful behavior, but this is still rare. These risky emotional states may be significant for some clients and are highly individualized. They may identify multiple emotions that precipitated their offending, and these emotions may or may not be continuing problems for them. One client may be able to describe how anger, resentment, disappointment, and feelings of entitlement contributed to a violent sexual act against a woman who had rejected him. Another may identify how sadness, loneliness, and fear of being alone led to a desperate and impulsive attempt to initiate a sexual relationship with a young child or adolescent who seemed to like him, albeit in a nonsexual way. These conversations help clients learn to identify and later monitor emotions that are difficult for them to successfully control. And because these emotions are all part of the normal human experience, we know that they will recur, which makes it all the more important for clients to learn to manage them in a healthy way.

Precursors to Risky Emotional States

After identifying their individual emotional "risks," clients must learn what triggers these emotional states. Earlier in this module, clients reviewed situational, cognitive, interpersonal, and other emotional factors that may lead to or trigger an emotional response. Return to that discussion, highlighting the precursors most related to the clients' risky emotional states. For some, this may mean finding triggers most likely to elicit anger. For others, the focus may be what causes boredom and prompts a need for excitement. Group discussions should focus on either one client or one emotion at a time to help clients learn what they should monitor and at what point they should attempt adaptive skills.

ALTERNATIVE FORMS OF COPING: BASIC TECHNIQUES (SESSIONS 23–25)

Basic Strategies

Clients may be able to decrease sexual offending and other maladaptive behaviors by learning and applying more adaptive regulatory strategies. The assumption is that they either lack the adaptive strategies needed, that the strategies do not work because of strong dysregulation, or because other, more maladaptive strategies have been more salient, available, and successful in regulating strong mood states. Thus, a clear goal of treatment is to help clients learn new strategies that are not only effective but also less harmful to themselves and others. (See Table 7.5 for a review of this section.)

Clients and treatment providers should be able to generate a lengthy list of alternative strategies. Many of these are designed to (1) decrease vulnerability to strong emotions (i.e., preventative strategies), (2) maintain a manageable level of emotional arousal (i.e., maintenance strategies),

TABLE 7.5. Alternative Forms of Coping: Basic Techniques (Sessions 23–25)

- Basic strategies
  - Review strategies for preventing emotional dysregulation, soothing intense emotions, and distracting from emotional distress
- Using alternative strategies
  - Include discussion of alternative strategies in weekly self-monitoring assignments

or (3) decrease dysregulated or uncomfortable emotions (i.e., crisis strategies). Some examples of these are listed below, several of which fall into more than one of these categories. Discuss these strategies and others with clients, identifying specifically how they may function to regulate emotional states. Some forms of treatment, such as DBT (Linehan, 1993), may already be familiar to clients and will include coping skills that clients can reference as part of this discussion.

1. Self-monitoring
2. Awareness of triggers
3. Reducing vulnerability to triggers (e.g., sleeping and eating as needed, managing stress)
4. Pleasurable replacement activities (e.g., hobbies, self-rewards)
5. Distracting yourself
6. Doing something inconsistent with the emotional state (e.g., anger = helping someone; sad = watching a comedy; lonely = calling a friend)
7. Taking a self-imposed "time-out": may include relaxation, breathing exercises, mindfulness, prayer, etc.
8. Calming activities meant to soothe strong emotions (e.g., listening to soft music, sitting in a dark or dimly lit room and breathing slowly, taking a hot shower or bath)
9. Physical activity or exercise
10. Intense physical sensations (e.g., breathing in very cold air, holding ice, listening to loud music, controlled muscle tension exercises)

Using Alternative Strategies

Because every client is different, some strategies will work better than others at regulating intense emotional states. Clients will need to practice these strategies both "in the moment" and also while not experiencing strong emotions in order to become more effective at using the skills. They will also need to determine which skills are ultimately more functional or effective for reducing dysregulation. Clients may find that some strategies do not work with some emotions. For example, when enraged, reading is unlikely to work as a distraction. Clients may also find that some strategies intensify certain emotions. Going to a crowded place may alleviate loneliness for some, while worsening it for others. Listening to loud music may exacerbate anger or provide an outlet for it.

Group facilitators should prepare clients for the fact that practicing and using unfamiliar or new strategies may feel uncomfortable at first. The strategies may not work, leading to frustration, hopelessness, or shame. There is a learning curve with new strategies. They may not be immediately functional or reinforcing but will become so following repeated use. If they do not, it is at this point that another strategy needs to be tried. Clients need to know this and go through this process as they are learning, for it will take time for these new strategies to become as useful, comfortable, and readily available as their more familiar, maladaptive ones.

Group members may have questions about more advanced skills that they can use to help regulate their emotions, urges, and behaviors. These skills may include interpersonal or cognitive regulation strategies. These will be addressed in greater detail in later modules, although some discussion of these skills (e.g., self-talk, thinking about pros and cons, interpersonal communication strategies) may be helpful during this module as well.

Finally, clients should describe their efforts to practice emotion regulation strategies during their self-monitoring discussion each time the group meets. This presents an opportunity for clients to identify and monitor those emotional states related to their offending behaviors and to practice new skills in response to those emotions. Feedback about their successes, frustrations, or expectations helps them learn to gradually replace maladaptive strategies with healthier, more adaptive ones. For clients who do not readily discuss their skills practice, treatment providers can prompt them during a review of self-monitoring activities or ask them specific questions about skills use related to other aspects of their treatment. Treatment providers may also have to assign specific skill activities or practice times to facilitate regular skills use. Though this represents only a small part of the overall module, it will remain an important component of self-monitoring and self-management, built upon throughout the remaining modules.

MODULE 3—CONCLUDING SESSIONS

Therapists should be sure to review the major topic points discussed during this module, including emotions, their intensity, the clients' sensitivity to certain triggers, self-monitoring, risky emotional states and their relationship to sexual offending, and adaptive replacement strategies. Clients can again use Form B1, "My Treatment Progress," in Appendix B to aid them in relating these concepts to their own goals and progress.

Emotions: Biology and Learning

Many of our feelings are things we are born with. They come hard-wired into our brains.

This includes emotions like anger, fear, sadness, or happiness. Even babies are able to feel these emotions. The body may react to one of these emotions automatically. For example, think about what your body does when you are very scared . . . or angry . . . or happy.

We also learn about emotions from the environment we live in. How we act when feeling some emotions is mostly learned. We learn from:

1. How others act when they feel that way.
   Family, friends, or others who are important to us. *(Ask clients how their family and friends act when angry, sad, or hurt.)*
2. Messages from our culture about that emotion.
   Television, movies, video games, and traditions. *(Ask clients what people in movies or video games do when they're angry, sad, or alone. What role does culture play?)*
3. How we are reinforced or rewarded in some way for our own emotional behavior.
   (Ask clients how others have reacted when they are upset, afraid, or happy. How do others react to what they do when they're emotional?)

What have you learned about each of these types of emotions?

Emotion	What I learned	How I learned it
_____	_____	_____
	_____	_____
_____	_____	_____
	_____	_____
_____	_____	_____
	_____	_____
_____	_____	_____
	_____	_____

FORM 7.2

Extreme Emotions and My Behavior

Think about specific examples from your past of how emotions led to impulsive behaviors, poor decisions, or behaviors that may have harmed you or other people.

Emotions	Behavior	Harm caused
1. Anger		
2. Anxiety		
3. Excited		
4. Sad		
5. _____		
6. _____		

CHAPTER 8

MODULE 4

Sexuality and Sexual Behavior

In Module 3, clients focused on dysregulated emotional states. Before moving on to other forms of dysregulation, it is necessary that clients discuss their sexuality, sexual behavior, and sexual development. These points will shape later modules that emphasize beliefs, perceptions, and interpersonal relationships. In this module, clients are not expected to divulge all aspects of their sexual lives and experiences. Instead, the focus is on how and what they learned about sex in the past, the role of sexuality in relationships, healthy and unhealthy sexual behaviors, and developing healthy and appropriate sexual boundaries.

The discussions and activities in this section may be awkward or difficult for some clients (and treatment providers). They are not meant to be. Clients have previously engaged in harmful, violent, or dangerous sexual behaviors, and discussing their sexuality may be viewed as a punishment. They expect that others will judge and criticize them. Unfortunately, many of them have probably been made to feel that they cannot have sexual relationships, or that sexual feelings are wrong, as the result of their past behaviors. And though clients are experienced in describing sexual details of their offenses, talking openly about non-offense-related sexual matters may be more difficult. Treatment providers should expect this reticence, acknowledge and normalize it, and attempt to alleviate the clients' anxieties to make this process smoother for everyone.

Goals for this module include (1) describing and understanding different types of relationships and associated interpersonal and sexual boundaries, (2) learning more about how early sexual experiences and messages about sexuality have shaped current beliefs and behaviors, (3) describing healthy sexuality and sexual arousal, and (4) understanding the role of sexual fantasies, masturbation, and pornography in past and current sexual practices. Upon completion of this module, clients will have learned something more about their own sexuality, including how it develops across the lifespan and the role that it plays in their lives and relationships with others.

The primary mode of teaching in this module is group discussion. Clients will describe their own experiences, give each other validation and feedback, and provide examples with minimal teaching from group facilitators. Here, the role of the treatment provider is to guide discussion, provide validation, promote education regarding healthy sexual beliefs and relationships, and help clients discover their own beliefs and preferences related to sexuality and sexual development. Due to the complex and often personal nature of the discussions in this module, we have provided numerous examples and guidance regarding potential areas of difficulty in communicating these concepts.

SEXUALITY AND RELATIONSHIPS: A REVIEW (SESSIONS 1–4)

In Module 2, clients briefly described a number of concepts related to sexual relationships and boundaries, including gender role stereotypes, types of relationships, relationship boundaries, and sexual health and education. It is worth revisiting these concepts again as you initiate this module (see Table 8.1), since their understanding of sexual relationships and boundaries, sexual stereotypes and expectations, and prior sex education will impact their responses throughout this section. This also presents an opportunity to go into greater depth, as clients may be more comfortable and open in treatment at this stage than they were in the earlier stages of SOS.

TABLE 8.1. Sexuality and Relationships: A Review (Sessions 1–4)

- Concept review
  - Clients review Module 2 concepts to lead into the rest of Module 4
    o Sexual relationships
    o Relationships and boundaries
- Sexual health and education
  - Review of concepts that may be essential for additional learning—sexual health, pregnancy and contraception, or other topics

---

Concept Review

Sexual Relationships

In Module 2, clients participated in activities designed to teach them about relationships, including how they are formed, how they differ, and what one can expect in these different types of relationships. Clients may find it helpful to review the following questions:

- What are some different kinds of "relationships"?
- How are sexual relationships different from other relationships (e.g., how you feel, expectations of the other person, goals in the relationship)?
- What makes a relationship healthy or unhealthy?

Relationships and Boundaries

Clients also described gender role stereotypes during early parts of Module 2. Revisit this discussion, asking them to relate these stereotypes to their expectations and behaviors. For example, if a client notes that women should obey men, how might this impact his own behavior toward women? If a client believes that a man should be stoic and not express his emotions, how will this influence his behavior and emotional expression in a relationship? (In this latter example, treatment providers may also find it helpful to draw on concepts from Module 3.) These stereotypes and beliefs, as well as other factors, contribute to the development of boundaries in relationships. Once again, have clients describe or demonstrate different types of boundaries. They should consider where boundaries come from, how they are communicated to others, and how they impact relationships and behavior. (We recommend that treatment providers revisit the activities and discussion points in Chapter 6 of this text for further detail.)

Sexual Health and Education

Finally, clients should review their experiences with sex education. Have them reconsider the importance of sex education in their own and others' lives. For clients who have spent a significant amount of time in institutions, it may be surprisingly common that they have had little sexual education. During pilot research, it was noted that many of the clients with the most significant histories of institutional or residential placement had the least amount of sex education, with the exception of learning about symptoms of sexually transmitted diseases. Treatment providers should gauge clients' level of understanding of some basic sexual concepts, and if needed, recommendations for further sex education can be made for those with very limited understanding of basic sexual functioning. Additional sex education could be incorporated into this module, if needed. This may include discussions of sexual health (see Form 8.1 at the end of the chapter for an informational handout for clients unfamiliar with sexually transmitted diseases and their prevention), facts versus myths about contraception and pregnancy (see Form 8.2 at the end of the chapter for a list of facts and myths for clients to discuss), or other topics as deemed necessary by treatment providers. (Several standardized protocols for sex education with different populations are commercially available, or publicly available on websites like *www.siecus.org*.) While the goal is not to presume that increased sexual knowledge will reduce recidivism, it is admittedly difficult to continue with discussions of sexuality without establishing some clear foundational knowledge of sexual processes. Therefore, treatment providers' decisions about needed areas of focus are meant to fill in gaps in knowledge that may impede further progress in this module.

HUMAN SEXUALITY (SESSIONS 5–10)

Learning about Sexuality

How do people learn about sex? Even in the absence of formal sexual education, people learn extensive information about sexual relationships and behaviors. In fact, most of what people learn about sexuality and sexual functioning stems from more informal educational opportunities. Clients will report various sources of sexual information, including those that were appropriate, accurate, and healthy, as well as those that were inappropriate or even abusive. Some clients may not have learned much about sexuality until they were arrested for a sexual offense. We want clients to identify who taught them about sexuality, how they learned, what was learned, and how it has impacted their beliefs and actions.

Treatment providers should facilitate a discussion involving the questions below (see Table 8.2). This is a less formal way of encouraging clients to reflect on their experiences and provides a great deal of information regarding the setting in which they learned about sexuality and relationships.

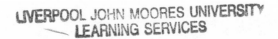

TABLE 8.2. Human Sexuality (Sessions 5–10)

- Learning about sexuality
  - Some questions for discussion
    - How old were you the first time you learned anything (or asked anyone) about sex?
    - Whom did you learn from?
    - How did you feel when you first learned about sex?
    - Was the information you received accurate? (And if not, how and when did you find out that it wasn't?)
    - Was the information helpful?
    - Did you get other information that conflicted with what you learned?
  - Discuss clients' perceptions of sexuality and aspects of their own sexual development (physical sexual development, impact on relationships, etc.)
- What makes something sexual?
  - Perceptual, situational, and experiential factors that define something as sexual
  - How people respond to something sexual
- Being sexual is being human
  - Review the four stages of the sexual response cycle
    - Sexual attraction
    - Arousal
    - Orgasm/ejaculation
    - Recovery period
  - Problems that can occur in each phase, and how well you can control your behavior in each phase

---

- *"How old were you the first time you learned anything (or asked anyone) about sex?"* The politically correct answer that many clients give is "in high school." But the reality is that the age of first exposure to sex or curiosity about sexual matters ranges widely. Some may have questioned a sexually explicit scene in a movie during late childhood or early adolescence. Others may remember asking others very early "Where do babies come from?" Others may have experienced sexual abuse at a young age and thus unfortunately learned about sexuality in a forced manner. Clients should offer a range of responses to this question. The point is not for them to describe the most formal or direct sources of sexual education (we know about those), but to think about early messages and interests in sex that may have shaped what they learned and how they later behaved.

- *"Whom did you learn from?"* This may include family members, friends, teachers, doctors or nurses, abusers, or movies or television shows, among other sources. Clients may offer a variety of anecdotes about these experiences. For example, one client at an SOS pilot site stated that when he was 7 or 8 years old, his older teenage cousins would tell one another dirty jokes while walking him home from school. He didn't understand why they were funny. When he later asked his grandmother what they meant, he received a quick lesson in male and female relationships (though he still didn't fully understand the jokes), and he recalled his cousins being punished for exposing him to such information. This can give a great deal of information though about the kinds of information that people received, and whether or not it was from a reputable and healthy source. In the example above, the client reported that even though he was told the rudimentary basics of sex, he still didn't understand the jokes, and he learned that sex is something not to be talked about openly (as he knew his cousins were punished).

- *"How did you feel when you first learned about sex?"* For some, early explorations of sexuality and sex education can invoke feelings of excitement or curiosity. For others, they elicit embarrassment or anxiety. Others are left feeling confused, hurt, or ambivalent. And for those whose first sexual learning occurred within the context of sexual abuse, more intense and long-lasting negative emotions may characterize their experiences. It is important to validate and normalize the feelings clients had in these early stages of sexual development. Clients sometimes hesitate to express positive emotions regarding sexual learning and development, given their past offending experiences. They either expect a negative reaction from others for doing so, or they have internalized the message that they should not associate sex with positive emotions or experiences as a form of self-punishment. However, this must be balanced with the need to maintain an awareness of the seriousness of their offending. This is a discussion of sexuality in a more normative context. We are not focusing on or normalizing offense-related behaviors.

- *"Was the information that you received accurate? (And if not, how and when did you find out that it wasn't?)"* The answer may already be obvious, given clients' responses to previous questions. This question allows clients to think about sexuality and sexual behaviors in a developmental context, challenging some of the sexual messages or facts that they received early on. Even though some of the information they received was inaccurate, they may not have learned this until much later. Some may still not realize that early sexual messages were false. This question can also introduce elements of their offending behaviors, as some clients committed offenses involving sexual "facts" or beliefs that they learned from others (e.g., " It is normal for parents to have sex with their children" or "Women just need to be told what to do").

• *"Was the information helpful?"* Clients may feel that information received was or wasn't helpful, maybe even regardless of whether or not the information was accurate. This often depends on the outcome or the specific situation. The question may be particularly sensitive for those who were victims of sexual abuse, or who acted on some of the information they learned only to discover that it was harmful to others (i.e., a sexual offense). For some, the information was accurate but unhelpful because of other problems, such as communication or social skills deficits that hindered the formation of healthy intimate relationships. In other words, some of what clients were taught was not sufficient to help them develop healthy sexual partnerships.

• *"Did you get other information that conflicted with what you learned?"* Clients were bombarded with sexual messages during their developmental years. Sexual information from media sources, like television or movies, or from family members and friends may conflict with what they learned from "official" sources, like formal sex education programs. Clients should be able to discuss how they resolved (or didn't resolve) these differences. Which source did they choose? Was information from their friends seen as more legitimate than information from their family members? If they were victims of sexual abuse, the emotionality associated with early sexual learning may have prevented them from adequately learning other sexual information later on. And how does this affect what they are learning now? Clients are gaining new insights into sexual relationships, and how does this compare with what they knew before, and how open are they to replacing long-held sexual beliefs?

Other issues are also relevant in the context of this discussion, including clients' overall perceptions of what they learned and who they learned it from (e.g., "Adults don't lie, so this must be true" or "This is how it always works"), how their early sexual learning influenced their relationships with others, and how their understanding of sexual behavior changed over time. Treatment providers may note that many clients learned very specific and rather clinical information regarding sexual anatomy and basic principles of reproduction, but comparatively little information about actual sexual relationships themselves. Others internalized strong messages of idealized sexual relationships—like fairy-tale relationships or those relationships that are "perfect"—that very seldom apply to real-world interactions with others.

As part of this discussion, clients may also wish to discuss their own sexual development and evolving identity as a sexual being. Understandably, some clients may have difficulty doing this or may feel uncomfortable discussing this topic as a group. Others will not have such difficulty. Treatment providers can gauge the group's readiness for such a topic. Some points to include are thoughts about their physical sexual development (e.g., how do they feel about their bodies, how they responded to changes in the body during puberty, feelings of self-consciousness about nudity, anatomical differences), their own comfort level as they matured and changed into more sexual beings (e.g., was sexuality something to be ashamed of, something to be hidden, or something to be flaunted), or how their changing sexuality affected their thoughts, emotions, and interactions with others.

What Makes Something Sexual?

By now, clients have voiced their beliefs about relationships and boundaries, sexual role expectations, and sexual behaviors. But to go back for a moment, have them think about how something is defined as "sexual." A person's views of sexuality and what makes something sexual are complex and varied. It depends on prior experiences, cultural background, wide-ranging expectations of behavior, and personal values and beliefs. Each client has different views and opinions of what sexuality is and how to define it. In this section, clients have the opportunity to explore their views and talk with one another about these topics. Treatment providers should encourage clients to be as nonjudgmental as possible with one another and to respect others' values, even if they disagree with them.

What is it about something—an interaction, a scene in a movie or television show, a picture, a comment or joke—that makes it sexual in nature? How do clients know? Have them think of specific examples from their everyday experience to illustrate these points. It may be hard to articulate just how you know something is sexual, particularly when it lacks some of the more overt elements of sexuality (e.g., nudity, sexual language). Other potential examples of sexual material include songs or music, styles of dancing, or flirtation. This last example, flirtation, can be especially hard for clients with social skills deficits. Flirtation is largely individual, and some will pick up on flirtatiousness quickly, whereas others don't. Likewise, some will read flirtatiousness in an interaction where it wasn't intended. Challenge clients to describe flirtation and how they would know when someone is being flirtatious. They should characterize the elements of that experience that communicate it as something sexual.

The next step is to identify how people respond to something sexual. (This step can help clients understand when something is sexual—they may not realize it until they get a certain reaction.) This step also depends on individual factors like culture, context, experience, or expectations. Potential responses to discuss are sexual arousal, shock or surprise, excitement, embarrassment, humor, disgust, curiosity, shame or guilt, fear or anxiety, or ambivalence. Treatment providers should be prepared with several examples to help initiate group discussion. Clients can express their own reactions to something sexual, whether it's a comment, an image on television, or an interaction with another person. These reactions depend on who is involved, the situation, how they feel at the time, or past experiences. How do they think others would react to the same thing?

Now is also an opportunity for treatment providers to validate client experiences. There are no "wrong" ways to respond to something, even if we implicitly know that sometimes the clients' responses have led to problematic behaviors. If something sexual elicits sexual arousal, this is still a normal human reaction. The client's decision to act on sexual arousal in a harmful or maladaptive way is the problem—not necessarily the arousal itself. A key point: we are including only normative sexual stimuli here, not things that some clients find sexual that are nonnormative or offense-related (e.g., children, animals, sadistic acts). When clients bring up these issues, treatment providers may need to remind them of the earlier discussions involving consent, dysregulated behaviors, and the like. Ultimately, we want them to transition into the next part of the discussion, learning about sexual reactions without leaping to judgment about past offending.

Being Sexual Is Being Human

Why are humans sexual beings? Some clients have never considered this question, whereas others can generate many explanations for the existence of sexual drive and sexuality. Sexuality is a normal part of being human. We want clients to understand this, and also to know that the goal of treatment is not a life without sexual interest or relationships. A goal of treatment is for clients to better understand and evaluate their past sexual experiences and make healthy decisions regarding future sexual behaviors. Because of the negative reactions and consequences surrounding their sex offending behaviors, some clients develop the perspective that sexuality itself is wrong or that they will withdraw from their sexuality as a self-imposed punishment. To such clients, abstinence seems easier than learning to make appropriate and healthy judgments about sexual relationships and behaviors. However, eliminating sexual urges and refraining from all sexual behaviors whatsoever is an unlikely reality for most people—sex offenders included.

Instead, clients will think about the process of sexuality, including sexual attraction and arousal, physiological sexual urges and responses, and the impact of sexual stimulation on the body. They can also see how these changes impact their thinking, moods, and interactions with others. The focus should be primarily on healthy sexual behaviors, though clients may mention examples from prior sexual experiences that were unhealthy or harmful to others. Whenever possible, try to keep group conversations about sexuality and sexual functioning focused on normative and appropriate relationships, validating and reinforcing these elements of their experiences.

Sexual Response Cycle

Clients should review the four stages of the sexual response cycle, made famous by the work of Masters and Johnson (1966). This is not a lesson in anatomy and physiology but instead a discussion of the thoughts, emotions, and other human experiences that characterize these stages, as well as sexual dysfunction or problems that may also occur. Below are listed the four stages, along with questions to guide group discussion.

1. *Sexual attraction.* What is sexual attraction? How do you know when you find someone attractive? What are you thinking? Feeling? Wanting to happen? What does your body do when you're attracted to someone?
2. *Arousal.* What does it mean to be aroused? What kinds of things happen to your body? As this is happening, what effect does it have on your thoughts? Your ability to problem-solve? How do you feel emotionally when you're highly aroused? How does it affect your interaction with another person? What are your expectations like? Or, what are you hoping will happen?
3. *Orgasm/ejaculation.* What is an orgasm? How does that feel? What are your emotions like at that moment? Are you thinking about anything when that happens? Are you able to control yourself or

your behavior during this phase? (In other words, are you going to be able to stop what you're doing?)

4. *Recovery period.* What happens after orgasm? How does your body feel? What are your emotions like? How do you feel about yourself and others? What types of thoughts are you having?

This should also involve a discussion of problems that can occur in each phase, such as lack of desire or obsessive desire in the attraction phase, difficulty getting an erection or hypersexual arousal in the arousal phase, or premature ejaculation or lack of ejaculation during orgasm. Similarly, clients should discuss the point at which they begin to "lose control" over their behaviors. This does not justify their offenses, as they were still able to control planning behaviors or other factors associated with offending. However, there is a degree of sexual arousal that clients may view as "the point of no return," so to speak, and the realization that they can do something before this point is helpful for clients. Waiting until the late arousal or orgasm phases, for example, before using skills to cope with sexual urges will be highly ineffective in controlling sexual behavior. Instead, clients should self-monitor these sexual phases and practice controlling their desire or urges at earlier phases of the process.

SEXUAL FANTASIES AND MASTURBATION (SESSIONS 11–15)

Sexual Fantasies

As sex offender treatment providers we take it for granted that clients know what a sexual fantasy is. While higher functioning clients may have a clear idea of this concept, those with cognitive deficits or limited sexual knowledge and experience may not understand them in the same way that we do. Confusing fantasies with urges, with behaviors, or with general sexual thoughts is common for many such individuals. Treatment providers should take some time to discuss fantasies, both general and sexual, to enable all clients to establish a common language and to learn about the role that they play in sexual interest, arousal, and behaviors, as is described in Table 8.3.

What Are Fantasies?

The first part of this step is learning what fantasies are. People routinely engage in fantasy, often described as day-dreaming. In thinking

TABLE 8.3. Sexual Fantasies and Masturbation (Sessions 11–15)

- Sexual fantasies
  - What are fantasies? Discuss THE nature and purpose of general and sexual fantasies.
  - How do fantasies affect behavior?
    - Can a fantasy become reality?
    - If a fantasy feels good, then will reality feel better? Do you expect it to?
    - What elements are not included in a fantasy?
    - Are you and other people different in your fantasies? How?
    - Examples of how fantasies can change your viewpoint
    - How might fantasy be reinforced over time? Does this have an effect on behavior?
- Masturbation
  - Perceptions and prior learning
  - Privacy and "rules" about masturbation
  - Sexual fantasies and masturbation

about their own experiences with fantasies or daydreams, clients should describe some of their common daydreams, along with why they have them, what purpose they may serve, and how they feel while they're doing this. Generally, fantasies serve as an escape, a way of improving one's mood, or a means of alleviating boredom. People usually fantasize about positive things rather than things that frighten, anger, or sadden them. There are times when fantasies are viewed as a problem, such as when they distract from necessary tasks, facilitate reality avoidance, or interfere with work, school, or relationships. Generally, however, people view fantasies as a normal, positive indulgence.

So what about sexual fantasies? They serve similar purposes, though they differ in that they also provide a sexual outlet and elicit sexual arousal. So what makes a fantasy sexual in nature, aside from the obvious sexual content? It could be situations or circumstances (e.g., where does it take place?), who is involved, the role of the self, and different physiological and emotional reactions to the fantasy. Have clients differentiate sexual and nonsexual fantasies by using these and other relevant factors. Clients should also briefly discuss who should and should not be included in a sexual fantasy. For example, most clients will agree that engaging in sexual fantasy about an attractive, similarly aged movie star is normal. However, sexual fantasies involving children or violence may elicit greater discussion—some clients will recognize that these elements of a sexual fantasy are inappropriate, even if it is only a fantasy.

How Do Fantasies Affect Behavior?

Though some clients are aware of the link between fantasy and behavior, others are not. The latter more actively deny that their fantasies have anything to do with their behaviors, and may even say that they can continue to fantasize about potential victims (e.g., children) without committing a sexual offense. But thinking about something in a positive light, as one does in a fantasy, may make it seem more real, more attainable, and more desirable. One goal of this section is for clients to understand a fantasy's effects on the body, the mind, and interactions with others. A related goal is to see how this can lead to behavior. Client discussion should include some of the following points:

- "Can a fantasy become reality?"
- "If a fantasy 'feels good,' will reality then 'feel better'? Do you expect it to?"
- "What elements are not included in a fantasy?" (This may be negative consequences, negative reactions by others, shame or guilt, etc.)
- "Are you different in your fantasies? Are other people different? How?"
- Give several examples of how a fantasized object may be viewed after positive fantasies. This may include food, a new car, or another person. Help clients understand how this fantasy view may be linked with actual behavior.
- How might the fantasy be reinforced over time? Does this have an effect on behavior?

Treatment providers will finish this discussion by emphasizing the point that sexual fantasy is a normative part of the human sexual experience. The nature of these fantasies, however, can impact behavior, and an important goal of treatment and of controlling sexual urges is to also learn to engage in adaptive and healthy forms of sexual fantasy.

Masturbation

Clients in a group setting may express some discomfort with openly discussing masturbation in front of others, including treatment providers. It is important to acknowledge and validate the clients' discomfort, and treatment providers may feel comfortable expressing their own feelings regarding leading such a discussion (e.g., "This is awkward for me too" or "This is something that we usually think of as a very private matter, and that includes talking about it"). It may also be helpful to relate this discomfort to social norms and the private versus public behaviors discussion in Module 2. The purpose is not for clients to divulge all the intimate details of their sexual or masturbatory lives but to examine their feelings and beliefs about masturbation, linking these with their sexual fantasies, urges, and behaviors.

Perceptions and Prior Learning

First, what have clients learned in the past about masturbation? Nearly everyone has an opinion about masturbation—who should or shouldn't masturbate, whether it is right or wrong, that it's a secret, what it will do to you, that you should never talk about it, and so on. Religious or spiritual beliefs, as well as standard cultural practices, guide these opinions. What are the positive and negative aspects of masturbation, coming from these different perspectives? And where did these beliefs come from? In addition to family, culture, religion, or early learning experiences, there could also be the effect of later sexual education or experience. As clients discuss these beliefs, be sure to encourage an open and nonjudgmental frame. This reflects clients' own opinions and values. There may be times when treatment providers disagree, but as long as the belief is not overtly harmful to others, the client should be given the opportunity to maintain his or her own values regarding masturbation. The discussion allows clients to articulate and define their own beliefs and how these beliefs originated. For some, the result of this discussion may lead to changes in their beliefs, as they examine early messages and feel that they no longer apply to their current lives. For others, such a discussion may solidify their beliefs. Regardless of specific client responses, treatment providers can use this discussion to measure clients' willingness and ability to discuss such issues, progress and insight, and their degree of self-control of sexual behaviors like masturbation.

Privacy and "Rules" about Masturbation

Second, clients will describe why masturbation is a private matter. (For those clients who have engaged in many acts of public masturbation, treatment providers will first need to establish that it is, in fact, a private behavior.) This may mean acknowledging that masturbation makes other people uncomfortable, that it is a very explicit sexual act, that people have strong beliefs about sexuality and the role of masturbation, and so on. A related consideration is how people would feel if someone masturbated in a public or open setting. People might witness such an act with embarrassment, fear, shame, anger, or disgust. Clients with more voyeuristic tendencies might respond with excitement. Allow group members to address each of these responses and any others they have thought of. And finally, what are the "rules" of masturbation in the clients' current lives? Some may live in a residential facility or institution with specific rules about masturbatory practices. Others may live in a community setting with restrictions on privacy (e.g., residential or transitional home) or the availability of masturbatory stimuli (e.g., restrictions on purchasing pornography). Clients' masturbatory practices can also change over time due to medical conditions, age, or the side effects of medications. Some clients will be uncomfortable providing details regarding the frequency or nature of their masturbation. Clients are not required to divulge such information here, as the purpose of the discussion is for them to identify situational factors that may hinder or facilitate these behaviors.

Sexual Fantasies and Masturbation

Third, clients should identify links between sexual fantasies and masturbation. This may seem obvious, but for clients with limited experience in describing sexual fantasies, or for whom masturbation represents a cultural, spiritual, or personal taboo, the association between sexual fantasies and masturbation may be less clear. Clients are typically able to understand that sexual fantasies are the thoughts or images associated with masturbatory behaviors. An important point is that masturbation, and its associated sexual gratification, will reinforce the sexual fantasy. This means that masturbation will make the sexual fantasy more rewarding, and will consequently reinforce the sexual content and persons involved in the fantasy itself. It could strengthen the desirability of persons in the fantasy (e.g., potential victims) and these persons' perceived willingness to engage in sexual behavior. Further, such reinforcement may also heighten one's willingness to engage in such behaviors in the future. Return to concepts discussed earlier in the module section related to fantasies, reminding clients that when fantasies are highly reinforcing, it makes the behavior seem more attainable and could potentially push someone from fantasy to behavior.

PORNOGRAPHY AND SEXUALLY EXPLICIT MATERIALS (SESSIONS 16–20)

As with many other topics related to sexual development and behavior, opinions about pornography are idiosyncratic and vary greatly. Some people view virtually any material depicting or describing sexual content as pornographic, including materials like lingerie catalogs, swimsuit magazines, or "dirty" jokes. Others may only categorize something as pornography if it depicts full nudity or explicit sexual acts. (This latter definition is generally the more accepted description of pornography.) In this section, clients will learn more about their own and others' perceptions of pornography so that they can think critically about the potential role of pornographic and sexually explicit materials in sexual behavior and offending (see Table 8.4).

What Makes Something Pornographic?

This discussion should help clients clarify their own definitions of pornography. Treatment providers can introduce these ideas by asking what clients think pornography is, what friends or family members think it is, or what others might consider pornographic (a sample worksheet for this and subsequent discussions of obscenity is provided in Form 8.3 at the end of the chapter). Pornography involves more than just nudity or explicit sexual acts, but also the purpose or function of the material.

TABLE 8.4. Pornography and Sexually Explicit Materials (Sessions 16–20)

- What makes something pornographic?
  - Client definitions of pornography
  - How others define pornography
  - What makes something obscene? Is all pornography obscene?
  - What are the legal standards of obscenity?
  - Why do people use pornography?
  - When does pornography use become a problem?
- Pornography, sexual fantasies, masturbation, and behavior
  - Clients link pornography with fantasies, masturbatory practices, and behavior
  - Clients describe how pornography has affected their own thoughts, arousal, and behavior

---

For example, are paintings or sculptures that portray nude figures pornographic? What about medical textbooks with graphic images of the human body? Depending on what the material is, how it is used, and how it is meant to be used, there may be greater or lesser degrees of ambiguity about its pornographic content.

Clients should also think about what makes some materials "obscene," or what makes some pornography illegal. Definitions of obscenity vary as much as definitions of pornography. Deciding that material is too offensive to too graphic depends largely on personal preference and values. In some areas, pornography is labeled "obscene" or illegal if it offends local standards of decency. These local standards vary widely, so that the same material might not be considered "obscene" or illegal in other locales. Other definitions of illegal pornography are more consistent and specific, regardless of community standards (e.g., child pornography). Still, clients have opinions about obscenity or whether or not certain pornographic materials should be illegal or prohibited. Societal norms, personal morals and experiences, and cultural beliefs all shape these opinions. As with other similar concepts within this module, clients should be prepared to articulate and examine the origins of their own beliefs.

Clients should also discuss why people use pornographic materials. Obviously, pornography is most often used for the purpose of eliciting sexual arousal. But given that sexually explicit materials are a more indirect or impersonal means of achieving sexual arousal, why might people choose to use pornography instead of or maybe in addition to direct sexual interactions with others? For some, pornography is a substitute for sexual relationships because pornography is more readily available and easily obtained, requires fewer social abilities, or is perhaps more consistently rewarding in light of social and sexual deficits. Some may experience greater sexual arousal with pornographic material, as the user can select preferred sexual stimuli or situations that are otherwise unavailable. Pornography is also a more immediate source of sexual gratification, and for those who struggle with delaying gratification is a more viable means of becoming sexually stimulated in the moment. Clients whose issues involve social skills deficits, body image or self-esteem problems, or sexual insecurity may identify more positive emotions associated with pornography use.

But when does pornography use become a problem? Clients who have strong moral, social, or cultural opinions regarding pornography may feel that any use of sexually explicit materials is problematic. For others, pornography is only problematic if they are caught and sanctioned for illegal pornography use. The majority of clients, however, will fall somewhere in between. Some points to consider include when others are bothered by pornography use, when the user is bothered by it, when it interferes with other aspects of the user's life, or when it negatively impacts relationships or behavior.

Pornography, Sexual Fantasies, Masturbation, and Behavior

The remaining discussions in this module link the concepts covered thus far. How does pornography affect sexual fantasies? How is masturbation linked to pornography use? How might this linkage ultimately impact behavior?

Clients have revealed their beliefs about the effects of pornography during these discussions. Some of these beliefs, though held by the majority of people, may actually be false. As clients review pornography's impact on fantasies, masturbation, and sexual behaviors, their beliefs should be addressed more fully (see Table 8.5 for an example of facts and myths to be discussed). For example, many believe that viewing pornographic materials will inevitably lead to sexual offending or problematic sexual behaviors. Research does not support this view, though there is support for the idea that frequent pornography use, and use of violent pornography, will change a person's expectations about sexual interactions and beliefs about sexual partners (women, in particular; e.g., Linz, Donnerstein, & Penrod, 1988; Malamuth & Check, 1981, 1985). A change in beliefs or expectations does not always perfectly correspond with changes in behavior, but in this case it could negatively impact interpersonal interactions and relationships (i.e., contribute to interpersonal dysregulation), and perhaps more indirectly impact behavior. On the other hand, some clients may think that their use of pornography has little impact on their patterns of sexual arousal. For example, clients may claim that their use of child pornography does not make them more likely to be sexually attracted to children, and that it will not influence their interactions with children. Obviously, this claim doesn't fit with what we already know regarding the relationships between sexual fantasy, masturbation, and reinforced patterns of sexual interest and arousal.

The goal of these final discussions in Module 4 is for clients to evaluate their own use of pornography and how it affects their thoughts, sexual urges, and sexual arousal. This will need to be balanced with the

TABLE 8.5. Effects of Pornography

Many people have differing beliefs about pornography and how it affects people. Some of these statements have been proven through research, while others have not. Remember that everyone has his or her own opinions and experiences. Use these topic points to start out client discussion.

1. Using pornography can change the way that a person feels about women, including how they should look, their role in a relationship, and expectations about sexual behavior.
2. Normal, nonaggressive, adult pornography does not really affect the behavior of the person viewing it.
3. People who view pornography are more likely to engage in risky sexual behaviors.
4. People can become "addicted" to pornography.
5. People who look at pornographic pictures or videos of children are more likely to molest a child.
6. The way sex is described or shown in pornographic media is not a realistic view of sexual relationships.
7. People who watch violent sexual films may become less sympathetic to victims of sexual assault.
8. People who view pornography are more likely to commit sexual offenses.
9. People use pornography because they don't have normal sexual relationships.
10. If people who have committed sexual offenses use pornography, it can keep them from offending again in the future.

rules and requirements of their current facility, institution, or release restrictions (e.g., probation or parole). The future use of pornographic materials will be an individualized decision. For some, pornography use has been so problematic that it cannot be safely continued, or only reflects illegal or deviant sexual interests. For others, pornography use may be occasional and more appropriate. Thus, a purely black-and-white approach to pornography (i.e., everyone should use it vs. it can never be used again) is unrealistic and perhaps unnecessary. Treatment providers are tasked with facilitating discussion in such a way that clients can make a balanced decision regarding their own use of sexually explicit materials, informed by what they have learned in this module, risk management strategies, and the legal or institutional requirements resulting from their prior sexual offending.

MODULE 4 CONCLUDING SESSIONS

Clients should be sure to review the major topic points discussed during this module, including sexuality, the body's sexual response, sexual fantasies, masturbation, and pornography. Again, treatment providers may find it helpful to refer to the "My Treatment Progress" worksheet in Appendix B to guide clients through a summary of these concepts and how they are associated with client goals and progress.

Sexually Transmitted Diseases:
Knowledge and Prevention

There are more than 30 types of sexually transmitted diseases (STDs). It is overwhelming to try to know about them all. There are five points you should be familiar with in order to keep yourself and others safe:

1. *Infection.* How does the STD pass from one person to another? Some require contact with bodily fluids, like blood or semen. Others can be spread through genital skin-to-skin contact.

2. *Symptoms.* Each STD has different symptoms. The best way to know something is different or wrong is to know what your body is like normally, when it is healthy. Talk to your doctor or nurse about any changes you've noticed.

3. *Treatment.* Some STD's can be treated with medication, which may or may not get rid of the infection. Others have no known treatment and may become a lifetime problem. Talk to your doctor or nurse about treatment options.

4. *Prevention.* Abstinence from sexual activity is the only 100% sure way to avoid STDs. You can reduce your risk by using condoms or having few sexual partners.

5. *Responsibility.* If you are worried that you might have an STD, get tested by your doctor. If you have an STD, it is your responsibility to talk to your doctor and tell any sexual partners before engaging in sexual activity.

Pregnancy and Contraception:
Fact versus Myth

Which of the following statements are facts about pregnancy and contraception, and which are myths, or false beliefs?

1. It is possible for a man to become pregnant.

2. A girl as young as age 9 can become pregnant.

3. A woman cannot get pregnant if it is the first time she has ever had sex.

4. A woman can get pregnant if she is raped.

5. Both people are responsible for birth control.

6. Sexual position can determine the baby's gender.

7. Birth control pills work after only one dose.

8. A woman can get pregnant without penile penetration.

9. There is no way to really tell if a man is the father of a child.

10. Oxygen can kill sperm once they leave the man's body.

11. Sperm can live up to five days after leaving the man's body.

12. A woman cannot get pregnant from anal sex.

13. Condoms are 100% effective at preventing pregnancy.

14. Having sex with a pregnant woman will cause her to have twins.

15. The male's sperm determines the baby's gender.

16. A woman cannot get pregnant if she's on her period.

What Makes Something Pornographic?

The dictionary defines pornography as:

1. Obscene writings, drawings, photographs, or the like, especially those having little or no artistic merit.
2. Sexually explicit pictures, writing, or other material whose primary purpose is to cause sexual arousal.
3. Lurid or sensational material.
4. Books, photographs, magazines, art, or music designed to excite sexual impulses and considered by public authorities or public opinion as in violation of accepted standards of sexuality.

What are some of the factors that make something pornographic?

1. _____
2. _____
3. _____

What is the definition of *obscene*? What would make pornography then *obscene*?

1. Obscene means: _____

   _____

2. Pornography is obscene when: _____

   _____

   _____

CHAPTER 9

Review of Motivation, Commitment to Treatment, and Treatment Goals

By now, clients have been in treatment for some time. They have developed initial treatment goals, learned important treatment concepts, discussed at least one problematic sexual behavior in detail (i.e., completed a behavioral chain analysis in Module 2), discussed the role of emotions and emotional regulation, and addressed concepts related to healthy sexuality and sexual development. Now, it is time for clients to review the goals they established in Module 1 and check in on their current level of motivation and commitment to treatment. The discussion in this module is similar to that in Module 1 but will reflect clients' progress in treatment thus far and reinforce already-learned concepts. We want clients to apply their knowledge to their continuing treatment goals. Clients are given the opportunity to reflect on their experiences and make changes to their treatment targets as needed.

Primary aims of this module are to evaluate client progress, to provide feedback to the clients regarding their progress and continuing needs, and to review important components of treatment. Clients should complete this module with an understanding of how what they have learned applies to their past behaviors, current efforts to self-manage dysregulation, and the development of more adaptive regulatory strategies. A related goal of this section is to reexamine client commitment, knowing that commitment and motivation vary significantly throughout the course of treatment. For some, the newness of treatment and early anticipation lead to initial bursts of motivation that may waiver and ultimately wane over time. For others, early resistance and struggles with commitment may transition into greater willingness, interest in treatment, and commitment to specific goals.

An additional goal of Module 5 is for treatment providers to measure the success of their interactions and efforts to develop a strong therapeutic alliance with clients. This effort includes the use of validation, motivational interviewing strategies and techniques, collaborative development of client goals, and responses to client behaviors and progress. These interventions will help guide client motivation and commitment throughout the treatment process, and the impact of such strategies should be readily apparent at this point in the treatment. Reviewing clients' perceptions of motivation and progress can signal needed adjustments in the therapeutic relationship.

BEING IN SEX OFFENDER TREATMENT (SESSIONS 1–5)

At the outset of SOS in Module 1, clients expressed their views and emotional reactions to participating in sex offender treatment, as well as their ambivalence about starting such treatment. This opening discussion was designed to assess their initial resistance to treatment, identify potential areas of concern and barriers to effective treatment relationships, provide opportunities for validation, and facilitate group cohesion among clients. Again in Module 5, we want to review with clients where they are in terms of their treatment commitment and motivation. This review includes a number of discussions or teaching points similar to those presented in Module 1, outlined further for the reader in Table 9.1.

TABLE 9.1. Being in Sex Offender Treatment (Sessions 1–5)

- Perceptions of treatment
  - Clients describe current emotional responses to treatment, now that they have been in treatment for some time.
    - How did they feel at the beginning?
    - How do they feel now?
    - What changed?
- Client ambivalence
  - How are clients still ambivalent? What questions do they have at this point?
  - Pros and cons of treatment
    - Review of important points from each module that were positive versus negative experiences for clients
  - Treatment provider ambivalence and use of radical genuineness (Level 6 Validation)

Treatment providers will note that this module relies more heavily on group or client process than earlier modules. The discussions here are formatted as a review of earlier concepts, but not so much for repetition or reinforcement of learning. Instead, clients are encouraged to describe the high and low points of treatment so that treatment providers and clients both can learn the right mix of treatment concepts and goals to assist progress. Key points throughout this module are understanding motivation and highlighting differences in clients' attitudes from the beginning of treatment to this midpoint. To do this, treatment providers may rely more on open or fluid discussion of the topic points mentioned in the following sections.

Perceptions of Treatment

In Module 1, clients discussed their emotional reactions to being included in sex offender treatment. These reactions included positive feelings like interest, hope, curiosity, or relief, as well as negative emotions like anger, fear, resentment, or disappointment. Then, clients' emotional reactions were probably informed by prior experiences with other forms of treatment, responses to being caught or sanctioned following their offenses, or their own perceptions and expectations concerning treatment. Some of these reactions may have been positive and reflected a desire to engage in therapy, whereas other reactions indicated anticipated problems or treatment resistance.

It is now time to have this discussion again. (Treatment providers may find it helpful to again use Form B2, "How Do I Feel about Being in Sex Offender Treatment," found in Appendix B.) How do clients feel now that they have been engaged in treatment for a period of many months or even years? We expect that their emotional responses to treatment have changed, whether for better or for worse. Evolving emotional responses in treatment are attributable to several factors. Clients who were initially fearful, anxious, or resistant to treatment may have discovered that the treatment process is not as painful as they had imagined. Similarly, clients who had a negative attitude at the outset may have since found benefit or meaning in their treatment experience. Therapeutic responses and strong alliances with treatment providers may have also shaped perceptions and emotional reactions. Conversely, some clients who were enthusiastic and confident at the beginning of treatment may have found that change was more difficult than they anticipated. Others may have experienced setbacks and engaged in continuing harmful or maladaptive behaviors, leaving them frustrated, ashamed, and angry. For these latter two types of clients, their initial positive feelings possibly soured, or left them more hesitant and doubtful regarding treatment success.

Within the context of this discussion, clients can compare their emotions at the outset of treatment to how they feel now. Treatment providers can help them recognize factors that shaped these differences and influenced their outlook, including treatment progress, interactions with others, new or old patterns of behavior, or changes in their personal circumstances. This discussion provides ample opportunity for treatment providers to use validation, highlight areas of continuing ambivalence, or even to explore conflicts between perceptions and emotional reactions. If clients feel safe and open in the treatment environment, even though they harbor negative emotions, they may struggle less with being honest about their emotions. Treatment providers should take this honesty and openness as a positive sign, even if they are not pleased with or optimistic about explicitly stated client frustration.

In this and subsequent discussions in this module, look for changes in clients' perceptions of treatment, their stated need for treatment, goals, interactions with one another and treatment providers, and the role of the treatment team or other agents involved in treatment planning. Point out these changes when appropriate, again tying them to the clients' current emotions or responses to treatment.

Client Ambivalence

As was noted in Module 1, clients are often ambivalent about engaging in sex offender treatment. Despite having been in treatment for the first four modules, clients may still find themselves ambivalent at times. Though the ambivalence is still present, its causes have likely changed. For example, clients who were unsure about treatment at the beginning but who still wanted to be involved might have struggled with the unknown: *What is treatment going to be like? Will I get better? What will people think of me when I'm in treatment?* Some of these uncertainties are now clearer, as clients have a better feel for how groups will proceed, what other group members are like, how they will be treated by group facilitators, and so on. However, other questions remain unanswered, even after a period of treatment. These questions relate to overall progress, what is left to address in treatment, or how well progress can be maintained. Now that clients see their progress, they may also see how far they still have to go, potential problems in the future, and doubts they have about treatment effectiveness.

In order to illustrate and embrace this ambivalence, treatment providers will again facilitate a discussion of the pros and cons of sex offender treatment. This discussion may feel different than the same discussion from Module 1, given that clients can base their impressions on events or learning opportunities from Modules 1 through 4. Some important talking points are as follows:

- How did clients feel completing a behavioral chain analysis of one or more of their sex offending behaviors? What did they learn from this analysis? What made it different from talking about an offense in another way? (In other words, was talking about the precursors to an offense in a step-by-step manner different than talking about the offense itself?)
- Did clients learn anything about their own dysregulation? How does this knowledge help them (or not) better understand their offending?
- How did clients feel discussing these issues in a group setting?
- Do clients like the format of treatment? (This issue is especially relevant for clients who have had prior forms of sex offender treatment.)
- Were there any surprises or disappointments?
- How do clients feel about the weekly self-monitoring activities?
- What is it like to learn and practice adaptive skills or strategies?
- How is this overall process different from sex offender treatment programming they have had in the past?
- What are clients' own perceptions of improvement, progress, or lack thereof? Have they gotten better? Is it easy for them to see progress?
- How do they feel about their goals? Is it more, or less, helpful to have input into their goals? (Note that some clients prefer for others to give them extensive direction and feedback in treatment.)

Clients may identify other advantages or disadvantages of treatment thus far. Treatment providers will want to ensure that clients have a fairly balanced view of treatment. We want to avoid the view that treatment is "all good" or "all bad," as such one-sided views leave clients little room for meaningful understanding of barriers to commitment or the nature of their treatment engagement and progress.

Another strategy is for treatment providers to reveal their own ambivalence about treatment. This is a form of validation called "radical genuineness" (Level 6 Validation; see Chapter 3) when the treatment provider responds to the client as a genuine person with equal feelings and equal respect. Here at this midpoint, treatment providers probably know their clients fairly well; they know what level of genuineness is beneficial, and how much therapeutic reality the clients can tolerate. It can be very useful for clients to see selected examples of therapeutic ambivalence. (Please note that this is *not* meant as a cathartic opportunity for therapists to voice frustration with particular clients or specific interactions in group or individual therapy.) Some examples of this ambivalence are briefly mentioned below:

• Think back on when the clients completed behavioral chain analyses of their offenses. Did that go more smoothly than anticipated? Was it difficult to identify incidents of dysregulation?

• The behaviors addressed in SOS are very complex. How does complexity impact treatment providers' motivation? Does this ever make the treatment provider feel frustrated or hopeless? Here, you want to make sure you don't make the clients feel guilty or ashamed. Instead, the goal is for them to see that you do have a realistic appreciation for the intricacies of treatment.

• Treatment providers will sometimes feel that group discussions are repetitive, or that it is really gratifying when everyone "gets it." This is how the clients feel as well.

• It may be sad, disappointing, or frightening when a client struggles with controlling his or her urges or behavior while in treatment. Clients may now be able to hear these feelings without judgment or shame, as the relationship between client and treatment provider is stronger and reflects a balance between concern for safety and interest in the client's well-being and progress.

STAGES OF CHANGE (SESSIONS 6–8)

Throughout treatment, a client's readiness and willingness to change will vary. This is a natural process, and it is expected that clients will feel differently about the change process during a treatment midpoint. This section is meant to make the process more transparent, to be discussed openly and without judgment of progress (or lack thereof). See Table 9.2 for a brief outline of topics in this section.

TABLE 9.2. Stages of Change (Sessions 6–8)

- Stages of change: A review
  - Clients will review the basic definitions of the five stages of change
  - Comparisons between initial and current stages of change
  - Question for clients and treatment providers to consider: Do goals need to be modified to reflect the current stage of change?

Stages of Change: A Review

Clients will return to the stages of change, which were introduced in the early sessions of Module 1. Then, clients were unfamiliar with the five stages or phases of the change process (Prochaska & DiClemente, 1983; Prochaska et al., 1992). It was important for them to initially understand the stages and apply them to their commitment to treatment. Now, clients have had greater experience with treatment and may have firsthand knowledge of what it is like to be "in" one or more of the stages, or to move between them. In Module 5, clients will briefly review the five stages of change, highlighting once again how these apply to sex offender treatment, and then identify their own current level of commitment. (Readers are referred again to Chapter 5 for additional details regarding each of these stages.)

Clients can now compare their current stage of change to that expressed in the first module of treatment. Those who have changed from one stage to another, regardless of direction, should take the opportunity to describe how this changed for them. This encompasses thoughts leading to change, emotions before and after, and also how this change has impacted their performance and role in treatment. Clients can also list important sources of support or skills that helped them in the commitment process. This facilitates their understanding of the therapy process and gives treatment providers information about what works for that particular client. Remember that learning basic treatment concepts is not the only goal—we must also get them involved and keep them motivated throughout the course of treatment.

Some clients may have progressed from earlier stages like precontemplation or contemplation to the later stages like planning or action. For these clients, it is easy to describe their progress, reinforce it, and anticipate continued success in treatment. Other clients may have struggled to move past the early stages of commitment, and some may have even moved from more advanced phases of treatment, like the action stage, back to precommitment. This can occur when clients experience a disappointing setback, such as an intense period of dysregulation, problems with maladaptive behaviors, or other situational difficulties like loss of social support or increased demands. In these cases, it is more difficult for treatment providers to offer support and validation. One must be cautious to avoid empty or superficial praises (e.g., "Oh, it will get better" or "But you know you can do it!"), as these may ring false to someone who has returned to a period of precontemplation or contemplation. Rather, it may be more effective and meaningful to the client to simply acknowledge his or her setback, accept a change in treatment commitment, and mourn the loss of it with him or her (e.g., "It feels so frustrating when you've worked that hard, only to do what you most wanted to *not* do. I get that it made you not care as much. Maybe it's the only way you could deal with the disappointment"). This use of Level 6 Validation—Radical Genuineness—can help treatment providers communicate their mutual grief.

As they think about change, clients will also think about the duration of treatment. How long does it take? How long do they have to maintain a commitment? If they are involved with an agency or institution as part of their sex offender treatment, how long will that last? And how long will risk management or supervisory restrictions be in place? Their frustrations with an indefinite or unknown duration of treatment can interfere with maintaining success and commitment to change, especially if clients have already made significant changes. Emphasizing such a long course ahead can invalidate current treatment gains. Clients may need to modify their goals to fit their current level of commitment. Looking at their stage of change and reflecting on their treatment commitment helps them design appropriate treatment goals for the current moment.

REVIEW OF TREATMENT GOALS (SESSIONS 9–12)

At the end of each module, or at least periodically throughout the prior four modules, clients have already reviewed their treatment goals and discussed how concepts in each module shape their goals and help them make progress. During this part of Module 5, clients will need to reexamine their strengths, their goals, their progress, and what they need from treatment from this point forward (see Table 9.3).

TABLE 9.3. Review of Treatment Goals (Sessions 9–12)

- Strengths and areas for improvement
  - Recognizing strengths—clients describe strengths that have aided their progress thus far
    - Which of these strengths are new?
    - How have these strengths contributed to progress? To commitment and motivation?
  - Areas for improvement
    - How have clients improved in some of the areas they identified for themselves in Module 1?
    - Have they gotten worse in some areas?
    - Clients generate a new list of areas for improvements.
- Treatment progress and review of goals
  - Review of goals set in Module 1
    - What progress has been made?
    - Opportunities for treatment provider and peer (client) feedback
  - Comparison with new "areas for improvement" just identified
  - Continue with prior goals (gradual progress) or set new ones

Strengths and Areas for Improvement

Recognizing Strengths

Client strengths are often overlooked in treatment, even by the clients themselves. Clients have been involved in treatment long enough that they can identify things that helped them pass through the first four modules of treatment. Clients may still define strengths in terms of major things, like breakthroughs in treatment, insight, or other markers of progress. However, success is also seen in the small strengths, such as regular group attendance, attentiveness during group discussion, appreciating the seriousness of sex offending behavior and treatment, positive relationships with group facilitators, commitment to treatment, efforts to self-monitor, and respect for others. Treatment providers and clients should examine these and other strengths and how they have contributed to client progress. They can also compare clients' strengths now to those they identified in Module 1. Are they the same? Have they learned or noticed new strengths? How have these new strengths or abilities helped them? Are there any strengths that they thought they had at that time, but now realize differently?

Areas for Improvement

In Module 1, clients also listed areas of improvement—both those that others think they should work on, and those that they themselves think are important. For many clients, these self-identified treatment needs were later formulated into the client's treatment goals. We assume that much has happened since Module 1. The client has shown improvement in some areas, and perhaps deterioration or new problems in others. Clients will need to generate a new list of "areas of improvement" to be addressed in sex offender treatment. In creating this list, treatment providers and clients should consider the following:

- Urges or behaviors that have worsened or emerged since the initial stages of treatment.
- Interactions with others or interpersonal relationships that have improved or worsened over time.
- Changes in the client's level of commitment to treatment or changes in his or her stage of change.
- Changes in group attendance, participation, and treatment behavior.
- Effects of the behavioral chain analysis in Module 2, in which clients discussed their offending behaviors and important precursors.
- The impact of self-monitoring activities on self-awareness and potential problems.
- Current ability to regulate or modulate emotional states.
- Discussions about healthy sexuality and sexual relationships.
- The client's current feelings regarding inclusion in group and perceptions of progress.
- Contributions of important others involved in treatment and risk management, including supervisory agents, other treatment providers, family members or other sources of support, and so on.

Treatment providers should be especially aware of clients who either under- or overestimate areas in which they need to improve. Providing supportive feedback, validation, and appropriate but gentle questioning can guide clients toward thinking about new areas in which they may need to focus treatment efforts.

Treatment Progress and Review of Goals

Have clients made progress toward achieving their goals? Prior to beginning this discussion with clients, treatment providers may find it helpful to refer back to the discussion of measuring and assessing progress from Chapter 4 of this text. As clients examine their progress, treatment providers should offer feedback to clients regarding their progress and perceptions of treatment success thus far.

For this discussion, clients must first review their long- and short-term goals identified in Module 1. Some may have difficulty remembering these specifically, but they have likely reviewed these or other related goals throughout the course of treatment, and others will have written them down for ease of review. Given the prior discussion of areas of improvement, some major goals and progress points will be readily apparent. Clients may want to ask themselves the following questions:

1. "Since I started this group, what are the things I've been working on?"
2. "How can I show others that I've made improvement?"
3. "What new behaviors or skills did I learn?"
4. "What kinds of things have been difficult for me since treatment began?"
5. "What kinds of feedback have others given me about my progress?"

Clients may also wish to give one another feedback about their progress in treatment. Treatment providers will want to facilitate this discussion between clients in a supportive and validating manner, particularly if progress has not been positive, or if problems with maladaptive behaviors have continued.

Clients will need to decide if their previous goals are still relevant and current, or if new goals need to be set. For some, new problems have emerged or become apparent through treatment discussion, and their goals may need to be revised or changed in order to accommodate these newly identified needs. Other clients have met some of their short-term goals and are ready to look at setting new goals as treatment progresses. These new short-term goals may still relate to the original long-term goals from Module 1. Treatment providers will want to be mindful of the concepts that will be addressed in Modules 6 through 9 (i.e., cognitive and interpersonal dysregulation in Modules 6 and 7, trauma and repairing damaged relationships in Module 8, and self-monitoring, self-management, and aftercare planning in Module 9). They can help clients develop goals that are consistent with some of these topic areas.

A problem that arises in this discussion is that clients sometimes feel like they have made so many changes, or shown so much behavioral improvement, that they are done with treatment. They may see themselves in a very active (or maintenance) stage of treatment commitment, but find it hard to set new goals. Treatment providers can challenge them to think of other areas of dysregulation that have not yet been addressed in treatment (i.e., cognitive and interpersonal), as well as any potential problems with maladaptive behaviors or behavioral dysregulation that could occur were they in a different environment, with different supports. Their difficulty seeing additional treatment needs may be born out of frustration with long-term treatment, limited insight into the complexity of their needs, or a desire to impress others with the progress they have made. Validating these components of their thinking as well as guiding them toward potential areas of treatment focus can help clients move past this point in the discussion.

REVIEW OF EXPECTATIONS AND GROUP RULES (SESSIONS 13–15)

It is useful for clients to again describe their expectations and review the rules of operation for their treatment group. This review may strengthen group cohesion and allow clients to process changes or problems in the treatment environment. Refer to Table 9.4 for a summary of these discussions.

Expectations

Clients will need to reexamine their expectations related to treatment, treatment progress, and the role of others. This was accomplished in Module 1 by having each client describe his or her expectations of themselves, their peers in group, treatment providers, and the treatment team or other supervisory and treatment agents. Clients should again generate such a list, this time emphasizing how their expectations might have changed since the onset of treatment. We want clients to articulate the nature of these changes. For example, clients who initially reported that their expectations of themselves were to simply attend group and learn

TABLE 9.4. Review of Expectations and Group Rules (Sessions 13–15)

- Expectations
  - Clients identify their expectations in treatment of:
    - Myself
    - My peers in group
    - My treatment providers/group facilitators
    - My case manager/treatment team
  - How have these expectations changed (if they have) since the beginning of treatment?
- Rules and rule violations
  - Review of rules and rule violations
    - Did any rule violations occur?
    - How did everyone feel?
    - What were the consequences?
    - How can such violations be avoided in the future?

from it may now have greater expectations, including self-monitoring, learning skills, and applying skills or strategies on a daily basis. Clients who had relatively lofty expectations of others (e.g., group leaders, peers, other supportive persons) may have since accepted a greater degree of responsibility for their own self-management and treatment progress. Comparing these past and current expectations in light of things that have been discussed thus far in treatment, and progress that they have made (or haven't), can help clients understand more about the change process and what they continue to need from treatment.

Rules and Rule Violations

It is again up to the clients to review and discuss group rules. These rules are specific to their expectations and their group, though treatment providers are always free to make suggestions or additions. Most commonly, group rules include concerns about confidentiality and respectful communication, and may also emphasize taking treatment seriously and being attentive and on-topic in group. Clients should also discuss any incidents involving violations or suspected violations of these rules that have occurred since the initiation of treatment. In most cases, these violations or allegations were made known and dealt with at the time of occurrence, but it is a good idea to review them anyway, as it may have been some time since they were last discussed. Treatment providers will need to proceed carefully so as to avoid ostracizing or continuing to punish those who have already made repairs to the group for such violations.

Clients should review several points about rule violations. First, the clients should review how this made everyone feel. With a violation of client confidentiality, for example, did people feel safe afterward when discussing personal information? Were they angry with the individual who had revealed client information? Were they frightened about what might happen as a result? If the problem was disrespectful or hostile treatment in group, how did this make people feel in group? Were they comfortable afterward? How did rule violations like these affect clients' progress? In other words, aside from how people felt, how did it affect their behavior, the nature of their discussions, and their commitment to treatment? Did people experience a setback as a result of group rule violations?

Second, what were the consequences for the person who violated the rules. Did it affect his or her group progress? Relationships with others in the group? Relationships with treatment providers? And what were the sanctions imposed so that the person could continue his or her participation in treatment? Again, it is helpful if group leaders provide concrete and specific instances for clients to consider in these discussions. Review those consequences and decide if changes need to be made for any similar violations in the future. Adjustments to rules and consequences can be made as needed. Clients should also review repairs that were made as a result of any violations. What were these repairs or reparations? Were they sufficient? How did they improve group relationships or heal mistrust?

Finally, how can group rule violations be avoided in the future? Some clients or groups of clients may not have yet struggled with these issues. But for others, even minor disagreements can feel like a violation of group trust and safety, or group rules regarding "honesty" or "taking things seriously" may be routinely broken. In all probability, there have been at least some incidents in which group rules and expectations have been ignored. Thus, group expectations and rules should again be clearly stated, and their importance made obvious (e.g., without confidentiality, clients will not feel safe to reveal information critical to their progress). Reviewing group rules periodically, perhaps with the introduction of new group members or when group cohesion is becoming fragile, is one proactive solution. Thinking about these issues in advance will at least raise their awareness of the issue, reassure them that group leaders are aware and keeping track of group dynamics, and highlight safety measures in place to ensure appropriate treatment behaviors.

MODULE 5 CONCLUDING SESSIONS

The purpose of this module is to check in with clients' commitment to treatment, feelings and ambivalence toward treatment, and progress, goals, and expectations of treatment. By now, clients have been engaged in treatment activities for quite some time, and they likely have questions regarding their own success and needed changes in goals and behavior. This is a good opportunity for clients to make needed changes to their treatment plan and to evaluate the effectiveness of their treatment participation thus far. From here, clients will return to discussions of dysregulation, adaptive regulatory strategies, and self-monitoring and self-management techniques that will enable more effective risk management.

CHAPTER 10

Expectations and Beliefs about Interpersonal Relationships

We now return to discussion of specific domains of self-regulation and the impact of dysregulation and self-regulatory deficits on maladaptive patterns of sexual behavior. In this module we review cognitive dysregulation as it relates to interpersonal relationships. We limit this review to the beliefs, expectations, and cognitive patterns associated with relationships, as these are the areas of cognition most likely to impact sex offending behaviors. While we recognize that there are other belief systems, patterns of thought, or perceptions and cognitive associations unrelated to interpersonal interactions, a comprehensive discussion of these are beyond the scope of this text.

Clients will draw heavily on prior discussions of sexuality, relationships, and boundaries from Modules 2 and 4, as well as components of Module 3, including the impact of thoughts, judgments, or perceptions on emotional experiences, or how strong emotional reactions can sometimes shape the way that we think. For clients with intellectual or developmental disabilities or other cognitive limitations, this module may be particularly challenging. The abstract nature of some materials may make it difficult for clients to comprehend and retain important treatment concepts. Additionally, clients with serious mental illness may struggle with recognizing the problematic or bizarre nature of their delusional thought content or perceptual processing. Throughout this module, we will provide fairly concrete and specific examples, as well as role-play opportunities, that may aid treatment providers in overcoming these obstacles to client understanding.

The activities and discussion topics in this module follow a consistent format (similar to that of Module 3, and to be seen again in Module

7). The module begins with a general discussion of cognitive principles and how beliefs and expectations shape our relationships. Next, clients examine cognitive dysregulation, with examples of how their own dysregulated thoughts can impact relationships. Clients then address ways that dysregulation facilitates sex offending or other maladaptive sexual behaviors. The final component of the module describes alternative adaptive strategies for modulating strong cognitive dysregulation.

The activities and concepts in this module are designed to accomplish several goals. One goal is for clients to better identify and understand their cognitive processes—including thoughts, expectations, perceptions, and beliefs—that contributed to past sex offending behaviors. A second and related goal is for clients to describe how these cognitive processes become dysregulated, and what poorly modulated thoughts "look" like. A third goal is for clients to recognize patterns of dysregulation and to relate these to their own sex offending behaviors. Finally, clients will develop and practice new adaptive strategies to aid them in more effectively managing their cognitive dysregulation. While these are relatively abstract concepts, they can be meaningfully described for persons who have cognitive deficits or active symptoms of serious mental illness through the use of specific examples, experiential explanations (e.g., "Think of a time when you were very judgmental. What did that look like? How did it feel?), and role plays. Even clients who struggle with cognitive examples can relate these to concretely identified experiences and use these examples throughout these discussions. Having already identified examples of their thoughts during the behavioral chain analysis process in Module 2 will certainly help.

BELIEFS: HOW WE VIEW OURSELVES, OTHERS, AND THE WORLD AROUND US (SESSIONS 1–10)

Beliefs are a basic and automatic component of our thought processes. They help us make sense of the world and guide our daily decisions. Cognitive therapies for any number of mental health or relationship problems (e.g., depression, anxiety, marital discord) focus on beliefs as a key underlying component of our behaviors, emotions, and interactions. These therapies assume that beliefs can be altered in order to change behavior. Whether or not one accepts that assumption, it is undeniably true that beliefs exert a strong influence on our perceptions and interpretations, interpersonal relationships, and behavior. To understand cognitive dysregulation and its relationship with maladaptive behavior, we must first examine the role of beliefs in our lives and interactions with others. An overview of these sessions is given in Table 10.1.

What Is a Belief?

Many people have difficulty distinguishing a belief from a fact. This is complicated because sometimes our beliefs are true—they are indeed facts. But just as our beliefs are sometimes true, they can also be nothing more than opinions or even false perceptions of ourselves or the world around us. So what is a belief? Clients will generate many definitions, most of which will include some variation of "a belief is something you *think* is true." This is the general definition we will use for this discussion.

Ask clients to list examples of their own thoughts. It could be something that the client has made up, or something that he or she is thinking at the moment. Go through each one of these examples and have clients determine whether the thought is a belief or a fact. Some examples may include the following:

"This is boring."—belief/opinion

"I don't understand. I'm lost."—fact/statement

"He's being rude."—belief/opinion

"That's not fair."—belief/opinion

"I am annoyed because he keeps interrupting me."—fact/statement

Clients should think about what helps them know if something is an opinion versus a fact. (Again, some beliefs are facts.) Typically, beliefs are characterized by judgments or opinions, whereas facts or factual statements may not carry judgmental or emotional connotations. However, these classifications are simply shortcuts, and we can also have judgments or emotional responses to factual beliefs. For example, I can believe that it is rush hour, or that it is snowing outside, and still have an emotional reaction to these factual statements. The primary purpose though is to start clients thinking about their beliefs in a more detached and objective way. It is an early step to monitoring cognitive dysregulation.

Where do beliefs come from? Human beings may be hard-wired to develop beliefs about their world, but specific beliefs are mostly learned from experience and the environment around us. Some points for clients to consider:

TABLE 10.1. Beliefs: How We View Ourselves, Others, and the World Around Us (Sessions 1–10)

- What is a belief?
  - Differences between beliefs and facts
    - Clients list thoughts, differentiating beliefs and facts
  - Where do beliefs come from?
  - Additional ideas for discussion:
    - You may not hold the same beliefs as the people you grew up with.
    - Your beliefs can change over time.
    - Some beliefs are associated with strong emotional responses.
    - How you behave, and how you see others behave, can impact what you believe.
    - You can still hold onto a belief, despite evidence that the belief may be untrue.
- Looking at our basic beliefs about ourselves
  - How clients define themselves
    - What things are most important to me?
    - What are things I like?
    - Things I don't like?
    - What am I most proud of?
    - If I could change anything about myself, what would it be?
    - What would I never want to change?
    - How would I describe myself?
    - How would others describe me?
- Looking at our basic beliefs about others
  - How clients define and view others (think about representative examples)
    - What things are most important to other people?
    - What types of things do others like or dislike?
    - What kinds of things are people proud of? Disappointed by?
    - If you could change one thing about others, what would it be?
    - Think of someone important to you—what things would you not want that person to change about him- or herself?
    - How do you describe other people in your life?
    - How would they describe themselves?
  - Clients compare views of themselves with others
  - Fundamental attribution error—client examples of when their own behaviors are due to circumstances and others' are due to personality characteristics or flaws
- What our beliefs say about our worldview
  - Tying together beliefs and how they view the world and others in it

• *You may not hold the same beliefs as the people you grew up with.* Were they the same at one point? When did they change? Why did they change? How did people react when they realized that you believed differently than they did? (It may help to have specific examples, like religion, politics, or opinions about other matters.)

• *You beliefs can change over time.* What makes this happen? Did you notice it? Was it a deliberate change? Are there beliefs you think will never change, no matter what?

• *Some beliefs are associated with strong emotional responses.* What beliefs do people get very emotional about? Why? How do they feel about others who do not hold the same beliefs, or who directly contradict or question their beliefs?

• *How you behave, and how you see others behave, can impact what you believe.* This is contrary to what most people think. Most assume that we act in a manner consistent with our beliefs, when in fact social psychology research tells us that we do the opposite: our beliefs are shaped by our behaviors. Help clients think of examples of this phenomenon. For example, perhaps attending group each week makes you believe it is important, or that giving money to charity makes you believe more strongly in altruism.

• *You can still hold onto a belief, despite evidence that the belief may be untrue.* Why do people continue to believe something, even after they've been challenged or maybe even proven wrong? Has this happened to you? What is it like when a fundamental belief is called into question? Why might it be hard to let go?

Looking at Our Basic Beliefs about Ourselves

People generally have a difficult time verbalizing beliefs about themselves. They may not be aware of them, or they may have biases that prevent them from really seeing their underlying beliefs. To help with this issue, client discussions should focus on the following questions: What things are most important to me? What are things I like? Things I don't like? What am I most proud of? If I could change anything about myself, what would it be? What would I never want to change? How would I describe myself? How would others describe me? Understandably, some of these questions may be so personal in nature that clients will not give complete responses in a group setting, nor will they always want to reveal the answers fully even to treatment providers. But coming up with at least one or two responses that reflect their own self-impressions will help conceptualize their beliefs about themselves, and they may continue to think about these concepts even after the session has ended.

Beliefs about the self fall into several categories, many of which will be evident from client participation thus far. They may express dichotomous or polarized beliefs, like "I am a good / bad person," or "I am a caring person / I don't care about others." Treatment providers may want clients to describe these beliefs in more balanced terms, though pushing for this may invalidate the person's real experience of him- or herself and beliefs about who he or she is. In other words, treatment providers can help clients consolidate and synthesize their self-perceptions into several coherent beliefs, but they should be cautious concerning their own urges to argue against negative self-beliefs. For some clients, this is truly how they feel about themselves, and while it may be painful or uncomfortable, this is an area to address in treatment rather than something the client should be "talked out of."

Looking at Our Basic Beliefs about Others

Clients have already described thoughts and beliefs precipitating their offending (from the behavioral chain analysis in Module 2), thoughts or beliefs related to their emotions (Module 3), and sexual beliefs (Module 4). Now, we want them to more generally discuss different types of beliefs that they hold about other people.

Return to the previous discussion on how they view themselves, and have them apply those same questions to others. What things are most important to other people? What types of things do others like or dislike? What kinds of things are people proud of? Disappointed by? If you could change one thing about others, what would it be? Think of someone important to you—what things would you not want that person to change about him- or herself? How do you describe other people in your life? How would they describe themselves? It may be helpful for clients to have a few representative persons in mind who embody different types of relationships. They may wish to apply these questions to family members, friends, enemies, authority figures, strangers, or other important groups.

How do these beliefs about others compare to their beliefs about themselves? They may be harder on themselves than on other people, or they may be less patient with others and more lenient and forgiving in their beliefs about themselves. This is an important distinction particularly when they move into later sections of treatment in which they discuss expectations and interpersonal dysregulation. For now, however, it is useful for them to articulate some of these basic beliefs about the self and others in order to better understand how they view the world around them and themselves in it.

Treatment providers will then introduce the "fundamental attribution error" (Jones & Harris, 1967; Ross, 1977) from social psychology research. This is the idea that we attribute the mistakes, errors, or negative behaviors by others to their own personal weaknesses or failures, whereas we attribute our own similar mistakes, errors, or negative behaviors to external and impersonal events. For example, if you are in a bad mood and say something overly hostile or critical, you may think, "I didn't get enough sleep last night" or "Everybody is so demanding and rude today." If someone else, however, is in a bad mood and snaps at or criticizes you, you might think, "She's always so mean to me" or "I wonder what his problem is? I didn't do anything wrong." One's own problematic behavior is attributed to situational factors and viewed as "out of character," whereas others' problematic behaviors are viewed as the result of their flawed character. The fundamental attribution error applies to everyone—not only clients. For clients, this way of thinking reinforces their beliefs about themselves and others and influences their expectations, their perceptions, and their behavior over time. When we think of important components of sex offender treatment progress in SOS or other modalities, like accepting responsibility, minimizing blame or rationalization, and balancing judgments, the fundamental attribution error plays a critical role in these processes. Form 10.1 at the end of the chapter is given as an illustration of how to discuss these seemingly abstract concepts in a concrete and specific way with clients.

What Our Beliefs Say about Our Worldview

How we think about ourselves and others shapes how we view the world. Whether we see others as friendly versus hostile, helpful versus selfish, or truthful versus dishonest affects our daily thoughts, emotions, and actions. Also, what the clients believe about themselves provides clues as to their own perceived role in the world around them. Do they see themselves as helpless victims, constantly plagued with problems beyond their control? Do they see themselves as bad people who cannot control or change their behaviors? Or maybe they are confused and isolated, believing that their problems are too overwhelming to face. The goal is for clients to tie together their beliefs about the self and others and identify how this influences their view of the world. Things that happen in their lives—Are they predictable? Personal? Changeable? Controllable? Negative or positive? Their responses depend on these beliefs and help define their worldview.

EXPECTATIONS (SESSIONS 11–15)

Our beliefs and worldview affect our expectations, or what we want from ourselves and other people. Just as they are shaped by our beliefs, our expectations shape our perceptions of others and interpersonal interactions. They also influence how we view ourselves within the context of important relationships. This section is outlined in Table 10.2.

Expectations and Relationships

Earlier in Modules 2 and 4, when clients discussed relationships and boundaries, they reviewed how expectations vary across different types of relationships. For example, clients may have reported greater expectations of close family members than friends, acquaintances, or strangers. These different expectations depend on the closeness of the relationship, whether or not the relationship is romantic or sexual in nature, or the other person's expectations and behaviors. They may also have noted that these diverse expectations shape their boundaries with different people. To expand on this point, clients will now consider how their expectations mold their relationships and interpersonal behaviors.

Clients, like everyone else, expect different things from different people. Their expectations are not always fair or realistic. Clients will need to identify at least one or more expectations of different relationships. Some examples are provided below.

TABLE 10.2. Expectations (Sessions 11–15)

- Expectations and relationships
  - Clients list expectations associated with different types of relationships
  - Compare and contrast different expectations
  - Highlight and discuss unhealthy boundaries from these expectations
  - Do clients apply these expectations to themselves?
- Expectations and behavior
  - Discussion of judgments; how expectations lead to judgment
  - Client examples of how expectations impact behavior

- *Stranger.* Basic expectations may be safety, privacy, or respect and civility.
- *Enemy.* An expectation of mistrust, secrecy, or deception may be valid.
- *Acquaintance.* One can expect simple acknowledgment of the relationship, civility, respect, or welcome.
- *Coworker.* Expectations may be of diligence, integrity, responsibility, or some trust.
- *Therapist.* Clients may expect respect, fairness, help, kindness, and interest.
- *Authority figure.* Clients may expect fairness and attentiveness while still expecting privacy and some guardedness in the relationship. Others, based on past experience, may have fairly negative expectations, such as criticism, abuse, or suspicion.
- *Friend.* Reasonable expectations may include mutual respect, willingness to help and listen, patience, and support.
- *Parent.* People generally expect much of their parents; identified expectations may be love, patience, help, compassion, and various forms of support (e.g., financial, emotional). For clients with histories of abusive parental relationships, they may additionally expect unpredictability, hostility, or criticism.
- *Other family member.* Less may be expected of other family members, though this is not always the case. Expectations such as love, assistance or aid, and support may also be present to a lesser or greater extent.
- *Romantic partner.* Here the expectations may be specific to the person, though often they will include things such as love, companionship, time, faithfulness, trust and intimacy, and respect. Some may also describe sexual expectations.

Clients may notice and discuss similarities and differences in one another's responses. Some will identify very few expectations in these relationships, while other clients may present a lengthy list. How do these correlate with their beliefs? For example, a client who believes that romantic partnerships should be characterized by trust, support, and respect will have different expectations than a client who believes the primary purpose of a relationship is obedience, loyalty, and service. Use these and other examples to help them openly articulate and see how beliefs do alter expectations. Clients will understandably have different expectations, and while they may give one another feedback regarding these differences, it is important that the discussion not characterize some expectations as either "right" or "wrong." These beliefs and expectations reflect where the client currently is, and though the nature of these discussions may help modify more dysfunctional, harmful, or unrealistic expectations and beliefs, this is a process that happens at the discretion of the client's commitment and readiness for change.

Some expectations reveal unhealthy boundaries or problems in relationships. When clients express these kinds of expectations, they may or may not be aware of such potential problems. Since they have been learning and using more self-monitoring techniques, they may already be more aware of such expectations, but if not, these expectations may need to be highlighted in discussion. Treatment providers can validate that there were (albeit unhealthy) antecedents or beliefs that may have caused these expectations to form (e.g., Level 4 Validation—"So because you've always felt put down or disrespected by women, you have higher expectations of them in relationships. . . . Like in order for them to have a relationship with you, they have to prove themselves to you and prove that they're not going to treat you like you've been treated in the past"). We don't want to agree with their expectations, but we do want them to be able to view them in a functional way so that they are aware and can evaluate them more objectively.

From here, clients will discuss how these expectations apply to themselves. Do others hold these same expectations of them? When applied to themselves, do they seem reasonable and fair? Or, based on their experiences, have others held them to a higher or lower standard? If others' expectations are different, how do they think that this has happened?

Expectations and Behavior

Our expectations of others work in complex ways to drive behavior. First, our expectations are associated with judgments, or ways of labeling something as good or bad. Judgments are merely shortcuts—we consolidate information to make faster and more efficient decisions, and we classify something as either positive or negative to expedite our decision making. These judgments are shortcuts that often reflect our expectations. For example, you may expect that traffic will be lighter if you leave home earlier than normal. If traffic is just as bad or worse than had you left at your regular time, you may think "This is terrible!" or "This isn't right!" These judgments reflect an expectation that there would be fewer cars on the road well before rush hour. Had you expected heavy traffic, or had you no expectations about the traffic, you may have made fewer judgments about your situation.

These expectations and judgments affect our other perceptions, shape our emotional responses and interpersonal interactions, and may ultimately motivate behavior. These connections occur regardless of one's values or the emotional valance of the judgment (i.e., good or bad). Thus, having beliefs, having expectations, forming judgments, and then translating these into decisions and behavior are normal human processes. The content of those thoughts and the resulting behavior may be maladaptive or harmful, but the process itself is not. As treatment providers, we want to ensure that clients understand this point. The goal is not to stop them from having expectations, or to prevent judgment. The goal is for them to be more aware of others' expectations and judgments, and of the impact of behavior with their relationships with other people.

A useful illustration of this is to have clients select several examples from the previous discussion of expectations in relationships and use these for further exploration. They should be able to identify thoughts, feelings, and behaviors related to these expectations. Also, clients can describe how these thoughts, feelings, and behaviors would change if their expectations were not met. So, for example:

Expectation: I should be treated with respect.
Thought: People should be nice to me.

Feeling: Hopeful, nervous.

Behavior: Being kind, talking to others.

If this expectation is not met, then the following:

Thought: That was unfair!

Feeling: Anger, disappointment, hurt.

Behavior: Being rude, making threats or demands.

Expectation: If I do a favor for a friend, then he/she should be willing to return the favor.
Thought: I'm glad to help out. This is someone I can rely on.

Feeling: Happy, proud.

Behavior: Doing a favor. May ask for a favor in the future.

If expectation is not met, then the following:

Thought: I was taken advantage of.

Feeling: Angry, hurt, betrayed.

Behavior: Complaining, being rude to friend, distancing self from friend.

This activity helps clients bring together the ideas that our thoughts and expectations influence our emotions, our decisions, and even our actions. These components are all interrelated, and other situational or interpersonal variables factor into behavioral outcomes. We must be aware of thoughts or expectations to better control their effect on behavior. If clients are ignorant of these underlying beliefs and expectations, then they will have little understanding of why they feel and act they way that they do.

COGNITIVE DYSREGULATION: GETTING STUCK (SESSIONS 16–20)

Our thoughts can sometimes be maladaptive, unhealthy, or cause problems for us. Traditionally viewed within a cognitive-behavioral framework as "thinking errors" (Beck et al., 1979; Yochelson & Samenow, 1976), certain thoughts may negatively impact our emotions, behaviors, and relationships with others, and are therefore potential targets for treatment. In SOS, these thoughts are not viewed as "errors." Labeling them as an "error" implies that they are wrong or unnatural. Instead, we choose to conceptualize these as dysregulated thoughts, or thoughts that may be uncomfortable for us and may drive us to action in order to alleviate that discomfort.

Sex offender research and treatment has strongly emphasized the role of cognitive distortions, or distorted beliefs that are often consistent with an offender's harmful sexual behaviors (e.g., Blumenthal et al., 1999; Bumby, 1996; Ward et al., 1997; Ward & Keenan, 1999). These cognitive distortions may serve as rationalizations or justifications for offending, or perhaps excuse the offender from culpability for his or her behaviors. These offense-supportive cognitive distortions represent only a part of the larger "thinking error" whole. So a logical question is this: Do you mean to say that these thoughts aren't wrong, and that we should accept them? *No.* In SOS, we view dysregulation as a natural and normal process. What is problematic is the intensity, frequency, uncontrollability, or content of the cognitive dysregulation, as well as the person's difficulties with managing it in an adaptive and functional manner.

Cognitive dysregulation, as described in greater depth in Chapter 2 of this text, is a normative process. When anyone engages in a behavior that harms others, it is natural to minimize this harmful behavior to alleviate cognitive dissonance or uncomfortable emotional and interpersonal responses prompted by the behavior. For example, most people believe that they are good, helpful people. A person who harms someone else but who still believes in his or her own fundamental "goodness" will think, "Well, it wasn't that bad." Or "I didn't really mean to do it. It wasn't intentional." Or maybe even "I wouldn't have done that if she wasn't pushing me so hard." Minimization, rationalization, and blame are all forms of cognitive dysregulation that we may see associated with maladaptive behavior. For some people, the cognitive dysregulation occurs in response to a low-level or less harmful behavior, whereas for others, it can lead to more serious and risky behaviors. The way in which this dysregulation is introduced to clients is described further below, with a summary given in Table 10.3.

Types of Cognitive Dysregulation

Sometimes clients (as well as treatment providers) get "stuck" in these dysregulated thinking patterns. We want clients to understand these types of thoughts, of which there are three major categories. The first includes some of the standard cognitive "errors" or distortions:

1. *Blaming.* Placing blame on someone else. *Example:* "It's her fault that this happened."
2. *All-or-nothing thinking.* Setting expectations too high; thinking that it has to be one way or that it won't work. *Example:* "If it's not going to be like this, then I might as well quit now."
3. *Catastrophizing.* Making a big deal out of something otherwise trivial. *Example:* "I got into trouble again. I'm never going to get out of here."
4. *Minimizing.* Making something seem unimportant; using the words "just" and "only." *Example:* "I only did that to annoy him. It wasn't that bad."
5. *Victim stance.* Feeling like no one understands, that others are making things hard for you, or that it was simply beyond your

TABLE 10.3. Cognitive Dysregulation: Getting Stuck (Sessions 16–20)

- Types of cognitive dysregulations
  - *Content dysregulation*—includes blaming, all-or-nothing thinking, catastrophizing, minimizing, victim stance, mind reading, judgment, etc.
  - *Process dysregulation*—includes racing thoughts, confusion, or blocked thoughts
  - *Pathological content dysregulation*—may include delusional beliefs, paranoia, magical thinking, or offense-supportive beliefs about victims or sexual behavior
- When are these thoughts dysregulated?
  - Discussions of discomfort or interpersonal distress, contrasted with how these thoughts impact others (i.e., Do they cause distress or frustration to others? Why?)
  - Can such thoughts be controlled?
  - Clients identify signs of cognitive dysregulation from their behavioral chain analyses and daily interactions with others.
- Cognitive dysregulation and relationships
  - Viewing cognitive dysregulation in the context of relationships
    - What happens when someone is highly judgmental of another person?
    - Does this improve the relationship, or does it cause damage?
    - How might one recognize this damage?
    - What happens when one person blames another for problems in life or problems in the relationship? How does that other person feel?

---

control. *Example:* "Everyone is against me. No one wants me to do well." "There just wasn't anything I could do about it."
6. *Mind reading.* Making judgments about what others are thinking; assuming you know what someone's motives or intentions are. *Example:* "She said that just to get to me."

Clients may need reminders that judgment is also a type of cognitive dysregulation. We all make judgments, but when we have difficulty letting them go or seeing them for what they are, they can have a negative effect on our emotions, self-esteem, and relationships with others. There are many more of these, including rationalization, justification, and the like. Clients should be able to list these, perhaps from other forms of treatment they have had that target such thoughts.

Other types of cognitive dysregulation describe how clients are thinking, or the process of their cognitive effort:

1. *Racing thoughts.* Clients may have times when they feel like their thoughts are moving too quickly for them to keep up or understand them. They may also have difficulty with maintaining attention and focus as a result.
2. *Confusion.* This exists on a broad continuum, ranging from momentary misunderstanding to a more pervasive sense of not knowing what is going on, not knowing what to do, or not being able to figure out what you want.
3. *Blocked thoughts.* Here, clients may feel like they simply "can't think," or that the thoughts aren't coming to them as quickly as they would expect. Some report this type of dysregulation as the result of substance use, psychiatric symptoms, or medication side effects.

Some clients will need to discuss a third form of cognitive dysregulation related more to mental illness or difficulties with managing reality. This third form includes delusions, or beliefs that are irrational and not shared by others: magical thinking; obsessive and irrational thinking; or paranoia, when they think others are trying to harm them or making things unusually difficult for them. Offense-supportive beliefs about victims and sexual behaviors may also fall into this category, particularly when those beliefs are not shared by others (e.g., "Sex with children is really not harmful to anyone" or "Every woman really fantasizes about being raped").

When Are These Thoughts Dysregulated?

Treatment providers should discuss these different forms of cognitive dysregulation with clients. Clients should recognize that the types of thoughts, beliefs, or thought processes discussed here are not always signs of acute dysregulation—for example, sometimes we just blame or judge others and then let it go. Like other forms of dysregulation, it is only when the thought or the cognitive processing is uncomfortable or distressing to the individual that we consider it dysregulated. These types of cognitive dysregulation commonly characterize clients' experiences, and in order to cope with them, they will first need to be able to identify and recognize them as dysregulation. Treatment providers can validate the experience of dysregulation without necessarily validating the dysregulated thought or belief itself. Offering specific, non-offense-based examples can help clients understand cognitive dysregulation without prompting denial or defensiveness. Opportunities may arise for validating hopelessness, frustration, or anxiety associated with blame and minimization, or for offering validation to those who feel intense confusion and an inability to make quick decisions. Viewing this as a normative process that can be taken to a maladaptive or problematic extreme (i.e., intense dysregulation) will help clients understand that the ultimate goal is not to criticize or judge their thoughts, or to keep them from having these thoughts altogether, but to learn to better monitor and manage them.

Cognitive Dysregulation and Relationships

Experiences of cognitive dysregulation or uncomfortable, unbalanced thinking can impact an individual in many domains, including relationship functioning. Clients will now view their own examples of cognitive dysregulation within the context of their own relationships. Clients should again describe how certain dysregulated thought patterns, such as judgment, blame, minimization, confusion, or paranoia, affect their relationships and interactions with other people. What happens when someone is highly judgmental of another person? Does this improve the relationship or does it cause damage? How might one recognize this damage? What happens when one person blames another for problems in life or problems in the relationship? How does that other person feel?

Address each form of cognitive dysregulation in turn. Some clients will feel comfortable sharing their own experiences. In some cases, treatment providers who have formed strong therapeutic relationships with clients can use their own experiences in treatment as an illustration. For example, referring to earlier stages of treatment when clients demonstrated blame and hostility can serve as an example of dysregulated thinking that may have hampered the development of treatment relationships. (This example should only be used if the blame and hostility are no longer present.) Specific and relatable examples can make learning more meaningful and allow clients to revisit their thoughts in relation to their own treatment relationships.

THOUGHTS, COGNITIVE DYSREGULATION, AND PROBLEMATIC SEXUAL BEHAVIORS (SESSIONS 20–22)

So now clients are ready for the big question: What does cognitive dysregulation have to do with sexual offending? Pose this as a challenge for them to think about. Now that they have discussed cognitive processes and dysregulation, how do they think it relates to their offending behaviors? (See Table 10.4 for an outline of these discussions.) To facilitate this discussion, treatment providers should refer back to prior discussions and activities that may have identified specific thoughts, beliefs, or patterns of thinking reflecting clients' dysregulation. Some sources of information may be the behavioral chain analysis of one or more offenses from Module 2; discussions of expectations in relationships and sexual beliefs from Modules 2, 4, and 6; thoughts related to intense emotional states from Module 3; and their weekly experiences with self-monitoring and reporting to the group.

Risky Thoughts and Sexual Offending

Much like the Module 3 discussion of risky emotional states and sexual offending, some types of cognitive dysregulation may be more associated with sexual offending than others.

1. *Idealized or exaggerated expectations of romantic partnerships.* Clients who believe in the "fairy tale" romance, the perfect romance, or the relationship with no problems are probably going to be disappointed. These expectations may occur when clients have rather limited experiences with healthy and balanced romantic partnerships (Marshall,

---

TABLE 10.4. Thoughts, Cognitive Dysregulation, and Problematic Sexual Behaviors (Sessions 20–22)

- Risky thoughts and sexual offending
  - What does cognitive dysregulation have to do with sexual offending?
    - o Idealized or exaggerated expectations of romantic partnerships
    - o Sexual stereotypes
    - o Blame and entitlement
    - o Sexual delusions
    - o Misperceptions of interpersonal cues
- Troubleshooting—some ideas to consider
  - Their thoughts may not be that different from "normal" people, so they have difficulty seeing this as dysregulated, or as leading to problem behavior.
  - Clients want to maintain harmful or offense-supportive beliefs, or they don't think their beliefs cause others harm.
  - Separating thoughts that preceded an offense from those that came after, like rationalization or blame.

1989). They expect these relationships to be perfect, largely because they are hopeful and idealistic. Unfortunately, such expectations may prevent them from forming positive and supportive, albeit realistic and sometimes "flawed," relationships with others. This may also increase their vulnerability to rejection, anger, and resentment (e.g., Baumeister et al., 2002).

2. *Sexual stereotypes*. Like the idealized versions of romantic relationships, strongly held sexual stereotypes or stereotypical beliefs about a person's gender role in relationships can hinder healthy relationship formation. Obviously, people who hold sexual stereotypes are still capable of forming strong, supportive relationships with others. However, some individuals will struggle when their stereotypical beliefs negatively impact potential friends or romantic partners. These often take the form of judgments and are most obvious when the judgment is combined with some expectation of how another person should behave in a relationship or interpersonal situation. (For a review of these stereotypes as cognitive distortions among sex offenders, we refer readers to Check & Malamuth, 1983; Johnson & Ward, 1996; Ward et al., 1997.)

3. *Blame and entitlement*. While we earlier described entitlement as an emotional state, it can also be classified as a thought. In this case, the person thinks or ruminates on his or her deservedness of something special, or that he or she sees him- or herself as deserving of attention and recognition. This can be closely associated with blame, as when a person places blame on someone or something for preventing him or her from getting or having what he or she rightly deserves. Sexual entitlement, blaming others for shortcomings, or thinking one is entitled to special treatment and consideration may all be relevant to this discussion (e.g., Baumeister et al., 2002; Hanson et al., 1994; Mihailides, Devilly, & Ward, 2004; Mills, Anderson, & Kroner, 2004; Ward, et al., 1997; Ward & Keenan, 1999).

4. *Sexual delusions*. Clients with delusional beliefs may, on occasion, harbor sexual delusions. Though relatively rare (e.g., Smith & Taylor, 1999), they do occur and can strongly influence perceptions of interpersonal relationships and drive behavior.

5. *Misperceptions of interpersonal cues*. Some individuals inappropriately or inaccurately assess interpersonal feedback, and if they do so frequently or consistently in certain types of interactions, this may relate to their maladaptive sexual behaviors. For example, clients who harbor

beliefs that others are sexually interested in them (e.g., children) will be more likely to misinterpret social cues in interactions with such persons in a sexual way (e.g., Jacques-Tiura, Abbey, Parkhill, & Zawacki, 2007; Ward et al., 1998; Ward & Keenan, 1999).

Troubleshooting

Some problems or difficulties may arise during the course of this discussion. Clients are not always be able to identify their cognitive dysregulation, describe its relationship to offending, or even acknowledge the potentially harmful nature of some of their thoughts. Similarly, treatment providers may struggle with addressing clients' thoughts, making the distinction between a "normal" example of cognitive dysregulation and one that may be harmful, or handling their own judgments and expectations of client behavior and progress.

First, clients' cognitive dysregulation (e.g., beliefs or judgments) from their behavioral chain analyses or other group discussions are not always that radically different from the thoughts of people who are not sex offenders. For example, a client who feels rejected might judge the person who rejected him or her. Another client may expect someone to share his or her very traditional values about sex and relationships, or what a normal course of courtship should look like. Thus, it may be difficult for them to see these beliefs as problematic, and it may even be challenging for treatment providers to demonstrate a clear or logical link between the dysregulated thought and the maladaptive behavior. Because this does happen, the similarities between their cognitive dysregulation and that of "normal" people should be made transparent. We don't want them to think that any dysregulated thought is associated with offending, or that we are expecting them to think differently than other people. Instead, they should be made aware of the complex relationship between thoughts and behavior, and how our thoughts can impact our emotions, relationships, and ultimately our decisions. Therefore, thoughts or beliefs that may seem "normal" and are at times dysregulated can lead to maladaptive behavior, or they may not, dependent on other circumstances. The goal therefore is for them to monitor and manage their thoughts more effectively than they have in the past.

A second problem arises when clients firmly believe in something truly harmful, or when they have little or no insight into the negative impact of their thoughts and thought processing. The challenge is twofold. On the one hand, clients have difficulty identifying and monitoring their dysregulation because they are so unaware of it. Instead of trying to force it, treatment providers may find it more helpful to simply note that lack of insight as another progress indicator and validate the client's frustration with treatment and difficulty with fully engaging. On the other hand, treatment providers will need to be cautious about their own response to clients' lack of insight or their persistence in maintaining problematic beliefs and expectations. The temptation is to confront minimization, denial, or blame, thinking that if the client would just sit and "listen to reason" that he or she would experience a magical burst of insight and awareness. This rarely happens. And while it may feel cathartic for the treatment provider, it can damage the therapeutic relationship and make the client defensive. This is not to imply that one can never question a client's beliefs or lack of awareness, but that doing so in a manner intended to forcefully elicit change is unlikely to be effective. Instead, treatment providers could say: "Well, I get that you don't see these thoughts as a problem. But others might. And that can cause you problems in the long run. You don't always have to think the way people want you to, but you do at least have to think about how your thoughts affect behavior, and how that behavior affects others." We again refer readers to Chapter 3 for further information about specific strategies to address client denial, minimization, or ambivalence.

A third issue is helping clients differentiate dysregulated thoughts like blame or rationalization that precipitated the offense from those that instead developed *after* it. The cognitive distortions traditionally targeted in sex offender treatment, for example, are often post hoc explanations or justifications of behavior. Though these may be important barriers to treatment commitment and progress, they are not clear precipitants of maladaptive sexual behavior. Treatment providers will need to help clients understand the difference between these two for clients to better understand the true precipitants of their behavior. As a form of radical genuineness in treatment (i.e., Level 6 Validation), treatment providers may decide to very openly discuss this dilemma. Explaining to clients that some blame, rationalization, or judgment may have developed following the offense to help them deal with the consequences (e.g., thinking "I did this, but I'm not a bad person, so really, what I did wasn't entirely my fault"). This allows clients to separate those thoughts from ones specific to the situation or interactions immediately prior to the offense. Again, returning to the thoughts described during the behavioral chain analysis can be a good starting point for this process.

ALTERNATIVE FORMS OF COPING: BASIC TECHNIQUES (SESSIONS 23–25)

Again, clients have reached a point in which it is crucial for them to begin evaluating alternative forms of coping to help them modulate and control their thoughts and cognitive dysregulation. As in the prior module addressing strategies for emotion regulation, treatment providers will find it helpful to refer to the Chapter 4 discussion of skills building to facilitate this process with clients. Please see Table 10.5 for an overview of this section.

Challenging Beliefs

Changing one's beliefs is not an easy task. Also, the beliefs that clients have identified as part of treatment are not always that radically different than those held by others. Therefore, the goal of treatment is not always to change their beliefs but only to help clients form a more balanced view given some beliefs that contribute to cognitive dysregulation or precipitate harmful behaviors. Beliefs and thoughts are problematic to clients if they become preoccupied with them, if their expectations are untenable or unrealistic, or if they lead to maladaptive patterns of behavior. SOS hopes to aid clients in identifying and self-monitoring cognitive dysregulation associated with their past maladaptive sexual behaviors

---

TABLE 10.5. Alternative Forms of Coping: Basic Techniques (Sessions 23–25)

- Challenging beliefs
  - Changing one's beliefs is not an easy task. Sometimes dysregulated beliefs are still "normal." They are a problem if:
    - ○ Clients become preoccupied with them.
    - ○ Client expectations are untenable or unrealistic.
    - ○ Client expectations or judgments lead to problematic patterns of behavior.
- Basic strategies
  - Review strategies for noticing or self-monitoring cognitive dysregulation, and distracting, accepting, or changing dysregulated thoughts
- Using alternative strategies
  - Clients identify scenarios in which they can use new skills for managing dysregulated thoughts
  - Include discussion of alternative strategies in weekly self-monitoring assignments

---

and that may continue to place them at risk of future maladaptive sexual behaviors.

Basic Strategies

Several basic strategies are needed to assist clients in better managing their dysregulated thoughts. A fundamental tenet of treatment is that these dysregulated thoughts will recur. Many types of cognitive dysregulation mentioned in this chapter are those characterizing the thoughts of offenders and nonoffenders alike. When this dysregulation is uncontrolled or combines with other factors (e.g., emotional or interpersonal dysregulation, situational variables), it will cause some individuals to struggle with effective and adaptive regulatory functioning.

Cognitive strategies are harder to conceptualize than emotional or interpersonal strategies. Clients may have greater difficulty with generating an unstructured list of cognitive skills. These are typically more abstract, and require more significant internal resources. For clients who struggle with cognitive or intellectual impairments, it may take greater effort and increased repetition and practice to learn and master some of these skills. However, treatment providers should be careful not to underestimate clients' abilities. These strategies function to increase awareness of cognitive dysregulation, distract from distressing thoughts, and work with or through problematic thought patterns.

1. Self-monitoring
2. Mindfulness—allowing a thought to be a thought: A great deal of emerging literature suggests that mindfulness activities can be highly effective in helping clients learn to effectively manage a variety of cognitive and other internal states. (For more on this topic, please refer to Hanh, 2010; Shapiro & Carlson, 2009)
3. Distracting yourself from your thoughts
4. Doing something kind for the person you're thinking negatively about
5. Thinking about pros and cons, or some other way of balancing a strong thought
6. Self-talk or self-encouragement
7. Acceptance of the thought
8. Medication and symptom management (for those who struggle with delusional beliefs or other difficulties with cognitive processing)

Using Alternative Strategies

As was the case with emotion regulation strategies, cognitive strategies are very specific to individual and situational factors. Because they are abstract and intangible, they may not be as immediately rewarding as other strategies they have used, nor will they always work. Practice is an important component of the treatment process. Clients will need to develop a list of several basic skills and strive to practice them both in neutral situations and in stressful situations involving experiences of cognitive dysregulation.

Treatment providers are responsible for helping clients identify and learn to self-manage their thoughts throughout the treatment process. One measure of progress is how quickly clients are able to recognize and "catch" themselves thinking in a dysregulated way. The goal is not for them to necessarily judge themselves or one another, but merely to notice and attempt to use skills in the moment. In the beginning, many clients will find this difficult, but if they are still able to recognize and acknowledge dysregulation, then this is acceptable progress. With regards to some of the more complex strategies, like mindfulness and acceptance, clients will need to recognize that mastering these strategies will take lengthy and prolonged practice.

During the initial minutes of each session, when clients share their self-monitoring progress from the past week, treatment providers can prompt them for dyresgulated thoughts and alternative strategies. This will also help reinforce these concepts and make them more immediately salient to clients in their everyday lives.

MODULE 6 CONCLUDING SESSIONS

Throughout this module, clients have learned about beliefs, expectations, cognitive dysregulation, and their impact on their relationships and behaviors. For many, this includes maladaptive sexual behaviors or problematic relationships. Clients should be sure to review these major topic points and progress toward treatment goals by referring again to Form B1 "My Treatment Progress," found in Appendix B.

FORM 10.1

"It's Not My Fault . . . It's Yours"

What we believe about our own behavior depends on the situation or environment. We look for other explanations for what we just did. But our beliefs about others' behavior depends on what we believe about them *personally*. This affects how we see others and their motives, and affects our judgments about them.

Some examples:

1. If you do badly on a group assignment, you might think:
   - It was too hard.
   - I didn't have enough time to finish it.
   - _____

   But if a peer does badly on a group assignment, you might think:
   - He is just lazy and didn't try.
   - He's just dumb.
   - _____

2. If you are in a bad mood and snap at someone who asks you a question, you might think:
   - I didn't get enough sleep last night.
   - He should see I'm in a bad mood and leave me alone.
   - _____

   But if someone is in a bad mood and snaps at you, you might think:
   - She's always mean to me.
   - What's his problem? He's just being rude.
   - _____

(cont.)

---

3. If you're late for an appointment, you might think:
   - Traffic was just terrible!
   - Too many people kept stopping me to ask questions, so I was late.
   - _____

   But if someone is late for an appointment with you, and you're left waiting on them, you might think:
   - He is *never* on time.
   - She is so irresponsible to leave me waiting like this.
   - _____

4. A friend asks you to help her move, and you say no. You think:
   - I have too much going on this weekend. I can't do it.
   - I have a bad back, so I really shouldn't be lifting heavy boxes.
   - _____

   You need help moving some furniture, and you ask a friend, who says no. You think:
   - She just doesn't like me.
   - I always help him out, and he never has time to pay me back.
   - _____

CHAPTER 11

Dysregulation and Interpersonal Relationships

So far, clients have learned about emotional and cognitive dysregulation and how they contribute to maladaptive sexual behavior. They have also worked to develop a set of adaptive regulatory strategies to aid them with effective self-regulation. One major domain of self-regulatory functioning remains: interpersonal regulation. Interpersonal regulation (or dysregulation) primarily centers on relationships. Relationships, and ways in which they can be maladaptive, unhealthy, or dysregulated, are key elements for understanding clients' problematic sexual behaviors. As noted in Chapter 1, the majority of perpetrators of sexual crimes were already known to their victims; they already had a relationship with that individual before the offense. That relationship was characterized by expectations, perceptions, and emotions, any of which could become dysregulated. Even those offenders who targeted strangers or persons relatively unknown to them likely had some expectations, beliefs, or emotions that preceded their offense against that particular victim.

This module focuses on the multifaceted nature of relationships, including relationship functioning, boundaries, communication and assertiveness, problematic or unhealthy relationship behaviors (i.e., dysregulation), and alternative coping strategies. Prior treatment discussions will be heavily referenced in this module, as many of the concepts discussed thus far are intimately related to relationship behaviors and sexual offenses. Treatment providers are encouraged to revisit and review previous concepts and discussions as needed. Goals for this module include improving clients' quality of relationships, helping them identify and change maladaptive relationship behaviors, and teaching them to be more effective at self-managing problematic aspects of relationships.

A related goal is for clients to begin looking at emotional and cognitive dysregulation—which they have continued to monitor on a weekly basis for reporting in group—within the context of their interpersonal relationships. So, for example, when clients discuss instances of emotional dysregulation like anger or loneliness, or cognitive dysregulation like blame or judgment, they can relate these to some of the relationship discussions in this module. This will provide a more comprehensive and integrated understanding of these concepts.

With greater familiarity between treatment providers and clients at this stage, many of the discussions may be more personal in nature for the clients. Validation, humor, and encouragement will reinforce clients for their treatment efforts and may help ease the sting of discussing behaviors that they may find deeply shameful. Treatment providers should be aware of the difficulties clients will have discussing their own role in unhealthy relationship behaviors and recognize their struggle in taking responsibility for them. Clinicians will need to monitor their own expectations of clients and maintain a collaborative approach in working toward client goals.

EXPECTATIONS AND BOUNDARIES (SESSIONS 1–5)

Discussions from Modules 2, 4, and 6 focused on different types of relationships, common expectations characteristic of these relationships, and boundaries. In Module 7, clients will expand these discussions, building on what they have already learned. The purpose is to ensure that clients have a basic understanding of what relationships are, how their thoughts or expectations shape these relationships, and what boundaries are and how they translate into behavior. An overview of these topics is provided in Table 11.1.

Relationships with Others

Before clients review prior discussions of different types of relationships, they should consider the basic components of relationships. Relevant questions include: What is a relationship? Why are relationships important to you? Why do people want to have relationships with others? Are there benefits to having relationships with other people? Have you ever had problems in a relationship? How did this affect you? How did it affect others? This discussion establishes the tone for the remainder of the module and gives treatment providers an understanding of

TABLE 11.1. Expectations and Boundaries (Sessions 1–5)

- Relationships with others
  - Clients discuss why relationships are important
    - What is a relationship?
    - Why are relationships important to you?
    - Why do people want to have relationships with others?
    - Are there benefits to having relationships with other people?
    - Have you ever had problems in a relationship? How did this affect you? How did it affect others?
  - Review of different types of relationships
    - Examples of different types
    - Ways in which they differ (e.g., trust/intimacy, expectations, power differential, their role in the relationship, common interactions, etc.)
- Boundaries
  - What is a boundary? Clients discuss different types and how they view these examples of boundaries.
  - Boundary violations
    - What does it mean when a boundary has been violated?
    - How do you feel when someone violates your boundaries?
    - How do you react to boundary violations?
    - How do others react?
    - How do you know what someone's boundaries are?
    - How do boundaries change over time?
    - How are your boundaries different when you're with different people, or in a different situation?

where clients are with regards to how they view relationships and what their needs are.

Clients with profoundly negative relationship experiences, or who believe that their history of sexual offending precludes them from forming or keeping relationships with others, may adopt an avoidance standpoint during this discussion. In other words, some clients may say they will refrain from all relationships, falsely believing that total avoidance will protect them from maladaptive behaviors or negative experiences. And while avoiding all human contact can reduce the likelihood of committing a violent sexual offense, it is impossible to completely sequester oneself from humanity, and few clients truly want to. This is also not the goal of treatment—to separate our clients from all human contact. Clients will need to work toward a more balanced understanding of relationships, their role in them, and how treatment can assist them in developing healthy relationships while simultaneously decreasing their maladaptive sexual behaviors.

Clients should now reexamine the different types of relationships. How many types of relationships can clients identify? They should be able to name various examples associated with each type. They will need to describe how these relationships differ with regards to how they develop, level of trust, expectations, type of communication, level of equality or power differential, their role in the relationship, common types of interaction, and so on. This discussion can inform client progress in several respects. First, treatment providers can get an idea of how well clients understand these concepts. But also, since these concepts have been reviewed at several points during the treatment program, providers can assess how much information the clients have retained, how their understanding has changed with time and new learning, whether or not new information has been internalized and integrated into the discussion, and if clients recognize the features of these relationships in their daily lives.

Boundaries

Concepts involving boundaries in relationships were introduced in Module 2 and then again in Module 4. Boundaries are broadly described as the separation between self and others, or more narrowly defined as the limits people set on their relationships. But what do clients think a relationship boundary is? Can they identify what their own boundaries are? Some examples of boundaries for them to discuss are (1) personal space, or how much physical space a person needs in different types of relationships or interactions; (2) communication and information sharing, or what types of information or intimate knowledge are characteristic of different types of relationships; (3) trust and emotional closeness, or how relationships differ with regards to trust and expectations of emotional intimacy; (4) privacy, or the preferences one has for how much others know and see about certain aspects of one's life; (5) role perceptions, or how self-expression through clothing, behavior, speech, or other means of self-presentation may reflects one's boundaries; (6) self-respect, or what types of treatment or interactions are expected or tolerated in relationships; and (7) time, or how one sets limits on time and personal involvement in activities and relationships with others. Obviously, these do not reflect all potential types of boundaries. Clients and treatment providers may be able to generate an even more exhaustive list, depending on the knowledge, experience, and comprehension levels of the clients involved in treatment. Clients should verbalize some of the different types of boundaries, along with examples of each, to illustrate the meaning of boundaries in relationships. Treatment providers can help illustrate these points with specific examples or in-group role plays so that clients who are less able to independently describe boundaries can at least recognize elements of boundaries and limits in the moment. For instance, treatment providers could provide examples of how boundaries differ by type of relationship (e.g., "Do you think he would loan me his car for the week if I asked? No? Why not? Why is that too much? We're coworkers, after all. Would it be different if I were his sister? How come?"), or give clear demonstrations of boundary violations in the moment, such as by asking (but not expecting) a client to empty the contents of his wallet for all to see (i.e., demonstrating expectations of privacy). Trust boundaries, which are sometimes fairly abstract, can be demonstrated by asking how much clients trust certain persons, like strangers, friends, ex-partners, close family members, distant family members, enemies, and so on. Clients may automatically say that they don't trust strangers, but they do in ways that are not immediately apparent. Asking, "Do you expect the cashier at the grocery store to steal from you? To hurt you?" can demonstrate that we all hold some basic social expectations concerning trust, even with regards to strangers.

As clients discuss different types of boundaries—and perhaps more importantly, violations of those boundaries—they should remain aware of how their own boundaries differ from those of other people, how those boundaries may have developed, and how people feel when their boundaries have been violated. To help with this discussion, clients can address the questions below.

1. "What does it mean when a boundary has been violated?" It may be helpful for clients to think of this **issue** in concrete and specific terms, using boundaries like trust, personal space, or privacy. Role plays staged between treatment providers, such as looking through someone's personal belongings (e.g., going through a purse, reading someone's notes), touching someone's clothing or hair, or pretending to reveal personal information to others, can all be good examples to assist clients in capturing the reality of a boundary violation. It can be hard to explain such an abstract idea as a "boundary violation," but seeing it in action prompts clients to recognize a violation and the actions, thoughts, and emotions it entails.

2. "How do you feel when someone violates your boundaries?" Again, in order to have this discussion, it will be helpful for clients to refer to specific examples. Violations of trust, for example, may call to

mind emotions such as betrayal, anger, fear, or humiliation. Violations of intimacy, such as someone revealing very personal information too soon in a relationship, may prompt feelings of discomfort, embarrassment, or suspicion.

3. "How do you react to boundary violations?" Clients' behavioral or interpersonal reactions to boundary violations often depend on their emotional responses. They may experience this variety of emotional reactions, or even feel mixed emotions following another's violation of their boundaries. They may react differently depending on whether they are scared, angry, surprised, disappointed, hurt, or disgusted. The seriousness, frequency, and intensity of the boundary violation, as well as their relationship history with the other person, also factors into the specific emotional reaction.

4. "How do others react?" Like their own reactions, others' reactions depend on their emotions or feelings related to the boundary violation, as well as their expectations and the nature of the violation itself. Clients should identify some of these factors as they discuss how others might respond. This exercise will offer some indication of their ability to understand others' emotions and perceptions, and to relate another person's behavior to his or her internal experiences.

5. "How do you know what someone's boundaries are?" This may be one of the most difficult questions for clients to answer. They may not know what their own boundaries are, so that makes it virtually impossible for them to figure out anyone else's. So how would they know? What signs do others give about their boundaries? What kinds of things might others expect from the client, and how might these expectations help them understand limits in relationships? People don't always explicitly state their boundaries, so clients will need to think of other ways to figure them out. Using prior examples either discussed or enacted in group sessions can be a helpful illustration.

6. "How do boundaries change over time?" We assume that as people change, and as relationships change, boundaries will change as well. Have clients think of specific examples from their own relationships. As they get to know a person better, how do boundaries become different? Thinking of boundaries like privacy, communication and intimacy, personal space, and trust can help them answer this question in the context of specific and known relationships.

7. "How are your boundaries different when you're with different people, or in a different situation?" Again, it always helps for clients to

have specific examples in mind. Think of boundaries with family members versus friends versus a supervisor or other authority figure. How do the types of information they share differ, depending on who they are with? How does their behavior, clothing, or speech differ when they are in public versus private places? Church versus a social gathering? Using these types of examples helps clients understand how boundaries sometimes depend on situational and historical factors. Treatment providers must help clients think through the nuances of social relationships, boundaries, and situational expectations. For example, most people would consider it a violation of personal space to be touched intimately by someone they barely know, though it is common practice in medical situations involving emergency care, necessary medical assistance, or when the physician performs an examination. These scenarios may justify differences in normal limits on privacy and personal space. And while many clients would agree that keeping secrets for friends is an important boundary, what if revealing that secret could prevent someone from harm? What other examples can treatment providers and clients generate? Clients will need to think about boundaries and boundary violations in situational or person-specific terms to illustrate the complexity of boundaries and interpersonal relationships.

COMMUNICATING IN INTERPERSONAL RELATIONSHIPS (SESSIONS 6–10)

Boundaries are surely one major issue in clients' interpersonal relationships, and communication is another. Entire treatment programs have been devoted to improving social and communication skills for clients with relationship problems, mental illness, intellectual and developmental disabilities, violent or aggressive behaviors, and so forth (e.g., Bellack, Mueser, Gingerich, & Agresta, 2004; Bloomquist, 2005). Therefore, it is simply impossible to teach clients everything they need to know to improve their communication with others in a few short weeks or months. Here, the goal is not just to make clients skilled communicators, but to help them understand relationships and relationship processes within the context of interpersonal dysregulation so that they can develop adaptive strategies and healthy relationship behaviors. Thus in this section we will focus on a few selected points related to communication difficulties that can impair effective self-management of interpersonal relationships, urges, and behavior (see Table 11.2).

TABLE 11.2. Communicating in Interpersonal Relationships (Sessions 6–10)

- Knowing yourself and stating your needs
  - Clients describe what they need from relationships
    - What kinds of relationships do they have?
    - What do they need from these other persons? What do others need from them?
    - How do expectations factor in?
  - Given this, how can they communicate needs?
  - What gets in the way of communicating their needs?—Intensity of emotions, types of emotions, dysregulated thoughts, perceptions and interpretations, importance of needs, ego, presentation style, and situational factors
  - Basic steps in this process
    - Identifying what you want
    - Stating the facts
    - Describing how it impacts you and the other person
    - Negotiating a decision
- Listening and validating others
  - Four components of interpersonal communication: words, tone, body language, and implied meaning
  - Clients practice guessing emotional valence of statements
  - Clients validate one anothers' emotions

Knowing Yourself and Stating Your Needs

Many communication skills interventions emphasize the importance of assertiveness training. However, good communication is more than just being assertive. It also involves knowing your needs, goals, and role in any given relationship, and then using that knowledge to effectively pursue those goals. It also requires awareness of the other person's needs, priorities, and limitations. This awareness involves self-respect as well as respect for others. A common problem is that clients often think in terms of their immediate needs. Remember that there is a hypothesized link between dysregulation and immediate gratification—an inability to effectively manage or modulate internal states leads to problems with delaying gratification. If you have little ability to control intense internal states, you have even less ability to tolerate them in the moment. This spills over into interpersonal communication, when a dysregulated person finds it challenging to accept refusals or cope with uncomfortable interactions.

As treatment providers, we need to assist clients in developing greater complexity in knowing themselves and then using that knowledge to inform their interactions with others. This can be most easily accomplished by starting with a specific task: have clients list important relationships along with what they and the other person need and want from the relationship, what their roles in the relationship are, what their expectations and boundaries are, and ultimately how they would like to see the relationship progress. In this way, clients and treatment providers can pull together concepts from the previous modules to better understand and conceptualize relationship functioning.

For example, for a client who has described problems in communicating with a work supervisor, the following questions are relevant to group discussion: What kind of relationship do you have with this person? What do you need from this relationship? What do you want? Are your needs and wants different? What do you think your work supervisor needs and wants from you? What is your role in the relationship? What kinds of expectations do you have of your supervisor, and what kinds of expectations does he or she have of you? How would you like to see this problem resolved? Where do you see this relationship going, or where do you want it to be? These kinds of questions lead to the ultimate issue, which is how clients can let others (e.g., this work supervisor) know what they want and ask for it while recognizing complex relationship factors.

When clients (or anyone for that matter) ask for something from another person, there is an expectation of how it will go, and how it will be resolved. If clients have not adequately considered the issues described above, they may ask for things that are irrelevant or inappropriate given the circumstances, or they may refuse requests that are a standard and appropriate expectation given the parameters of that relationship. This is why it is so important for them to have an understanding of these principles before they begin practicing assertiveness and other communication skills techniques.

The next step is for clients to know what prevents them from effectively stating their needs or communicating with others in a helpful way. To put it simply, what gets in the way? Some common obstacles are described below.

• *The intensity of one's emotions.* A client's fear, anger, impatience, or hopelessness, or these emotions in the other person with whom they're interacting, have an effect. These emotions can become so intense, or their impact on thoughts, urges, and behaviors so profound, that they prevent effective communication.

• *Emotional valence.* Responses like anger, entitlement, or defiance have a very different impact on interpersonal interactions than emotions like fear, sadness, or guilt. One's own emotional valence can therefore shape the nature of the interaction and influence one's ability to communicate with another person in that moment.

• *Dysregulated thought processes.* Experiencing judgment, blame, or rationalization can affect how we view an interaction and consequently deal with the other person. Expectations of the other person, whether fair or not, can also implicitly shape our patterns of communication.

• *Perceptions and interpretations.* Our assumptions, perceptions, and interpretations of situations and behavior also contribute to ongoing communication with others. These perceptions can be dysregulated, but even regulated or balanced assumptions about others change the nature of an interaction.

• *Importance.* The importance of a request may also affect one's ability and willingness to communicate it. This can be either positive or negative, depending on the circumstances. In some cases, the importance of a request drives us to pursue it, whereas in other cases, its importance may cause reluctance if there is a fear of rejection or denial.

• *Egocentricity.* While clients may not understand what egocentricity is, treatment providers do. Help clients understand how their own self-importance, entitlement, or egocentricity can complicate interpersonal communication.

• *Presentation style.* How you present or deny a request does matter. Behaviors like arguing, demeaning others, making demands, or manipulating shape whether or not others will do what we want. Some clients have had success in using these methods to accomplish their goals, but they may interfere with other goals, like maintaining self-respect or maintaining the relationship over time.

• *Situational factors.* Idiosyncratic situational factors can also affect communication and its outcome. Communicating at a time when the other person is busy or distracted, in a setting that does not allow for privacy for personal requests, or at an otherwise inappropriate time or place will also prevent someone from effectively making his or her needs known.

When reviewing these factors, clients should be able to generate examples from their own experiences. Thinking about interactions with family members, friends, treatment providers, case managers, supervisors, attorneys and judges, or even victims can help them better conceptualize the barriers that prevent them from more effectively stating their needs and having those needs met. Again, they should think of these examples in terms of the nature of their relationships; whether or not their goals, wants, and needs are reasonable and appropriate; and how their expectations shape interpersonal interactions.

Clients may already know a number of strategies for asserting themselves and making their needs known. Basic steps in this process include identifying what you want (which they have already discussed in some detail in the first part of this section), stating the facts, describing how it impacts you and the other person, and negotiating a decision. Returning to earlier examples, have clients mimic or role-play what they would do in a given scenario where they must state their needs or establish healthy boundaries with others. It may help to have clients attempt this process by using another client's example. Being removed from a situation can help them think critically about it, while allowing the person who is actually involved in the situation the opportunity to hear others' opinions and approaches.

Listening and Validating Others

How do you listen to someone? As treatment providers, you are already aware of the validation techniques discussed in Chapter 4 of this text and how they are used to listen therapeutically and help the client feel heard or understood. It is also important for clients to learn how to listen and validate to improve their relationships with others. Clients are typically less aware of how to listen and truly hear what others are saying. Their relationships may be hampered by focusing too much on their own needs or demands, making assumptions or one-sided interpretations of what others say, or simply not attending to the conversation. Granted, listening attentively is not the only solution to interpersonal skill deficits, but improvement in listening and communication abilities can facilitate healthier relationships overall. Thus, better listening is important for clients to learn, especially in anticipation of more complex skills, such as resolving interpersonal conflict.

To more effectively listen to others and validate them, clients will need to consider four important components of interpersonal communication:

words, tone, body language, and implied meaning. Words are the most obvious. This is what people directly say. For some clients, this component is the easiest to attend to, or the most obvious. For others, the words get lost as they try to think of what they want to say next, what the person means, or how this impacts them. These latter such individuals don't really hear what the other person has said. The second component, tone, helps us understand the emotional context of someone's words. Some people focus so much on tone that they don't focus on what is actually being said, whereas others focus very little on tone and miss emotional connotations or the intended effect of the words. The third part, body language, is an extension of tone. This is how the person actually presents themselves physically as they speak. This presentation can communicate emotion and intent. It can also communicate something about the nature of the relationship between speaker and listener. And finally, implied meaning brings these three components together. It involves the other person's emotions, thoughts, and expectations, which are made evident through their words, tone, and body language.

Understanding what another person actually means requires higher order listening skills and maybe knowledge of the other person. Obviously, there are times when the person's actual words and their implied meaning are the same. But in established relationships, there is a history between the persons involved in an interaction. This history leads to deeper meanings and more unspoken communication, and clients will have to listen carefully and mindfully. Clients must balance words, tone, body language, and implied meaning to more meaningfully communicate with others in their relationships.

A group activity can help clients understand and practice these concepts. For this exercise, treatment providers should prepare a number of sentences or statements that lend themselves to different implied meanings and emotional connotations (see Table 11.3 for suggestions). Have each client read a statement with several different implied meanings and emotions. For example, the statement "I've been in treatment for a while now" could be presented as frustrated, indifferent, proud, or defeated. The client can communicate one of these meanings to the group through tone, body language, or other words that may help. Other group members should guess what is really being said (i.e., implied meaning), identifying components of the other person's communication that led them to this conclusion. This exercise will help them better listen and observe, also getting feedback from others when they have difficulty with these concepts. It may make them more conscious of their own communication style as well. Another beneficial activity could include recorded television

TABLE 11.3. The Listening Game

Make a number of index cards for the clients to select from, each containing a statement and several meanings or emotions. Each client selects a card to read aloud, using tone of voice, body language, and other nonverbal cues to convey the emotions listed. Other clients will guess what is meant and describe how they decided on an answer.

1. My sister never wrote me back. (angry) (sad, lonely)
2. I have a treatment team meeting next week. (nervous) (hopeful)
3. I don't have my homework assignment. (silly, playful) (embarrassed)
4. I need to go see the doctor. (scared) (annoyed)
5. I have a lot of work to do before then! (excited) (overwhelmed, stressed)
6. He didn't talk to me when I saw him at work. (worried) (hurt)
7. She wasn't supposed to be here today. (confused) (angry)
8. Why do I have to do that? (defensive) (concerned)
9. It's been raining all day. (disappointed) (interested, happy)
10. The phone isn't working. (frustrated) (surprised)
11. I don't have anything to do today. (relieved) (bored)
12. I've been in treatment for a while now. (proud) (tired, defeated)
13. We have somebody new in group. (paranoid, suspicious) (curious)
14. I don't think you're listening to me. (annoyed (amused, entertained)
15. Can somebody help me with this? (desperate) (confused)

shows involving different relationships (e.g., soap operas, *telenovelas*) where many meanings are conveyed through tone, body language, and implied meaning. Clients can watch such programs and interpret the communication between different characters in the program.

After listening, the next step is to validate. Clients are not expected to validate at the same level that therapists do, nor is the goal for them to promote healing in the other person. Instead, we want clients to listen and meaningfully communicate. An important precursor to using validation is for clients to monitor their own emotional and cognitive dysregulation. Without keeping track of their own emotional responses, judgments, and expectations, they will find it difficult to really listen and validate someone else. Then they must attend to what is said (and what isn't being said) and place this in the context of the relationship. What is being implied? What is the expectation here? What are the consequences for the client (listener) and the other person (speaker)? Using the first few levels of validation (i.e., listening and observing, reflecting, and articulating unspoken thoughts or emotions) can be a good way for clients to improve their ability to communicate understanding and to help the other person feel that his or her input is valued.

INTERPERSONAL DYSREGULATION (SESSIONS 11–15)

Clients should now think about how interpersonal interactions can become dysregulated and how this dysregulation can lead to maladaptive behaviors (see Table 11.4 for an outline of these discussions). Interpersonal dysregulation is often manifested as maladaptive behavior, and the early cues of interpersonal dysregulation may be emotional or cognitive—the dysregulated thoughts and feelings that they have already discussed in prior modules. In some ways, this makes interpersonal dysregulation the most complex and the most difficult to change. In the spirit of validation and radical genuineness (i.e., Level 6 Validation), treatment providers may want to make clients aware of this complexity prior to beginning this section of treatment. Doing so may prepare them for their frustration with self-monitoring and using new strategies.

Monitoring Your Own Dysregulation

How does one know when an interaction is dysregulated? Put another way, how do you know when things have gone awry? Treatment providers will want to review some of the maladaptive relationship behaviors that clients identified in Module 2, along with their earlier discussions of healthy and unhealthy relationships. Clients will be able to provide examples of times when their relationships have not gone well, or interactions that made them feel uncomfortable or upset. Have them differentiate the components of a "normal" or regulated interpersonal interaction (e.g., honesty, openness, comfort level, willingness to engage in an interaction) from those which are not "normal" or may be dysregulated.

TABLE 11.4. Interpersonal Dysregulation (Sessions 11–15)

- Monitoring your own dysregulation
  - Treatment providers and clients review maladaptive relationship behaviors, as well as characteristics of healthy and unhealthy relationships
  - Clients list characteristics of regulated versus dysregulated interactions, and examples of dysregulated interactions or relationship behaviors
  - Identify how other forms of dysregulation may be related to these
- Interpersonal dysregulation and maladaptive behavior
  - Clients refer back to their list of dysregulated interactions—how are these related to their offending behaviors?
    - o Clients identify emotions, thoughts, or urges associated with these
    - o What triggered these interactions or relationship behaviors?

Have the clients list as many dysregulated or uncomfortable interpersonal behaviors they can think of. These may include, but are not limited to, the following:

1. Arguing, insulting, or yelling at others.
2. Being overtly or implicitly hostile.
3. Making demands or threats; issuing ultimatums.
4. Lying.
5. Manipulating others so that you can get your way.
6. Isolating yourself from others.
7. Giving others the "silent treatment."
8. Being generally disrespectful or rude.
9. Hiding important emotions, thoughts, or urges; shutting down.
10. Being defensive.

Within this discussion, it may be helpful for clients to articulate why these are dysregulated behaviors. This may be stated in terms of their emotions during the interaction, how it may have made the other person feel, whether or not they want to have these kinds of interactions with others, and the like. Also, how would they characterize this as dysregulation in the context of their relationship goals? Does it help them maintain a relationship with another person? Do they want to remain in a relationship with someone who does this to them?

As we have already noted, early cues of interpersonal dysregulation are often emotional or cognitive. In many cases, their expectations, judgments, and other thoughts may be dysregulated within the context of these problematic interactions. Similarly, they may experience emotional dysregulation, when they feel badly about a particular individual or interaction. For each of the examples of interpersonal dysregulation listed above, also have clients identify other forms of related dysregulation. How do they feel when they are making a demand (e.g., entitled, angry, defiant, scared)? How do they feel when someone else refuses to talk to them (e.g., angry, confused, ashamed)?

Obviously, some of these dysregulated behaviors are common and at times unavoidable. We don't want to normalize pathological or dangerous behaviors, but we do want to validate and help clients understand how their dysregulated behaviors can be taken to extremes. For example, clients should not have an expectation that they will never argue again. This is unrealistic and only sets them up for failure. Clients will want to idealize their future relationships. They want their romantic partnerships to be perfect, their day-to-day interactions to be stress-free, and their own behaviors to be without fault. Again though these are all unlikely, and failing to realize the normative aspects of interpersonal dysregulation may prevent them from effectively dealing with it. The dysregulation itself is not necessarily the problem, though frequent and uncontrolled interpersonal dysregulation can obviously cause problems and make people feel quite uncomfortable. The problem targeted in treatment is when clients use maladaptive strategies to cope with their interpersonal dysregulation. Helping them see this connection gives clients a better sense of what is expected, and what exactly they will need to monitor and manage in order to be successful in treatment.

Interpersonal Dysregulation and Maladaptive Behavior

There are individualized links between interpersonal dysregulation and maladaptive strategies, and clients will need to examine their problematic behaviors across the spectrum, including sexual offending, aggression, criminal activity, or substance abuse. Other behaviors, including general irresponsibility or impulsivity, are also relevant. How did manipulation, for example, play a role in their sexual offending? Were they violent or threatening toward someone whom they thought was rude or disrespectful? What types of interactions cause them to go out and drink or use drugs (e.g., someone insulting them, feeling ignored and isolated)?

For each of these behaviors, have clients identify relevant emotions, thoughts, or urges. The important part here is for clients to link these relationship behaviors or dysregulated interaction patterns with specific experiences. These examples don't necessarily have to be an offense; they might give examples like offense-supportive sexual fantasies (e.g., arguing with a woman and then fantasizing about raping or humiliating her) or urges related to sexual or other maladaptive behaviors. Treatment providers will need to emphasize the point that clients may not be able to inhibit interpersonal dysregulation, but that the intensity, duration, and behavior resulting from the dysregulation is something that the client can ultimately control.

WORKING WITH INTERPERSONAL DYSREGULATION (SESSIONS 16–22)

Learning to regulate relationship functioning can be a slow and difficult progress. Because interpersonal dysregulation involves many other factors, like intense emotions, judgments and assumptions, expectations, and others' behaviors, one must first understand sources of interpersonal dysregulation and basic problem-solving strategies. From here, clients can move into more specific discussions regarding adaptive interpersonal skills. We refer readers to Table 11.5 for an overview of this section.

Handling Conflict in Interpersonal Relationships

Not all relationships go smoothly. Clients have already discussed differences between healthy and unhealthy relationships in Module 2. Questions that can be used to review include: What makes a relationship healthy? What makes it unhealthy? How do you know if you're involved in an unhealthy relationship (e.g., emotional reactions, expectations, physical sensations, self-esteem)? What are some of the negative consequences of being in an unhealthy relationship? Treatment providers should note any all-or-nothing thinking that arises. Clients, like anyone else, may expect that healthy relationships are always happy and conflict-free, or that those in unhealthy relationships cannot possibly love one another. We want clients to adopt a more balanced view of healthy and unhealthy relationships, recognizing that they may share important characteristics, or that they can change over time to become healthier or unhealthier.

TABLE 11.5. Working with Interpersonal Dysregulation (Sessions 16–22)

- Handling conflict in interpersonal relationships
  - Clients again review healthy versus unhealthy relationships
    - What makes a relationship healthy?
    - What makes it unhealthy?
    - How do you know if you're involved in an unhealthy relationship (e.g., emotional reactions, expectations, physical sensations, self-esteem)?
    - What are some of the negative consequences of being in an unhealthy relationship?
  - Clients review and discuss sources of conflict in interpersonal relationships
- Problem-solving strategies
  - Clients review basic steps for problem solving and apply these to several examples from their own experiences
    - Define the problem
    - Gather information
    - Look at timing
    - Weigh the pros and cons
    - Seek help or advice
    - Negotiate
    - Take it to someone else

There are many sources of conflict in interpersonal relationships. Some examples with client responses are given below in Figure 11.1. (A blank version is provided for client use in Form 11.1 at the end of the chapter.) Treatment providers will want to review these causes of conflict and have clients provide relevant examples from their own experiences. These examples can inform subsequent discussions related to problem solving and interpersonal skill building.

Problem-Solving Strategies

Interpersonal dysregulation or conflict in relationships can reach a breaking point, when something simply must be done. This forces a decision: What type of behavior will ultimately improve or end the dysregulation or conflict? Clients have engaged in a variety of both adaptive and maladaptive behaviors, including sexual offending, in order to change a conflictual relationship or alleviate their distress following interpersonal dysregulation.

Each client should generate an example of a problem he or she has encountered in one or more of their relationships. The example could be chosen from the previous discussion on sources of interpersonal conflict, or could be something that has recently occurred in their personal, professional, or therapeutic relationships with others. Then proceed through the questions below to help them more clearly conceptualize the problem.

1. *Define the problem.* What is the conflict about? How did it start?
2. *Gather information.* What are the facts? What are your opinions? What are the other person's opinions? What could be causing the conflict?
3. *Look at timing.* Can it be resolved right now? If not, when? What could be gained by waiting?
4. *Weigh the pros and cons.* What risks or benefits are involved? How does this positively or negatively affect you and others?
5. *Seek help or advice.* What do others think? Do others have ideas about the problem, or maybe even the solution?
6. *Negotiate.* Do you understand the other person's side? Does he or she understand yours? Can you reach an agreement through communication and give-and-take?
7. *Take it to someone else.* Sometimes the conflict cannot be resolved through negotiation. Strong beliefs or opinions, or unwillingness to negotiate, may necessitate taking the decision to another person.

Below is a wheel representing 12 factors that can lead to differences of opinion, disagreements, or actual interpersonal problems.

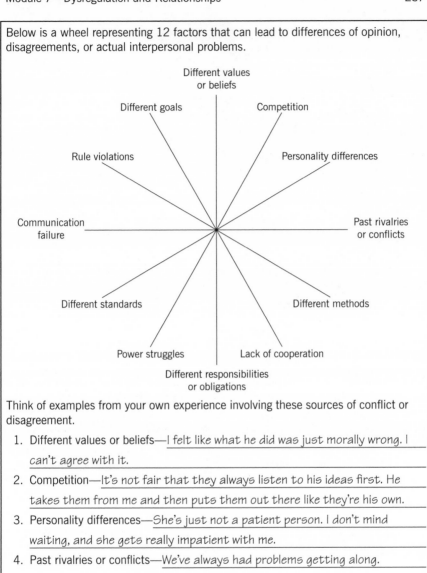

Think of examples from your own experience involving these sources of conflict or disagreement.

1. Different values or beliefs—I felt like what he did was just morally wrong. I can't agree with it.

2. Competition—It's not fair that they always listen to his ideas first. He takes them from me and then puts them out there like they're his own.

3. Personality differences—She's just not a patient person. I don't mind waiting, and she gets really impatient with me.

4. Past rivalries or conflicts—We've always had problems getting along.

5. Different methods—That's not how I would do it.

(cont.)

FIGURE 11.1. Sample client worksheet—"Sources of Interpersonal Conflict."

6. Lack of cooperation—I can't get anyone to help me. I'm tired of doing it all by myself while she just sits there.

7. Different responsibilities or obligations—He is so demanding. He doesn't understand that I have a lot of other things on my mind right now.

8. Power struggles—I'm the one in charge here, so I should be the one making the decisions. She keeps trying to take over.

9. Different standards—He may be okay with doing something sloppy like that, but it's not acceptable to me.

10. Communication failure—She never listens to what I'm saying, and then doesn't follow through on what I want her to do.

11. Rule violations—I know they said not to do that, but it's a stupid rule. It's not like others have to follow that rule.

12. Different goals—I really don't care whether or not they think I'm doing a good job.

FIGURE 11.1. (*cont.*)

These are only first steps in the problem-solving process. In many cases, once clients have carefully thought through the problem or conflict, opportunities for resolving the issue will naturally present themselves. In other cases, seeking help or consultation from others provides alternative viewpoints and strategies as well. For clients who struggle with generating solutions on their own or accepting the available alternatives, treatment providers may need to brainstorm specific persons clients could consult for additional help. Taking the time to go through this process can also help alleviate strong emotions or temper firmly held opinions that may be negatively impacting the client's ability to effectively resolve the issue.

ALTERNATIVE FORMS OF COPING: BASIC TECHNIQUES (SESSIONS 23–24)

Adaptive coping strategies for dealing with interpersonal dysregulation are complex and varied. Developing and using such strategies calls upon other areas of adaptive coping. Learning to modulate strong emotions and negative emotionality, expectations and judgments of others, and deficits in interpersonal functioning necessarily precedes the use of some of these interpersonal coping skills. Thus, clients will need to rely on information they learned in previous modules to help them better manage their interpersonal dysregulation. (See Table 11.6 for an overview of this section.)

Alternative Coping Strategies

Mastering these strategies will take time and practice. As always, clients should expect that they will struggle with these strategies at first, and that they may not feel as comfortable or automatic as familiar strategies, many of which may be maladaptive or harmful.

1. Self-monitoring of emotions, thoughts, and urges—It may be more important for them to monitor these than the actual relationship or interpersonal behaviors, as these often feed into interpersonal dysregulation.
2. Monitoring judgments and striving to be nonjudgmental
3. Willingness—This may mean willingness to compromise or negotiate, work with others, maintain the relationship, or to let go of an unhealthy relationship
4. Acceptance and letting go of self-righteousness, anger, defensiveness, or being "right"
5. Exercising kindness to others
6. Prioritizing interpersonal needs
7. Nondefensively communicating your needs to others
8. Listening to and validating others

TABLE 11.6. Alternative Forms of Coping: Basic Techniques (Sessions 23–24)

- Alternative coping strategies
  - Clients learn new ways of coping with interpersonal dysregulation and using adaptive interpersonal skills
  - Review of how interpersonal coping is related to other areas of dysregulation
- Using alternative strategies
  - Clients monitor and discuss interpersonal dysregulation, conflict, and skills practice each week

---

Using Alternative Strategies

Clients will need to practice these strategies in various settings and situations, and with people in different types of relationships. Only practicing or using them in high-stress, important relationships can lead to disappointment and perceived failure when uncomfortable or unfamiliar strategies are either unsuccessful or not reinforcing. Practice over time lets clients decide which strategies work best and in what situations, and with which relationships or people. Clients will eventually become more automatic and effective in managing dysregulation and can gradually replace old, maladaptive patterns of behavior.

Clients may also find it useful to begin monitoring interpersonal conflict or dysregulation on their weekly self-monitoring homework for group. This exercise also gives them more opportunities to practice the skills as they heighten their awareness of dysregulated emotions, thoughts, and interactions with others.

MODULE 7 CONCLUDING SESSIONS

In this module, clients have completed their discussion of the three types of dysregulation—emotional, cognitive, and interpersonal—that can lead to behavioral dysregulation and maladaptive behavior. They have reviewed communication in relationships, understanding their own needs and expectations in relationships, interpersonal dysregulation, conflict and problem solving, and adaptive replacement skills. Clients can again refer to the "My Treatment Progress" worksheet found in Appendix B for a review of these concepts in relation to their goals and progress.

Sources of Interpersonal Conflict

Below is a wheel representing 12 factors that can lead to differences of opinion, disagreements, or actual interpersonal problems.

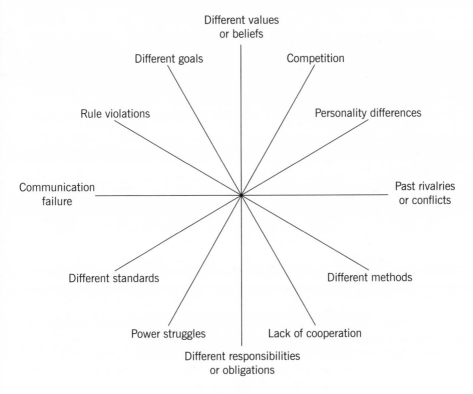

Think of examples from your own experience involving these sources of conflict or disagreement.

1. Different values or beliefs—_____

_____

2. Competition—_____

_____

(cont.)

3. Personality differences—_____

_____

4. Past rivalries or conflicts—_____

_____

5. Different methods—_____

_____

6. Lack of cooperation—_____

_____

7. Different responsibilities or obligations—_____

_____

8. Power struggles—_____

_____

9. Different standards—_____

_____

10. Communication failure—_____

_____

11. Rule violations—_____

_____

12. Different goals—_____

_____

CHAPTER 12

Coping with the Past

Clients who have committed sexual offenses or engaged in serious problematic sexual behaviors will need to cope with their own past experiences, including both negative life events and their own harmful behaviors toward others. In this chapter, we consider the role of trauma in SOS, as well as client discussions, activities, and treatment targets that can assist them in addressing significant events from the past.

This chapter begins with a discussion for treatment providers concerning the role of trauma in clients' lives, how to address traumatic experiences in treatment, and how to conceptualize past events within the context of SOS and the Multimodal Self-Regulation Theory. We also make recommendations with regards to assessment and treatment interventions for providers to consider should clients present with significant trauma needs. Following this introductory discussion, we present activities and discussions emphasizing the impact of trauma, acceptance and forgiveness, and repairing relationships or damage caused by sexual offending.

Important goals for this module include familiarizing clients with the relationships between traumatic experiences, dysregulation, and self-regulatory deficits; helping them recognize their own dysregulation related to stressful or traumatic life events; describing the impact of trauma or harmful behaviors on victims; and helping clients come to terms with and accept their own behaviors. Descriptions of client sessions include suggestions and activities to aid clients in reaching these goals and understanding the key concepts in this module. Treatment providers will also notice suggestions for addressing additional client needs that may be beyond the scope of standard sex offender treatment interventions.

243

WORKING WITH TRAUMA

Many clients with a history of sexual offending also have their own histories of victimization or maltreatment, including emotional abuse, physical abuse, sexual abuse, neglect, or another form of major life loss. Research estimates of the prevalence of childhood and adolescent maltreatment in sexual offenders varies widely, ranging from 20 to 90% (e.g., Haapasalo & Kankkonen, 1997; Jonson-Reid & Way, 2001; Stinson & Becker, 2011; Stinson, Becker, & Sales, 2008; Worling, 1995). This variation depends on the accuracy of reporting, characteristics of the population sampled, and definitions of maltreatment. Little is known regarding the rates of maltreatment or abuse once these offenders reach adulthood, but sexual assaults in prison and other facilities as far-too-common occurrences (e.g., Crossmaker, 1991; Guerino & Beck, 2011). Sex offenders who also present with symptoms of mental illness, cognitive or intellectual deficits, or backgrounds characterized by impoverished relationships and limited social support are even more likely to have encountered significant experiences of maltreatment (e.g., Firth et al., 2001; Stinson & Becker, 2011). Many individuals involved in sex offender treatment programming are also struggling with their own problems related to trauma and traumatic experiences.

Some clients find it difficult to deal with other aspects of sex offender treatment because of their own trauma issues. This appears to be particularly salient when an offender is asked to consider the impact of his or her behavior on his or her victims. Repeated emphasis on the harm they have caused to others can make them more aware of their own trauma, the impact of that trauma, and the guilt that they may feel as the result of causing another person to experience a similar event. Also, the repeated emphasis on the wrongness of their behaviors that characterizes many sex offender treatment approaches may in fact heighten their own awareness of the seriousness of what happened to them. This does not mean that clients with histories of trauma are to be excluded from treatment, but that treatment providers should at least be aware of potential problems and make early efforts to limit the aversiveness of treatment interventions. In rarer cases, it may not be possible for clients to fully engage in sex offender treatment until they have learned to more consistently cope with the thoughts, emotions, and urges associated with their trauma. Treatment providers will need to assess whether or not any individual client's trauma history is so pervasive and impactful as to render him or her unable to complete treatment until he or she has sufficient skills in place.

Should sex offender treatment include trauma work? Some SOS clients with histories of maltreatment will want to address trauma in therapy along with their sex offending issues. However, this is not a straightforward or easy process. Some clients do not want to discuss histories of abuse or maltreatment. They should not be forced to do so, as this could retraumatize some individuals. Some clients may want to discuss traumatic experiences, though they might lack the skills needed to cope with the resulting dysregulation. This point has also been made with regards to other forms of cognitive-behavioral intervention with populations sensitive to trauma issues (e.g., DBT for individuals with characteristics of borderline personality disorder) in that not all clients are immediately able to cope with the guilt, shame, anger, or other emotional responses in a functional and adaptive way at the outset of treatment. Clients must have the appropriate skills base to adequately monitor and self-manage trauma reactions before treatment providers presume to work with them in addressing their trauma.

So what should we do for clients with serious histories of trauma? First, treatment providers and other involved clinicians should complete a thorough assessment, not only related to the client's sexual offense, psychiatric needs, or other relevant criminogenic needs or responsivity factors, but also of (1) the nature of any abuse, maltreatment, or trauma that may have occurred in childhood, adolescence, or adulthood; (2) the seriousness and extent of such aversive experiences; (3) how this impacted the individual at the time and its continued impact today; (4) how this will affect participation in sex offender treatment; (5) whether or not being in a group of other similar sex offending individuals will exacerbate any lasting effects of traumatic experiences; (6) their willingness to engage in treatment interventions potentially related to their trauma history; (7) their own perceptions of how being a victim affects their behavior, interpersonal functioning, and treatment readiness; and (8) areas of skills deficits that may leave them vulnerable in dealing with trauma issues. Clearly, this is a highly individualized assessment process, and the majority of clients will still be able to participate meaningfully in treatment despite a history of abuse or maltreatment. Treatment providers should carefully evaluate each case prior to making decisions about treatment inclusion, appropriate group placement, therapist choice, and other factors related to the speed, length, and focus of sex offender treatment. Some helpful instruments to guide providers include the Trauma Symptom Inventory (Briere, 1995) and the Detailed Assessment of Posttraumatic Stress (DAPS; Briere, 2001).

Second, what do we do when clients want to address their trauma in treatment? SOS is a treatment that teaches clients about dysregulation and self-regulatory deficits to foster the development of more adaptive regulatory abilities, but does not specifically address trauma. Many of the modules assist clients in effectively self-monitoring and self-managing problematic moods, thinking patterns, interpersonal interactions, and urges and behaviors, some of which may result from traumatic experiences, though the emphasis is still primarily on sexual offending and other maladaptive behaviors. Individuals who want trauma therapy will have an additional set of treatment needs that are beyond the scope of sex offender treatment. If treatment providers feel that such therapy is appropriate, or that a client may eventually be ready for such an intervention, they may need to identify additional sources of support for such matters. We do not recommend supplemental sex offender treatment, but that individual therapy, group therapy, or other supportive group experiences may be offered in tandem with SOS to aid clients in coping more effectively with their trauma (e.g., trauma-focused CBT; Goodyear-Brown, Fitzgerald, & Cohen, 2012). Clients should also be allowed to voice their own preferences with regards to how trauma would best be addressed, though there will understandably be occasions (such as when clients have been told by others that they have to address their trauma) when treatment providers and clients disagree about their readiness for trauma work. In cases when a client feels he or she must work on trauma but seems emotionally unprepared or ill-equipped to cope with the resulting dysregulation, treatment providers can suggest a "wait and see" approach, encouraging clients to work on SOS skills development prior to making further decisions about their trauma needs.

IMPACT OF TRAUMA (SESSIONS 1–10)

Here clients will review what trauma is, its role in sexual offending, and general and specific impacts of traumatic experiences to learn how harmful or aversive experiences can facilitate dysregulation and interfere with adaptive coping. Treatment providers will be challenged to strike a balance between validating and normalizing reactions to trauma while not normalizing the actual event itself. It may be helpful to review the validation strategies described in Chapter 3 before proceeding with these discussions.

Clients will also have the opportunity to reflect upon and verbalize the impact of sex offending behaviors on their victims—often a component of measuring treatment progress and release planning. Remember that victim empathy is not necessarily a determinant of risk (e.g., Hanson & Harris, 1998; Hanson et al., 2007). Just because a client can appreciate the impact of sexual abuse on a victim does not lessen risk, though a client who is completely unable to understand the negative affects of sexual victimization might cause concern. An overview of these sessions is provided in Table 12.1.

The Basics of Trauma

We often take for granted the impression that clients know what trauma actually is. "Trauma" is often used synonymously with abuse or neglect, but there are many other types of traumatic experiences. Also, simply because an event or situation has the potential to be traumatic does not mean that everyone experiences a trauma reaction. The first step then is to discuss stress and experiences that the clients find stressful.

TABLE 12.1. Impact of Trauma (Sessions 1–10)

- The basics of trauma
  - Discussion of stress and stressful experiences
    - o Differences between positive and negative stressors
    - o Which types of negative stressors could also be traumatic?
    - o What differentiates traumatic from nontraumatic negative stressors?
  - What are characteristics of stressful or traumatic events?
- Being a victim of a traumatic experience
  - Clients list categories of traumatic experiences
  - General effects of trauma and victimization
    - o Who can be a victim?
    - o What are trauma's effects on a person's emotions, thoughts or beliefs, self-image or self-esteem, relationships, physical health, or behaviors?
    - o How long do these effects last?
    - o Can some people be okay after a traumatic event?
  - Personal reactions to trauma
    - o Clients reflect on their own experiences of trauma or extreme stress
      - □ Consequences of trauma on their overall functioning and other specific areas
      - □ Hypothetical effects (for those without substantive histories)
- Trauma and dysregulation
  - Clients relate specific types of dysregulation (emotions, thoughts, physiological sensations, interpersonal interactions, and urges or behaviors) with experiences of trauma or extreme stress
  - Treatment providers reinforce individualized nature of the trauma response

Obviously, not all stressful experiences are traumatic. But if clients can first conceptualize trauma as the result of certain intensely stressful experiences, they may more readily identify dysregulation within the context of a traumatic experience.

A useful activity is for clients to complete and discuss the Life Experiences Survey (Sarason, Johnson & Siegel, 1978), typically available online or in compilations of paper-and-pencil psychological self-assessments. (See Form 12.1 at the end of the chapter for a sample of this instrument for client use.) In this assessment, both positive and negative stressful experiences are described. Important life changes that are typically viewed as positive, like the birth of a child, finding a new job, or marriage, can still cause stress. Clients may have difficulty relating to this idea; many idealize or overvalue positive life events and minimize the stressors associated with them. Negative events, such as accidents, natural disasters, or victimization, are more easily viewed as stressful and potentially traumatic. The following topics can help lead this discussion: differences between positive and negative stressors, how a positive event can be stressful, which types of negative stressors could also be traumatic, and what differentiates traumatic from nontraumatic negative stressors (e.g., controllability, impact on the person, whether or not the experience is "normal").

It may also help for clients to discuss important characteristics of traumatic or stressful events, like whether or not the event is an acute or chronic stressor, relationships with other persons involved in the stressful or traumatic event, special circumstances that made it a more serious stressor (e.g., being homeless after a natural disaster vs. being temporarily relocated vs. being seriously injured), and other factors like perceived controllability, predictability, or preventability. Considering these variables will help clients decide if any given stressor is traumatic, or if people can suffer long-term effects of such an incident.

Being a Victim of a Traumatic Experience

In Module 2 clients briefly discussed the effect of sexual trauma on victims. We now expand that discussion to include other forms of abuse, neglect, trauma, or maltreatment, many of which have been described in the previous discussion of stressful life events and traumatic experiences. Clients should again name several major categories of traumatic events, such as physical or sexual abuse, neglect, crime victimization, natural disasters, witnessing a violent act, sudden and unexpected loss of a loved one through violence, or other catastrophic experiences.

General effects of trauma and victimization. Clients should address the following questions or discussion points with regards to the examples they have listed:

1. *Who can be a victim?* Make sure clients understand that children, adolescents, adults, relationships partners, and so on, can be victims of abuse, neglect, or other traumatic experiences. Clients may assume that only young children, for example, are victims of abuse, forgetting that adults can be attacked and victimized by friends, family members, or even strangers, and that people residing within institutions who are victims of violence or sexual assault are also victims of trauma.

2. *What are trauma's effects on a person's emotions, thoughts or beliefs, self-image or self-esteem, relationships, physical health, or behaviors?* These points will be discussed at greater length later, within the context of dysregulation. But for now, it is important for clients to brainstorm the many areas of functioning that may be affected by different forms of traumatic experience. Clients may also need to think of these as a "domino effect." For example, physical violence that causes damage to the victim's health and physical well-being may also have a financial, occupational, or recreational impact in the long term, which can also affect relationships, self-esteem, and emotions.

3. *How long do these effects last?* This is highly variable and depends on any number of unique factors, including the circumstances of the traumatic experience, support, the person's resilience, and available resources. Clients should have some basic understanding that some experiences affect people rather acutely, or in the short term, while others affect them for many years to come.

4. *Can some people be okay after a traumatic event?* Obviously, yes. However, this question must be approached with caution. A key point is that reactions to trauma are highly individualized. We don't want to communicate the idea that trauma is okay or inconsequential, or that people do not suffer long-term effects from experiencing traumatic events. But the reality is that some people are more resilient than others, and that such persons may suffer few functional, emotional, or relationship impairments following traumatic stressors. Giving clients the impression that people are permanently or irreparably damaged after a negative life event can be very invalidating, particularly when clients have experienced such events themselves. While one would not necessarily argue that an individual now in sex offender treatment has successfully weathered a traumatic experience, we also do not want to negate hope. Helping

clients understand resilience factors, including available resources and support, therapeutic interventions, removal of an ongoing negative stressor, or unique strengths and self-regulatory abilities, can help them better conceptualize recovery or resilience following a traumatic event.

Personal Reactions to Trauma

If possible, have clients think about their own experiences that have been negative, aversive, or traumatic. Many clients in sex offender treatment have been victims of trauma during childhood or adolescence, or even as adults within the legal or mental health system. It is not necessary for clients to disclose their own experiences in any detail if they feel uncomfortable doing so. There may be additional reasons why they should not specifically describe their experiences, ranging from personal discomfort, to inability to cope, to potentially upsetting other clients who have experienced similar trauma but who are less able or willing to discuss it. Treatment providers should work with clients to determine their ability to participate in this section.

Willing clients should briefly list some of the consequences of their own trauma or victimization. Such consequences may include effects on their overall functioning, thinking, emotions, relationships, or other important areas. Clients who have not had experiences with trauma or maltreatment may choose to simply support others who voice such effects, or they may feel more comfortable supplying additional hypothetical examples of how trauma could impact them, were they to experience it.

This section of the module is not intended to serve as therapy for those with trauma. The goal is to highlight responses to trauma and help clients understand how it affects them. Referring clients for additional and supplemental treatment may be the outcome of these discussions. Clients who express a greater need to work on these issues in treatment should be given resources to help them do this. While this is not a major component of SOS, it may be relevant to behavioral improvement, enhancing their progress in treatment, and more effective functioning in other areas of their lives.

Trauma and Dysregulation

How do we link traumatic experiences to sexual offending and other forms of maladaptive behavior? Some clients will in fact ask, "Why would someone who suffered sexual abuse go on to abuse others themselves?

Don't they know better than anyone else how bad it is?" Clients have already discussed the different forms of dysregulation, and more recently have considered the effects of trauma that signal dysregulation or deficits in self-regulatory functioning. Clients should now think of dysregulation that occurs during and after the traumatic event: types of emotional responses a person has, his or her thoughts or self-perceptions, how he or she interacts with others, and urges or behaviors that may be associated with abuse. Some examples are provided below to facilitate client discussion:

- *Emotions*—fear, disgust, shame, guilt, anger, sadness, betrayal, or resentment.
- *Thoughts*—blame, judgment, confusion, worry, dissociation, or self-criticism.
- *Physiological sensations*—pain, numbness, shakiness, nausea, edginess, or extreme sympathetic nervous system responses like accelerated heartbeat, hyperventilation, or hyperarousal.
- *Interpersonal interactions*—isolation, hostility, irritability, overly sexual or promiscuous behavior, or aggression.
- *Urges and behaviors*—aggression, suicidality or self-harm, disordered eating or sleeping behaviors, substance abuse, or sexual acting out.

This kind of discussion more concretely links prior discussions of trauma and its effects with dysregulation and specific maladaptive behaviors. It aids clients in appreciating how trauma contributed to their own dysregulation, self-regulatory deficits, and patterns of maladaptive behavior. It will also help them better understand the individualized nature of responding to trauma, in that they will see that not everyone responds to trauma or dysregulation in the same manner, and that for some individuals maladaptive sexual behaviors or unhealthy relationship behaviors may result.

THINKING OF YOUR OWN PROBLEMATIC BEHAVIOR (SESSIONS 11–17)

This section of the module is divided into three basic areas: reactions to sexual offending, forgiveness, and acceptance. An outline of these areas is further described in Table 12.2. These discussions may be particularly difficult for many clients. Clients often enter treatment with

TABLE 12.2. Thinking of Your Own Problematic Behavior (Sessions 11–17)

Reactions to sexual offending
- Clients discuss their own and others' reactions to their sex offending behaviors
  - Why do you and others have that reaction?
  - Is that normal? Did you expect that? Is it fair?
  - Do you have any ability to change it?
  - Does it need to be changed, and if so, why?
  - Is it something you can learn to live with?

Forgiveness
- Clients discuss different meanings of forgiveness and how they view the concept
- Clients discuss beliefs about forgiveness that may interfere with treatment
  - Is forgiveness necessary?
  - What does it mean if someone does or does not forgive you?
  - Does forgiveness change the past?

Acceptance
- What is acceptance? What are different meanings of acceptance?
- Using examples from their own pasts, clients contrast acceptance with nonacceptance.
  - Long-term client goal: accept their past faults and behaviors.
- Discussion of ways to reach acceptance

an expectation that in order to feel better about themselves or to reduce their future risk, they must seek and obtain forgiveness. Few of them really understand the dynamics of forgiveness, or what is involved in learning to accept their past behaviors. Thus, the focus of this section of Module 8 guides them through this process but may leave them feeling even more ambivalent, and perhaps dysregulated, about themselves and their behaviors than before.

Reactions to Sexual Offending

In Module 1 clients compared societal perceptions of sexual offenders (e.g., only bad people do that, they should be punished, they're sick, they need treatment) with their own (e.g., it was a bad decision, they need treatment, they were victims of abuse). The purpose at that time was to give clients a chance to express their feelings and perceptions in a safe and validating environment, and also to cue treatment providers to potential barriers to openness in treatment for individual clients. In this module, we want clients to revisit this earlier **discussion**, focusing instead on reactions to their own offending rather than general societal views or their own nonspecific perceptions.

Clients will list emotions, beliefs, behaviors, or other reactions that people have had in response to their sexual offending. This list may include victims, victims' families, their own family members, friends, employers, educators, law enforcement agents, members of the criminal justice and correctional systems, or other people aware of their sex offending background. Similarly, clients will also list their emotions, beliefs, behaviors, or other reactions to their own offending. It may be helpful to compare lists, as there may be similarities. Also invite clients to compare what they have described with one another. The following questions may help them understand their own and others' reactions:

1. *Why do you and others have that reaction?* Reactions may be based on many factors, including prior experiences, societal norms, one's own beliefs or expectations of behavior, others' beliefs or expectations of behavior, specific features of the offense (e.g., severity or identity of the victim), whether or not such behavior has happened before, a history of other problematic behaviors, or things that the client may have said or done in response to being caught following the offense (e.g., justifications, blame toward the victim or others, denial of responsibility).

2. *Is that normal? In other words, did you expect that? Is it fair?* Sometimes people have reactions to an event that are fairly expected or normal. Being shocked, angry, disappointed, or afraid are common reactions that others have following sexual victimization, either as victims or as those who know victims. For clients, reactions of shame, guilt, self-directed anger or disappointment, or hopelessness might be typical. Believing that such a thing shouldn't have happened, that someone is to blame, or that someone should be punished are also common societal responses to sexual abuse. Clients may be more easily able to accept expected reactions, even though they are still painful in the moment. They may in fact be suspicious or feel greater shame when people do not react in an expected manner (e.g., a family member who forgives them rather easily). Also, clients in a group setting may react to others' offenses in an expected way. Have them articulate what this was like. For example, a client who describes his or her offense with indifference or little remorse may receive hostility or frustration from others. This is probably normal, though the client may not realize it in the moment.

3. *Do you have any ability to change it?* Clients typically want to "make it better." This could be making others less angry with them, decreasing their own sense of guilt and shame, or trying to avoid reminders or forget what happened. Clients may also want to solicit contact with victims to explain themselves, alleviate negative feelings, or ask for forgiveness. But the reality is that they have no control over how others feel, think, or otherwise react. And while they do have some control over their own reactions, there is still some inevitability in how they respond. They will (hopefully) feel guilt. This at least cues treatment providers that they can minimally appreciate the wrongfulness of their behaviors, even though they may engage in seemingly contradictory behaviors like denial or minimization of harm. They will also feel angry at themselves, or disappointed by consequences and damaged relationships. Though the impact of these feelings may diminish over time, one cannot forcibly change them.

4. *Does it need to be changed? If so, why?* This question is particularly difficult. Some common responses to sexual victimization are functional in terms of helping clients realize the impact of their behaviors, motivating them to change, and encouraging them to be respectful of victims' or others' boundaries. At times, however, their own extreme reactions may hamper their efforts to change, worsen the ability to effectively manage dysregulation, or increase dysregulation. Clients would need to address strong reactions that persist over time, become maladaptive, or are grossly disproportionate to what is expected. Excessive shame, depression, self-harm behaviors or suicidality, isolation or failure to form supportive relationships, or other similar reactions or outcomes may need to be addressed in treatment.

5. *Is it something you can learn to live with?* Some reactions are simply normative and expected, and may not be amenable to change. Clients cannot change how others feel, or whether or not their behaviors have irreparably damaged relationships. In that case, they will have to learn to live with it. Their own guilt is similar—they will need to learn to live with the knowledge of what they have done (i.e., acceptance). If change is possible, then they will need to consider repairing these relationships, a topic discussed at further length later in this module.

Forgiveness

When clients think about how their behavior affects others and their own self-esteem and emotional state, it is natural for them to hope that others will forgive them, and to want to solicit forgiveness from victims. They may struggle with understanding that victims don't want to forgive them, or that forgiveness does not absolve them of responsibility for their offending.

Forgiveness means many different things to different people, and in different cultures. Definitions or conceptualizations of forgiveness may involve religious or spiritual messages, or qualities and expectations associated with human relationships. Below are some interpretations or definitions of forgiveness—based on different cultural, spiritual, or religious beliefs—for clients to consider. (These same points are summarized in Form 12.2 at the end of the chapter.)

- Letting go of anger or resentment when you, or when someone else, does something that you think is wrong.
- Accepting that you, and others, are not perfect, and not dwelling on the imperfections.
- Letting go of hatred, or the desire for revenge.
- Showing mercy, compassion, and understanding.
- Peace and contentment with what you or others have, and what you or others have done in the past.
- Accepting someone's apology.
- Accepting someone's attempt to right a wrong.
- A sense of spiritual peace and acceptance toward yourself or another person after a wrong has been committed.
- Letting go of negative feelings toward yourself or another person.

Many clients will already have their own expectations about forgiveness, including what it means, why we do it, and how to forgive. Be sure to include these expectations in the discussion of the above statements.

Despite discussing these different viewpoints and aspects of forgiveness, many clients will likely maintain one or more fundamental beliefs about forgiveness related to their own sexual offending—that others should forgive them if they are sorry, that forgiveness absolves them of responsibility for future risk, or that they can never fully forgive themselves. These beliefs are problematic (or even dysregulated) since they can interfere with relationships, self-esteem, emotional state, and overall progress in treatment. Thus, several issues are still relevant. Is forgiveness necessary? What does it mean if someone does or does not forgive you? Does forgiveness change the past? Treatment providers need to adapt these discussions to the level of comprehension, responsivity, commitment and willingness, or progress of their clients. These are elemental beliefs about forgiveness that will influence acceptance and relationships with others. For clients who struggle with cognitive dysregulation in this area, pointing out examples of times when others have hurt them and expected forgiveness can illustrate the complexity of this process.

Acceptance

Acceptance is different from forgiveness. Acceptance is part of forgiveness; you have to accept in order to truly forgive. However, you don't have to forgive in order to accept. This is an important distinction for clients, especially as some will find it impossible to forgive themselves for their behaviors, or will acknowledge that they are unlikely to ever be forgiven by victims or others. Despite this situation, they can still develop acceptance. (This section is summarized in Form 12.3 at the end of the chapter.)

So what is acceptance? It can be several things, such as taking something as it is given to you, tolerating the moment for what it is, believing something to be true, or completely accepting or understanding reality as it is. Acceptance is without judgment, blame, or strong emotion. Acceptance is taking a situation for what it is. This is contrasted with what acceptance is *not:* trying to change the way things are, refusing to believe reality, or feeling strong emotions or judgments about the way something is.

Understanding the meaning of acceptance versus not acceptance may be easier if clients and treatment providers generate specific examples of real-world events that must be simply accepted, regardless of whether they feel right or wrong. On a basic level, you have to accept that you cannot control what other people do. Or that you can't accomplish all that you would like to do. On a more complex level, you may have to accept that bad things happen for no reason, that you can't go back and change the past, or that others may treat you unfairly or dislike you. Acceptance is a process, and clients will have to work toward this with time and effort.

A goal is for clients to learn to accept their past behaviors and past faults. Some people believe that sex offenders should continually dwell on the wrongs they have done, but this does not necessarily lead to lasting change or improvement in self-regulatory ability, and may in fact increase dysregulation and isolation from effective social support. Improved self-regulation and social support are known factors in the prevention of future sexually violent behaviors (e.g., Hanson & Harris, 1998; Hanson et al., 2007) and are goals of SOS. Acceptance of past offending does not mean that it did not happen, that it wasn't wrong, or that clients are not responsible for their behaviors. Treatment providers may have to work on their own acceptance, as we often struggle with telling clients to accept their past offending behaviors. Again, this does not mean that we believe their behaviors are acceptable in a moral sense, but only that we accept that they happened and must be dealt with in treatment.

Reaching acceptance involves new skills and abilities. These may seem fairly abstract and highly cognitive, but clients should be able to relate to at least a few of them.

- Look at what you have in the present, without dwelling on the past or worrying about the future.
- Find your compassion.
- Look for your denial and unwillingness, and let go of it.
- Be open to what others can teach you.
- Separate acceptance from your emotions. Getting "stuck" in a state of anger will prevent you from being able to accept reality as it is.
- Let go of your judgment, blame, and resentment.
- Let go of shame, even if the guilt remains.
- Practice humility.
- Let go of being "right."
- Embrace the parts of you that are flawed, imperfect, or unique.

Acceptance is a major step for most clients. It may take much longer to accept themselves and their offenses than they have time for in active treatment. There will be frustrations for treatment providers as well—some clients do not see anything wrong with their behavior and can therefore easily "accept" it. For others, they readily accept offenses because they have internally minimized the harm caused to others. It may take reminders that this does not negate responsibility, imply that they are "cured," or mean that their victims have forgiven or forgotten past hurts. These frustrations and expressions of client "acceptance" are further indicators of a client's level of willingness to change and progress in treatment. Do not let this detract from the others' treatment gains.

REPAIRING RELATIONSHIPS (SESSIONS 18–20)

By now, most clients should have some awareness of the damage caused by sexual crimes and harmful sexual behaviors. Though some may still deny or minimize the full impact of their behaviors, others are more aware of how they have hurt others and of the need for trying to mend

TABLE 12.3. Repairing Relationships (Sessions 18–20)

- The damage of sexual offending
  - Clients describe ways that their sex offending behaviors have damaged others (e.g., victims, family members, friends, community)
- Why repair relationships?
  - Clients think of reasons why it is important to repair a relationship that has been damaged, using both non-sex-offending and sex offending examples
  - Review of some Module 7 concepts, like why relationships are important, different types of relationships, and characteristics of healthy and unhealthy relationships
- How do we repair relationships?
  - Clients describe what they think repairs are, and what this process would look like
  - Ideally, who would clients address to make repairs to these relationships?
  - Clients review several methods of repairing family and community relationships

internal, interpersonal, and community damage. (See Table 12.3 for an overview of this process.)

The Damage of Sexual Offending

Before discussing reparations, clients will need to briefly review the impact of their sex offending behaviors on relationships with others. These discussions may be difficult for clients. Some do not value relationships with others, some minimize the damage or harm they have caused, and some experience intense feelings of shame and guilt that hamper their ability to openly address these issues. Furthermore, some clients may have to accept the reality that they can never truly repair certain relationships or fix the damage they have done. Treatment providers can use several techniques to facilitate such discussions, including motivational interviewing strategies, validation, extending, playing the devil's advocate, and other such methods. This will help clients manage their own emotional and cognitive dysregulation and gently challenge their "stuckness" or defensiveness in talking about their own role in causing damage to important relationships.

Why Repair Relationships?

Clients will present with different levels of willingness to repair relationships. First, think of reasons why they might want to repair damaged relationships. How important is the relationship? How serious was the behavior or harm done? What are the implications of the relationship remaining damaged? What are the potential benefits of trying to restore the relationship? Clients may be better able to answer these questions with a neutral example at first, such as one unrelated to their sexual offending. Thinking of relationship repair using a less personal serious behavior may decrease defensiveness, shame, and hostility.

It may also help to reference Module 7 (Chapter 11) discussions describing why relationships are important, characteristics of healthy versus unhealthy relationships, and different types of relationships. Sometimes, for example, the need to repair a relationship depends on the type of relationship, whether or not it was healthy, or if it is worth repairing. This becomes more complicated when clients provide an example in which they and the other person both need to repair damage (i.e., the victim or other person affected also engaged in some unhealthy behavior). This is an important distinction, as clients are not always responsible for every negative interaction that occurs in a relationship. However, some clients will take this too far, saying the victim "owes" them an apology for reporting their offending behavior, or should apologize for "prompting" the offense. If this should happen, it will be difficult for treatment providers and other clients to tolerate such statements. Keep in mind that this is an example of cognitive dysregulation, and serves as a measure of the client's treatment progress, or lack thereof. To respond, treatment providers should emphasize negative feelings still remaining as a result of damage to the relationship (e.g., "It sounds like you're still pretty angry at them for what happened, and that may interfere with your willingness to make repairs"), and remind clients that we can only repair our own behaviors. We cannot force others to repair what we think has been damaged. Depending on the client's openness and commitment, it can also be helpful to provide feedback about how much he or she is able to accept responsibility for unhealthy relationship behavior.

How Do We Repair Relationships?

Clients need to think about what this process will look like. Will it take time? How will trust, others' feelings about them and their behaviors, their own feelings, and others' expectations change as they try to make amends? What are realistic expectations concerning this process? Are there times when they cannot repair the damage, or when it won't be possible to ever address the person or persons toward whom they have caused damage?

At this stage of treatment, we may need to challenge clients' perceptions of forgiveness and repairing relationships. Clients can have a rather simplistic expectation that apologizing for their behavior makes amends or reduces harm. Apologizing to the victim is encouraged in other forms of treatment, frequently in the way of an apology letter, in order to demonstrate empathy and to take responsibility for one's behavior. Clients then expect that this is both necessary and sufficient for victim forgiveness. In reality, an apology means more to the offender than to the victim, and may in fact cause more damage. The behaviors are often too extreme for a mere apology. And most apologies include some element of an explanation, which may fall flat to someone who has been seriously harmed. So overall, an apology is not going to serve as reparation. However, the desire to apologize is not completely irrelevant. If a client feels no need to apologize, this tells us a great deal about that individual's progress in treatment, potential risk to others, interpersonal dysregulation, and ability to develop healthy relationships. Developing an apology can also be an important step toward self-forgiveness. Moreover, when clients have victimized family members who later desire reunification, such efforts to apologize may be an important component of this process.

On occasion, clients will be able to make repairs directly to their victims, particularly if the victims were family members or somehow associated with members of the offenders' families. However, as is often the case, victims will sever any ties or communication with the clients. This could be because they were strangers prior to the offense, but more often it is as a result of the severity and harmfulness of their behavior. Clients may also need to make repairs to society in general, as many are impacted by sexual violence in indirect ways and can be reassured or comforted by methods of reducing harm. Some suggestions are listed below for clients to consider, and they should be encouraged to think of other reparations.

- *Participate and work in treatment.* This demonstrates an appreciation of the harm that was caused and an effort to ensure that such behavior does not recur.

- *Strive for adaptive and healthy behavior.* This can demonstrate a sincere effort to change and an appreciation for harm caused to others.

- *Give others time, distance, or space.* Sometimes victims or others impacted by sexual violence want separation from the offender, even if they indicate that it's not a permanent separation (e.g., family members who were victimized but who wish to maintain minimal contact).

Respecting this desire for time to heal, distance, or psychological space can show victims that the offender is trying to be considerate of their needs and desires.

• *Give back to the community.* In cases when it is not possible, advisable, or desirable to repair relationships with specific victims, clients may wish to do something beneficial for the community. It may be meaningful for them to give back to those who are victims of other trauma, such as contributing to a domestic violence shelter, providing supplies for disaster relief organizations, or other such efforts. In one agency for adolescent sexual offenders in New Jersey, for example, clients sew quilts and blankets for children in domestic violence shelters, and learn about victims of domestic violence and child abuse (DonGiovanni & Travia, 2007).

• *Educate others.* Clients can educate others about relevant topics, including mental illness, violence, seeking treatment or help, substance abuse, or victimization. This does not necessarily have to be an educational effort in which they identify themselves as sex offenders, but as persons who wish others to understand the impact of relevant behaviors or conditions.

Clients may need to make multiple efforts to repair damage to others, and it still might not result in actual improvement in their relationships or help for the victims. It is not, however, an empty effort. Such efforts highlight the importance of relationships, ways in which relationships and other persons are damaged by their behaviors, and the sometimes laborious efforts needed to heal others' wounds and hurts. Clients will also find that healing takes time, and it may never result in completely restored trust or a fully repaired relationship. Nor will working toward self-forgiveness ever completely absolve them of guilt. But moving toward acceptance, forgiveness, and repaired relationships fosters adaptive emotional, cognitive, interpersonal, and behavioral regulatory strategies.

MODULE 8 CONCLUDING SESSIONS

In this module, clients have addressed issues related to stress and trauma, acceptance and forgiveness, and repairing damaged relationships. This module is critical for helping them understand and come to terms with their behaviors and recognizing the impact of their behaviors on others.

Also, realizing limitations in their ability to solicit acceptance and forgiveness from others, or to change the past, assists them in using adaptive strategies in a more focused and skillful way. Again, we recommend reviewing the "My Treatment Progress" handout in Appendix B to help clients relate Module 8 concepts to their progress and goals. Clients who do not value the concepts in this module will present with more limited insight into their own risk, suggesting that they may be at greater risk of future problematic or maladaptive sexual behaviors. Treatment providers may also complete this module with recommendations for additional trauma therapy for clients in need of such intervention.

Stressful Life Experiences

Below are listed a number of life experiences that may cause some people stress. Some of these are negative life events, while some of them are positive life changes. Even positive changes may cause some people to feel stress. Think about your own life and check whether or not this is a current or past stressor, or both.

	In the past year	More than 1 year ago
Death of a close family member (e.g., parent, spouse, child, or sibling)		
Divorce or marital separation		
Detention in jail or other institution		
Major personal injury, illness, or change in mental health status		
Marriage		
Being fired from work		
Major change in health or behavior of a family member		
Sexual difficulties		
Major change in financial state		
Death of a close friend		
Moving or changing living conditions		
Having troubles with family members		
Major change in type or amount of recreation		
Major change in church or spiritual activities		
Major change in social activities		
Change in medications or daily schedule		
Major change in sleeping habits		
Major change in eating habits		
Being a victim of violent behavior		
Witnessing violent behavior		

What Is Forgiveness?

Many different cultures have defined forgiveness—sometimes using religious or spiritual meaning and sometimes focusing on human relationships. Some thoughts on forgiveness are described below. Discuss these as a group and learn what forgiveness means to you.

- Letting go of anger or resentment when you or someone else does something you think is wrong

- Accepting that you and others are not perfect, and not dwelling on their imperfections

- Letting go of hatred or the desire for revenge

- Showing mercy, compassion, and understanding

- Peace and contentment with what you or others have and have not done

- Accepting the apology of another

- Accepting someone's attempt to right a wrong

- A sense of spiritual peace and acceptance toward yourself or another after a wrong has been committed

- To let go of negative feelings toward yourself or another person

How Can I Reach Acceptance?

Many forms of therapy and treatment, as well as spiritual traditions, suggest that healing happens through a process of *acceptance*. But there are varying beliefs about what acceptance is and how to get there. Below is a discussion of what acceptance is, as well as what it isn't—removing many of the value judgments (good vs. bad) that are linked to this concept. This discussion can help you figure out how to reach acceptance about your own past and past behaviors.

What *is* acceptance?
- Taking something that has been given to you
- Believing something to be true
- Completely understanding and accepting reality as it is

What *isn't* acceptance?
- Trying to change the way things are
- Refusing to believe reality or what you have been given
- Feeling good or bad about the way something is

How is acceptance different from forgiveness?
- Acceptance is part of forgiveness. You have to accept in order to truly forgive. But you don't have to forgive in order to accept.

How do I get there?
- Look at what you have in the present, without dwelling on the past or worrying about the future.
- Find your compassion.
- Look for your denial, and let go of it.
- Be open to what others have to teach you.
- Separate acceptance from the emotions you may feel about the situation. Getting "stuck" in a state of anger will prevent you from being able to accept the situation by itself.
- Let go of judgment and accept the situation as it is.

CHAPTER 13

MODULE 9

Making Good Choices

Managing Urges and Behavior in a Healthy Way

Once clients and treatment providers have completed Modules 1 through 8, clients have explored their commitment to treatment; learned basic treatment concepts; discussed dysregulation and self-regulatory deficits within the context of their problematic sexual behaviors; learned about emotional, cognitive, and interpersonal dysregulation; discussed sexual development and relationships; and addressed the impact of their behaviors on themselves and others. Now, prior to the conclusion of current treatment programming or decisions about ongoing treatment, clients will review and integrate new self-monitoring and self-regulatory strategies learned through treatment.

In this chapter, clients will focus on several broad goals. One such goal is to evaluate their decision-making processes, including how decisions impact behavior, and how their decision making has changed since the initiation of treatment efforts. Another goal is for clients to update their self-monitoring needs and progress toward adaptive skills building. This goal also directs them toward the final components of treatment, when they develop continuing treatment goals and an aftercare plan. Clients will also learn how to cope ahead. This module helps clients integrate strategies that they have learned throughout treatment. Thinking of these concepts and accomplishments together, along with describing their ongoing commitment, encourages them to maintain important changes, build a support system consistent with their goals and life changes, and seek additional forms of intervention and help.

OUR DECISIONS, OUR BEHAVIOR (SESSIONS 1–10)

By now, clients have a fairly good idea of the behaviors being targeted for change. These include a variety of sexual behaviors, as well as interpersonal relationship behaviors and improved use of strategies or skills to help them better cope with dysregulation. Clients are also describing and discussing these behaviors on a weekly basis as part of their self-monitoring activities, and reviewing their progress at the end of each module. They can now discuss these behaviors within the context of decisions and decision making. We have consistently conceptualized their sexual offending and other harmful or unhealthy behaviors as maladaptive strategies. But these behaviors also represent decisions reinforced over time, and reflect the many decisions involved in their attempts to self-regulate. The activities and discussions in this section are summarized in Table 13.1.

TABLE 13.1. Our Decisions, Our Behavior (Sessions 1–10)

- Decisions and behavior
  - Clients give examples of recent decisions and how they have impacted others
  - What affects decision making?
    - Clients discuss factors that influence their everyday decisions, including experiences, past choices, past and current emotions, self-perceptions, perceptions and judgments of others, beliefs about how others view them, expectations, urges, opportunities, and available resources and support.
  - How do decisions affect behavior?
    - Clients describe how urges are related to decisions and behavior.
    - Clients should give examples of both good and bad decision making. What were the intended consequences of those decisions? What were the unintended consequences? How did these decisions have positive or negative effects on others?
    - Clients describe their behaviors that were the most positive/helpful and the most negative/harmful.
  - Relationships and decision making—clients give examples of role models for both adaptive and maladaptive decision making and behavior.
- Role of self-monitoring in decisions and behavior
  - As clients review their self-monitoring activities throughout treatment, think about each area of dysregulation they monitored. Did they make changes or achieve noticeable progress?

Decisions and Behavior

Every decision we make impacts our own behavior and sometimes the behaviors of others. Have each client give an example of a decision that he or she made today and how it impacted him or her and other people. For example, clients made the decision to come to group, or to attend a therapy session. How does that decision affect the client, the group leader or treatment provider, other clients, or members of the client's support group? How does that decision affect persons in charge of monitoring their progress and risk? How does that decision influence future behaviors, or impact potential victims? Group leaders can also give examples from their own experiences to help illustrate these points. So, for example, group leaders may talk about their own decision to provide treatment that day, and how this decision affects the client, those who depend on treatment being available, and others. During the course of this exercise, clients will give examples of decisions that had a positive effect on others, as well as examples of decisions that may have had a negative or harmful effect. Importantly, they should recognize that not all "positive" decisions are positive for everyone, just as not all "negative" decisions result in negative outcomes or harm to others.

What Affects Decision Making?

So far in treatment, we have heavily emphasized the role of dysregulation, self-regulatory deficits, and reinforcement or functionality (i.e., whether or not a behavior "works") in understanding how clients have acted in the past as well as how they continue to behave in the present. But how do they ultimately make decisions? How do these same factors—dysregulation; deficits in emotional, cognitive, interpersonal, and behavioral self-regulation; and environmental opportunities and reinforcement—contribute to their everyday decision making? Now is when clients will tie these concepts together and start thinking about how they will mindfully choose adaptive strategies over more maladaptive ones. Knowing how they made past decisions can help them make better decisions in the present and future. Some points to include are listed in Table 13.2.

For the above discussion, have clients share their experiences with making both good and bad decisions, as well as how these decisions have impacted others. Each client should be able to give an example of a good decision he or she has recently made, and a bad decision he or she made in the past. What were the intended consequences of those decisions? What were the unintended consequences? How did these decisions have

TABLE 13.2. What Affects Decision Making?

- *Past experiences.* How do their past experiences with relationships, sexual behavior, dysregulation, or other factors impact the decisions that they make now?

- *Past choices.* Sometimes clients may make a choice or decision simply because this is what they have "always" done, or because it is what has worked for them before.

- *Past and current emotions.* Emotional experiences can be very powerful. Refer to Module 3 discussions of emotions and risky emotional states as a resource for helping clients see how their emotional states influence decision making.

- *Self-perceptions.* Clients' views of themselves, whether in a negative, neutral, or inflated and overly positive light, impact their decisions about interpersonal interactions and relationships.

- *Perceptions and judgments of others.* How they view others, including their judgments of others' behaviors and choices as good versus bad, can also influence their decisions in relationships.

- *Beliefs about how others view them.* Clients also have ideas about how others view them, and these ideas can have a strong hold on how they treat others and what they ultimately decide to do. If they think others view them negatively, don't trust them, or don't care about them, clients will make choices accordingly. Their choices will be vastly different than if they think the other person loves, trusts, and wants the best for them.

- *Expectations.* Clearly, what you expect is going to play a significant role in your decisions and related behaviors. This also affects your perceptions of yourself and others, and how you think others should view you.

- *Urges in the moment.* People often underestimate the strength of urges, including urges of a sexual, aggressive, hostile, avoidant, or controlling nature. These urges could be very strong, or they may be so automatic as to be rarely noticed in relation to decisions and behaviors.

- *Opportunity.* Many rational decisions are based on an internal survey of available opportunities. Perceived opportunity is based on prior experiences and goals and is therefore highly idiosyncratic to the individual. What one person perceives as an opportunity may appear irrational, bizarre, or problematic to another person.

- *Available resources and support.* Knowing that you have alternative resources or sources of support available can dramatically change your decisions, or at least influence your perception of available options.

positive or negative effects on others? As they reflect upon what influenced their decision making, ask them to consider how much forethought they gave to the potential impact of such decisions? Obviously, we think that potential consequences should influence our choices. However, in the moment, the consequences of a decision may seem more remote or less salient than potential gain or other factors.

How Do Decisions Affect Behavior?

Clients should also think about how their decisions ultimately lead to their behavior. How are decisions related to urges? In some cases, urges precede and strongly influence decisions. In others, making a decision solidifies or intensifies an urge. Often, then, an urge combined with a strong decision and other related factors (like intense emotions, prior experience, or potential reinforcement) leads to behavior. For example, if a client decides that he or she wants to "get back" at someone, this decision, combined with a strong sexual urge or an urge to humiliate or hurt someone, facilitates harmful behavior directed toward that person. On the other hand, a decision to be helpful, combined with the urge to talk to someone or do him or her a favor, can lead to more adaptive behaviors or healthy contributions to a relationship.

Which behaviors do clients feel are their most positive, or the most beneficial? This choice could include behaviors that are helpful, supportive, or productive, or that demonstrate adaptive and skillful regulatory strategies. They probably reflect the client's healthy decision-making processes, and the client may be able to describe these processes more specifically by using examples. Likewise, what behaviors do they think have been the most negative, or the most harmful to themselves and others? (They are most likely to name offenses or other problematic behaviors, including those that led to their inclusion in treatment, though treatment providers can encourage them to think more broadly in terms of other negative behaviors.) How are these negative or harmful behaviors linked to negative or harmful decision making? Again, tying their decisions to specific behavioral examples will more clearly illustrate such concepts.

Relationships and Decision Making

Clients should also prepare themselves to think about the influence of interpersonal relationships on their decisions and behaviors. They can do this by answering the following questions:

1. "What persons in your life have been positive role models for good decision making?"
2. "Who are the people in your life who served as role models for harmful behaviors?"
3. "Did some people model both helpful and harmful decision making?"
4. "How did these relationships impact the decisions and behaviors related to your sexual offending?"

This discussion again helps clients consolidate what they have learned about the interactions between emotions, thoughts or decisions, relationships, urges, and ultimately, behavior.

During such discussions of decisions and behavior, treatment providers may find it necessary to troubleshoot certain problem areas. First, some clients will categorize their decisions and behaviors as either "all good" or "all bad." Although we have collapsed these outcomes into similar categories during this section of the module, this was done mostly for ease of communication. Rarely is it ever so simple that decisions are either just bad or just good. Some appear inherently bad, particularly when they involve harm toward the self or others. But the "badness" of a decision rests on a continuum, and some decisions are worse than others, and some will have a more negative impact than others. Clients will find that many decisions are neutral or ambiguous. This finding will prompt them to think about other variables that factor into their decision-making and behavioral choices. Second, clients can oversimplify what to do about decisions that lead to problematic behaviors—just don't have them. This view of how to improve decision making and behavior is too one-dimensional. Treatment providers will need to emphasize the idea that clients will always make bad decisions—this is just normal human behavior. It is more effective to think about how to make better (though maybe still imperfect) decisions and how to control other environmental, interpersonal, and internal factors in the process. Third, clients will point out that making better decisions is not the only solution to improving behavior. This is true. Clients may have every intention of making better decisions, but if they lack the resources, knowledge, and opportunity to do so, this will not work. Clients will need to learn new strategies and develop sources of social support in tandem with their desire to improve decision-making processes. Fourth, we have emphasized the importance of positive and negative role models. As some clients will note, they may perceive little choice in their role models. If they come from highly dysfunctional families or interact most often with those who make poor decisions or engage in maladaptive behavior, they may have limited ability or willingness to disengage from such relationships. It may also be true that they have few opportunities for developing strong prosocial bonds, given their own self-regulatory deficits, interpersonal skills deficits, and the stigma associated with sexual offending, mental illness, disabilities, or the like. An important treatment goal for such persons is to develop strong boundaries in unhealthy relationships with family members or persons in their primary support group, develop a strong sense of self (including values, goals, etc.), and to foster prosocial and healthy sources of support.

Role of Self-Monitoring in Decisions and Behavior

Important components of SOS are self-monitoring and self-management. As clients have progressed through modules describing emotional, cognitive, and interpersonal dysregulation, as well as sexual urges and behaviors, they have likely made changes to their self-monitoring practices that reflect changes in their treatment needs and goals. For this part of the module, clients will need to review their self-monitoring activities throughout treatment. Which risky emotional states did they monitor? Types of cognitive dysregulation? Problematic interpersonal behaviors or boundaries? How have these shaped their personal goals throughout the treatment process, and where are they with those goals and self-monitoring activities now? Treatment providers will want to help clients relate their self-monitoring practices to actual changes in behavior, ways of thinking about behavior, or daily decision making. Clients should also describe how self-monitoring has improved their ability to recognize and work with strong emotions, uncomfortable thoughts, or unhealthy relationship behaviors (i.e., dysregulation).

SKILLS BUILDING: RECOGNIZING ADAPTIVE VERSUS MALADAPTIVE SKILLS (SESSIONS 11–13)

By now, clients understand important differences between adaptive and maladaptive skills. To review, adaptive skills are functional, effective, and do not cause harm to oneself or others, whereas maladaptive skills may also be functional and effective but at the same time they present the possibility of harm. Both types of strategies promise the alleviation of intense emotional, cognitive, or interpersonal discomfort, but only one of them results in adaptive and truly healthy behavior. Clients can give examples of both kinds of strategies—adaptive and maladaptive—from their own experiences and discussions throughout the course of SOS. (This exercise is outlined in Table 13.3.)

Maladaptive Strategies

To more easily recognize and categorize their maladaptive skills, clients should list examples of maladaptive strategies related to strong emotions, interpersonal stress, or cognitive dysregulation. For example, strong emotions like anger, paranoia, sadness, boredom, or loneliness may elicit physical aggression, sexual coercion, or substance abuse. Problematic thoughts like blame, judgment, racing thoughts, or delusional beliefs may lead to verbal aggression or threats, impulsive behaviors, and self-harm. Uncomfortable interpersonal interactions or unhealthy relationship behaviors, like lying, manipulation, arguing, or isolation from others, could lead to sexual aggression or impulsive behaviors meant to cause harm to someone else. Finally, intense or uncomfortable urges—often classified as behavioral dysregulation—like sexual urges, aggressive urges, or self-harm urges, can facilitate problem behaviors or offense-supportive behaviors. These urges can also prompt other maladaptive strategies, such as deviant sexual fantasies or substance abuse, that subsequently disinhibit the client and precipitate harmful behavior. (A sample client handout to facilitate this discussion is provided in

---

TABLE 13.3. Skills Building: Recognizing Adaptive versus Maladaptive Skills (Sessions 11–13)

- Maladaptive strategies
  - Clients list examples of maladaptive strategies related to strong emotions, interpersonal stress, or cognitive dysregulation.
  - How do dysregulated behavioral urges lead to the use of maladaptive strategies?
  - What are the characteristics of maladaptive strategies?
- Adaptive strategies
  - What are the characteristics of adaptive strategies?
  - Role models for adaptive skills use
    - o Who are people in your past who are like this?
    - o What adaptive skills or strategies did you learn from them?
    - o Who are the people in your current environment or support system who are like this and who use adaptive skills?
  - Clients discuss role models who may use both adaptive and maladaptive skills

---

Figure 13.1, with a blank version for the client in Form 13.1 at the end of the chapter.)

What are the characteristics of maladaptive strategies? In other words, how do we know that a strategy is maladaptive? Factors like harm to self or others, increased negative emotions or interactions, boundary violations, negative responses from the environment, and so on, are all relevant signs. When clients are able to clearly and specifically describe the features of maladaptive strategies that actually make them maladaptive, they will be better prepared to recognize maladaptive strategies in the future. The reality is that even if they use adaptive over maladaptive strategies on a regular basis, they will still be exposed to new strategies all the time. Some of these new strategies will be maladaptive, and because they are unfamiliar, clients may not immediately recognize them as such. We want to equip clients with the ability to make better decisions and use more adaptive skills both now and in the future.

Adaptive Strategies

Similarly, what are the characteristics of adaptive strategies? These characteristics are more abstract because one cannot simply define them as "not harmful." But generally, adaptive skills improve self-image, strengthen supportive relationships with others, facilitate stable and positive emotions, and gradually increase tolerance of dysregulation over time. This is another opportunity for clients to review many of the strategies that they have learned throughout treatment, and to describe how they have applied and practiced these strategies over time. Group leaders can validate clients' continuing feelings of frustration with strong urges related to maladaptive behaviors, or any lingering sense of unfamiliarity with newly learned adaptive strategies.

The development of adaptive skills requires effort as well as exposure to people who are positive and healthy role models. One way to learn adaptive skills is to view and model the behaviors of those people who are respected, liked by their peers, and who are helpful and show empathy and compassion for others. Have clients discuss the following: Who are people in your past who are like this? What adaptive skills or strategies did you learn from them? Who are the people in your current environment or support system who are like this and who use adaptive skills?

Clients should also be aware of those persons from whom they have learned maladaptive skills or behaviors. In some cases, these are the same

Sometimes people do harmful, dangerous, or risky things when they feel strong emotions, are in unhealthy relationships, have problems with their thoughts, or experience intense urges. Below, list several maladaptive or problematic behaviors from your past that may be connected to these. Some examples are provided from prior modules to help you out.

Strong emotions—anger, loneliness, boredom, paranoia, etc.

- Physical aggression
- Drug abuse
- Masturbating while peeping in the neighbors' windows

Problems with my thoughts—blame, judgment, racing thoughts, or delusional beliefs

- Making threats or ultimatums
- Self-harm or suicide attempts
- Isolating myself from others

Uncomfortable interactions or unhealthy relationships—arguing, manipulation, lying, or isolation

- Doing something impulsive, like property destruction, to hurt somebody
- Being sexually violent
- Making threats of violence

Intense or uncomfortable urges—sexual urges, aggressive urges, self-harm urges, etc.

- Drug abuse
- Sexual fantasies about children
- Sleeping all the time

FIGURE 13.1. Sample client worksheet—"On the Lookout for Maladaptive Behaviors."

people from whom they learned adaptive strategies, too. (Clients sometimes want to put people in only one, black-and-white category.) Treatment providers should keep in mind that this is common—many people engage in a combination of both adaptive and maladaptive strategies, but that just how adaptive or maladaptive the strategies are, and the balance between them, exists on a continuum and is highly individualized. For clients, this is a complex problem. Think about their developmental history: important caregivers and family members, peers, and others have evidenced both adaptive and maladaptive coping strategies. Because of these relationships, they are likely to have continued contact with such individuals. This will make it difficult for them to continue learning and using adaptive strategies in their primary environment, to refrain from falling into old habits with maladaptive behaviors, and to be reinforced for adopting healthier and more skillful behaviors.

REVIEWING SKILLFUL BEHAVIOR (SESSIONS 14–18)

In Modules 3, 6, and 7, clients reviewed emotional, cognitive, and interpersonal dysregulation. Along the way, they also learned other valuable concepts related to sexuality (e.g., sexual development and expression), boundaries and healthy relationships, and acceptance and forgiveness related to past harm. Our goal now is to consolidate what clients have learned about skillful behavior and adaptive regulatory strategies from these discussions (see Table 13.4 for an overview).

Emotion Regulation Strategies

Emotional dysregulation is a common and normal occurrence, though some people struggle more with the intensity of their emotions, sensitivity to negative emotionality, and coping with strong emotions in a skillful manner. Earlier in Module 3, we identified three primary types of emotion regulation skills: those that prevent or protect from vulnerability to strong emotions, those that help distract you from your emotions in the moment, and those designed to soothe or diminish intense emotional experiences. Specific strategies described in Chapter 7 include the following:

1. Self-monitoring
2. Awareness of triggers

TABLE 13.4. Reviewing Skillful Behavior (Sessions 14–18)

- Emotion regulation strategies
  - Clients review the emotion regulation strategies from Chapter 7, including those that they generally use.
  - Skills practice
    - Which skills worked? Which ones didn't? Under what circumstances were these emotion regulation skills more or less effective?
- Cognitive regulation strategies
  - Clients review the cognitive regulation strategies from Chapter 10, including those that they generally use.
  - Skills practice
    - What worked? What didn't? Why? How did these strategies "feel" different than using emotion regulation strategies?
- Interpersonal regulation strategies
  - Clients review the interpersonal strategies discussed in Chapter 11, including others that they tried.
    - What worked? What didn't? What happened when the other person did not react like you wanted? Did these strategies help maintain important relationships or improve stressful interactions with others?
- Behavioral regulation strategies
  - How did clients deal with strong behavioral urges, or dysregulated behaviors? What strategies did they use to cope?

3. Reducing vulnerability to triggers (e.g., sleeping and eating as needed, managing stress)
4. Pleasurable replacement activities (e.g., hobbies, self-rewards)
5. Distracting yourself
6. Doing something inconsistent with the emotional state (e.g., anger = helping someone; sad = watching a comedy; lonely = calling a friend)
7. Taking a self-imposed "time-out": may include relaxation, breathing exercises, mindfulness, prayer, etc.
8. Calming activities meant to soothe strong emotions (e.g., listening to soft music, sitting in a dark or dimly lit room and breathing slowly, taking a hot shower or warm bath)
9. Physical activity or exercise
10. Intense physical sensations (e.g., breathing in very cold air, holding ice, listening to loud music, controlled muscle tension exercises)

Clients should review their experiences with practicing and using these skills. Which skills worked? Which ones didn't? Under what circumstances were these emotion regulation skills more or less effective? Also, have clients identify additional skills that they have found useful in modulating their strong emotional states.

Cognitive Regulation Strategies

In Module 6, clients reviewed various types of cognitive dysregulation, ranging from distressing or problematic thought content to difficulties with thought processing. Some experiences of cognitive dysregulation are more common than others, thus making them a challenge for clients to recognize, monitor, and address through skillful coping. Adaptive regulatory strategies for cognitive dysregulation also involved three types of skills: recognizing and monitoring cognitive dysregulation, distracting from dysregulated thoughts, or working through problematic thought patterns in a logical way (i.e., cognitive restructuring). The strategies described in Chapter 10 include the following:

1. Self-monitoring
2. Mindfulness—allowing a thought to be a thought: A great deal of emerging literature suggests that mindfulness activities can be highly effective in helping clients learn to effectively manage a variety of cognitive and other internal states.
3. Distracting yourself from your thoughts
4. Doing something kind for the person you're thinking negatively about
5. Thinking about pros and cons, or some other way of balancing a strong thought
6. Self-talk or self-encouragement
7. Acceptance of the thought
8. Medication and symptom management (for those who struggle with delusional beliefs or other difficulties with cognitive processing)

Again, clients should review these and other relevant strategies that they either did or did not find useful in addressing cognitive dysregulation. What worked? What didn't? Why? How did these strategies "feel" different than using emotion regulation strategies? Encourage clients to think of alternative strategies not listed here that were also helpful to them as they improved their cognitive regulatory abilities.

Interpersonal Regulation Strategies

Interpersonal dysregulation is most often characterized as unhealthy or uncomfortable relationship and interpersonal behaviors, which could also include violation of others' boundaries. These range from hostile and aggressive interpersonal behaviors to avoidance and withdrawal from relationships. In Module 7 we discussed a variety of problem-solving strategies for resolving interpersonal conflict, but there were also more basic skills designed to regulate problematic interactions.

1. Self-monitoring of emotions, thoughts, and urges—It may be more important for them to monitor these than the actual relationship or interpersonal behaviors, as these often feed into interpersonal dysregulation.
2. Monitoring judgments and striving to be nonjudgmental
3. Willingness—This may mean willingness to compromise or negotiate, work with others, maintain the relationship, or to let go of an unhealthy relationship
4. Acceptance and letting go of self-righteousness, anger, defensiveness, or being "right"
5. Exercising kindness to others
6. Prioritizing interpersonal needs
7. Nondefensively communicating your needs to others
8. Listening to and validating others

It was also noted within the discussion of these skills in Chapter 11 that clients would need to practice these skills in the context of multiple types of relationships and interactions. In having done so, they should now be prepared to describe their successes and frustrations with using these and other related interpersonal problem-solving strategies. Beyond the questions of what worked and what didn't, client should also discuss additional troubleshooting efforts when the other person did not react in an expected way. Did these strategies allow them to maintain important relationships or to improve stressful interactions with others?

Behavioral Regulation Strategies

Though we did not specifically address strong physiological urges and behavioral impulses in a specific chapter or module of SOS, these ideas were interwoven throughout all treatment activities. Behavioral urges and dysregulated behaviors are often seen as outcomes—these are the maladaptive strategies targeted in SOS and other treatment programming.

These urges and behaviors arise from other types of dysregulated states, including emotions, thoughts, and interactions with others. Important themes presented throughout SOS that lend themselves to behavioral dysregulation skills include:

1. Self-monitoring important urges and physiological states (e.g., sexual arousal)
2. Mindful awareness of urges—knowing the urge is there but not reacting to it. Allowing an urge to be an urge, and nothing more.
3. Distracting yourself from intense urges
4. Reminding yourself of personal goals and how these conflict with certain urges or behaviors
5. Removing self-judgment—trying not to judge yourself because you still struggle with certain urges
6. Using skills to adaptively cope with emotions, persons, situations, or thoughts that may precipitate your urges or behaviors
7. Doing something inconsistent with an urge (e.g., being nice to the person you want to yell at, thinking about how that person must feel)
8. Intense physical sensations that may remove the focus from your own physical state (e.g., holding ice, immersing your face into cold water, intense physical activity)
9. Willingness—includes willingness to accept urges, to stay focused on goals, and to use adaptive skills

Clients will have strong opinions about the effectiveness of such strategies. Once dysregulation has reached the point of a noticeable physical urge, or a near-behavior, using skills effectively is more challenging. Encouraging skills practice earlier can sometimes alleviate the pressure of using these skills in the moment, but clients should also be aware that urges and problematic behaviors may still occur, despite relative success in treatment.

SELF-MANAGEMENT AND COPING AHEAD (SESSIONS 19–20)

Clients should complete this module, and the treatment itself, with an understanding that they will need to continue self-monitoring and self-management and develop a plan for coping ahead (see Table 13.5). In

TABLE 13.5. Self-Management and Coping Ahead (Sessions 19–20)

- What is coping ahead?
  - Clients discuss the need to cope ahead, and the reality of continued problems (i.e., you can't avoid everything).
- What is involved in coping ahead?
  - Identify common forms of dysregulation that clients are still dealing with.
    o How are they related?
  - Identify common sources of this dysregulation.
  - Describe how (and which) skills help with dysregulation.
  - Identify expected challenges or obstacles to adaptive skills use.
  - List specific people who will facilitate dysregulation and maladaptive skills versus people who will facilitate adaptive skills use.

this way, clients can demonstrate what they have learned, plan ahead, and express the importance of continued self-monitoring and management of dysregulation and maladaptive regulatory behaviors. (It is also informative for treatment providers if clients have learned little, see no need for planning ahead, and minimize their need for continued self-management.) Since **an** important indicator of potential risk is the client's insight into his or her risk of future sexual offending (e.g., Hanson & Harris, 1998), this section of treatment can help treatment providers make final decisions regarding client dangerousness, the success of treatment efforts, and continued treatment needs. Clients who demonstrate a fairly good understanding of their need for coping ahead and self-management will look very different from those who believe that the end of treatment means an end to their need to monitor dysregulation and work on adaptive skills development. (These principles in relation to assessing dynamic risk are further discussed in Chapters 2 and 15.)

What Is Coping Ahead?

A plan for "coping ahead" is very different from the traditional relapse prevention plan that is more familiar to some clients and treatment providers. Within the context of relapse prevention, clients develop a plan for identifying high-risk situations; triggers for sexual behavior; patterns of distorted thinking, grooming, or planning behaviors; and avoidance strategies to reduce risk and keep them from returning to prior deviant sexual patterns. Whereas such a plan encourages clients to avoid high-risk situations, or characterizes certain urges and experiences as a "lapse," in SOS we expect that such risks, urges, or internal experiences are unavoidable, everyday experiences for some clients in sex offender treatment. Sexual urges; contact with potential victims; cognitive processes like blame, rationalization, and minimization; and strong negative affect will continue to occur in clients' (as well as anyone else's) lives. The reality (from an SOS perspective) is that everyone becomes dysregulated in emotional, cognitive, interpersonal, and behavioral ways. Even sexual urges are normative human experiences, though for some the content may be nonnormative or associated with offense behaviors (e.g., sexual urges for children or coercive sexuality).

Therefore, clients instead create a plan for coping ahead. Here, they identify their most common forms of dysregulation, how they typically respond to this dysregulation in both adaptive and maladaptive ways, what they have learned in treatment, what they need to monitor on a daily basis to manage this dysregulation most effectively, and possible strategies to aid them with more effective self-regulation and self-management. The coping plan is intended to deter maladaptive or harmful sexual behaviors, but from a perspective of acceptance and alternative strategy development. The assumption is that clients can be successful at managing their sexual urges and behaviors.

Clients must think of this plan in advance. The goal is to cope ahead of time. If they wait until the moment that strong urges, intense emotions, dysregulated thoughts, or uncomfortable and unhealthy interpersonal interactions occur, their dysregulation may be too strong for them to manage. They will need to plan ahead and practice their anticipated skills and responses so that when these situations do occur, the new skills and strategies will be more automatic and easily used despite strong dysregulation and a history of self-regulatory deficits.

What Is Involved in Coping Ahead?

This plan to cope ahead includes several key elements. First, clients should identify common forms of dysregulation with which they still struggle. This may include a review of their self-monitoring targets throughout treatment, as well as a discussion of specific kinds of dysregulation identified in Modules 2, 3, 6, and 7. In doing so, they can specifically identify how this dysregulation typically manifests itself. Do they have strong emotions? What are they? What about persistent or problematic thoughts? Are there unhealthy relationship behaviors that continue to be an issue? How do these relate to strong behavioral urges, like sexual urges, urges for self-harm or suicidal ideation, aggressive urges, or the desire to use illicit substances?

Second, clients should describe common sources of this dysregulation. How are such strong emotional, cognitive, or interpersonal states elicited? How do situational, emotional, experiential, interpretive or perceptual, and other factors impact dysregulated states? How are they related to one another? By now, clients and treatment providers have probably noticed individualized patterns or consistent responses. For example, some clients will have strong associations between anger and entitlement, blame and judgment, and manipulative or hostile relationship behaviors. These states may also be associated with strong urges for aggression or sexual violence, as well as similar maladaptive behaviors. Each client should be able to describe these processes in some detail at this point in treatment.

A third discussion point is how skills help with these dysregulated states. Earlier in this module, clients described all of the strategies learned and used throughout treatment. Here, they are focusing on areas of dysregulation in which they are in greatest need of adaptive skills use. Once clients have identified specific types and sources of dysregulation, they should review related skills in all three major domains of dysregulation, focusing on (1) preventative strategies to maintain stability and reduce vulnerability to strong internal states; (2) skills to help distract from strong emotions, thoughts, or urges; (3) strategies for soothing intense emotions and judgments; (4) problem-solving and conflict-resolution methods; (5) ways of developing and maintaining relationships; (6) acceptance; and (7) self-monitoring. They should also recognize and acknowledge a need for skills practice. Clients may feel that these discussions are repetitive, but it always helpful for them to review what has been most effective (or ineffective) for them. Further, it allows treatment providers another glimpse into their sincerity and the depth of their appreciation for needed improvements in their self-regulatory abilities. Clients who are willing to undergo these discussions and review concepts are those who may be more likely to benefit from and appreciate them, whereas clients who feel that they have already learned and covered this information in treatment—who also feel they no longer need it—are potentially at greater risk of continuing to engage in maladaptive behaviors.

A fourth component of coping ahead is to identify specific barriers and challenges they may face in implementing effective and adaptive coping strategies. For example, some clients may report that their emotions are still fairly unpredictable, that their moods vacillate so quickly that they feel they have little control over them. Others may note (correctly) that not all interpersonal interactions, particularly unhealthy ones, are fully within their control—others also have some part in the direction of an interpersonal relationship. They will need to think of some specific examples to help them plan ahead for such obstacles. If they always think about the future in abstract terms, such as "I might be really emotional," it will not be as effective as thinking, "Sometimes I get really angry when I feel someone is belittling or rejecting me, and I might lash out at them without thinking first." Detailed descriptions of these barriers could include people, situations, personal characteristics (e.g., stubbornness, impatience), or other factors that might inhibit effective self-regulation.

Finally, they will again need to identify specific persons who could be involved in creating or facilitating dysregulation, using adaptive strategies, contributing to maladaptive strategies, or helping them stay focused in their efforts to change. Knowing, for example, that some family members are generally supportive but will also encourage or enable maladaptive behavior (e.g., excessive use of alcohol, unhealthy relationship behaviors) can help clients achieve balance in their self-monitoring, reliance on others, and recognition of potential sources of continued dysregulation. Additionally, thinking about how to seek and develop relationships with others who are better at self-regulation can help proactively pursue these relationships.

This results in a plan to cope ahead, regardless of whether or not clients are soon done with sex offender treatment. For those who anticipate future treatment (to be discussed further in Module 10), this plan will aid them in maintaining success and progress that they have made thus far and in developing continued treatment goals. For those who may be completing a term of treatment for now, this plan will have a more immediate significance, as it may be their primary source of support and maintenance in the future.

MODULE 9 CONCLUDING SESSIONS

In this module, clients reviewed their decision-making processes, how their decisions impact behavior, and how relationships with others shape their decisions and behaviors over time. These decisions and behaviors are associated with self-monitoring, self-management, and the use of adaptive versus maladaptive skills. Listing types of emotional, cognitive, interpersonal, and behavioral dysregulation targeted in treatment will also help clients better conceptualize their progress and treatment needs. Wrapping up with a comprehensive review of adaptive coping strategies and plans for coping ahead will help them as they move into Module 10, which focuses more on their ongoing commitment to change, feelings about completing sex offender treatment, and determining their future course of treatment and self-management. Clients may face a great deal of uncertainty as they move into the final module of treatment. Not knowing what will happen to them, how others will react to them, or whether or not they will continue to receive needed support will greatly impact their likelihood of continued success.

FORM 13.1

On the Lookout for Maladaptive Behaviors

Sometimes people do harmful, dangerous, or risky things when they feel strong emotions, are in unhealthy relationships, have problems with their thoughts, or experience intense urges. Below, list several maladaptive or problematic behaviors from your past that may be connected to these. Some examples are provided from prior modules to help you out.

Strong emotions—anger, loneliness, boredom, paranoia, etc.

- _____
- _____
- _____

Problems with my thoughts—blame, judgment, racing thoughts, or delusional beliefs

- _____
- _____
- _____

Uncomfortable interactions or unhealthy relationships—arguing, manipulation, lying, or isolation

- _____
- _____
- _____

Intense or uncomfortable urges—sexual urges, aggressive urges, self-harm urges, etc.

- _____
- _____
- _____

CHAPTER 14

MODULE 10

Motivation, Commitment, and Treatment Goals

This is the final module of SOS. In Module 10, clients and treatment providers will review clients' progress, describe struggles with commitment to treatment, and identify goals for continuing behavioral change. These discussions will review earlier concepts and help clients integrate them into final closure on their work in sex offender treatment. Clients will also need to process the therapy experience. By the end of Module 10, clients have been involved in therapy for quite some time—in some cases, perhaps years. They have formed relationships with treatment providers and fellow clients in treatment, and the very treatment itself has become part of their routine and support system. As with the termination of any therapeutic relationship or process, clients (and treatment providers) will need some devoted time to adjust to this ending and to reflect upon their experiences.

This module also emphasizes the development of an aftercare plan. While some clients may be in the position to continue SOS by starting again and formulating new goals, the majority will move on to different environments, different treatment activities, and even different lives. An important part of this transition is preparing clients for aftercare support, supervision, and risk management. Aftercare planning is individualized and unique to each client. Clients will need to leave treatment with a specific plan to ensure continued success and to instill a sense of confidence as they move on with their lives. The concluding sessions of treatment will therefore emphasize these transitions.

Goals of this module include reviewing clients' progress, emphasizing the importance of maintaining a commitment to therapeutic change, and preparing clients for the emotional and interpersonal aspects of concluding long-term treatment. Additional goals are to help clients make decisions about future treatment needs, comply with supervision and risk management requirements, and plan aftercare. Treatment providers may want to refer ahead to discussions in Chapter 15 related to transitioning from SOS into other forms of treatment, and how to translate SOS principles into dynamic indicators of community risk.

BEING IN TREATMENT (SESSIONS 1–8)

Since SOS has no specific time frame, clients present with different needs and unique situations and will therefore require varying lengths of treatment involvement. While those who receive more intensive sex offender treatment services (e.g., longer groups, groups that meet more frequently) are likely to finish sooner, it will still reflect a lengthy journey of self-management and adaptive skills development. We refer readers to Table 14.1 for a review of how to structure client reflection on treatment experiences.

Looking Back

Clients began treatment in Module 1 with a discussion of their feelings about treatment. (Refer to Form B2, "How Do I Feel about Being in Sex Offender Treatment?" in Appendix B.) At that time, they might have endorsed negative emotions, like anger, resentment, or anxiety, along with positive emotions like hope, curiosity, or relief. These feelings were again reviewed in Module 5, once clients had already identified important areas of dysregulation and self-regulatory deficit and thought about new strategies for adaptive coping. First, clients should describe changes in

---

TABLE 14.1. Being in Treatment (Sessions 1–8)

- Looking back
  - Clients reflect on changes in their feelings about treatment; beliefs, thoughts, and expectations; and relationships and interpersonal interactions throughout the treatment process.
  - Clients describe the process of developing new skills.
  - What strengths did they rely on or develop during treatment?
- Looking forward
  - Clients review their long- and short-term goals throughout treatment and set long-term goals for the future.

their emotions throughout the entire treatment process. These changes include their feelings about being involved in sex offender treatment, the treatment itself, their future, and themselves. They will need to consider how these emotions in each of these categories have changed since the beginning of their treatment experience. What (or who) was responsible for these changes? How did they affect the clients' commitment and motivation? How did making progress change the clients' emotional response to treatment, and at the same time, how did their emotions impact their progress overall? Clients may wish to discuss other feelings associated with treatment, such as feelings about treatment providers or supportive persons involved in their treatment, and how they feel or have felt about their own behaviors. Those with dramatic emotional changes since the initiation of treatment may show particularly salient differences in their commitment, perceptions of their own and others' behaviors, and views of themselves during this time.

A second area of reflection relates to their beliefs, thoughts, and expectations. Initially, the clients discussed their perceptions of sex offenders and contrasted these with societal perceptions of the same. They also identified pros and cons, or advantages and disadvantages, of sex offender treatment, which likely reflected many of their beliefs during the early stages of treatment involvement. In both Modules 1 and 5, clients described expectations of themselves, their peers, treatment providers, and treatment team members or others involved in their treatment. It is useful for them to review these points, and to identify their expectations now: What do they expect of themselves in these final stages of the current treatment sessions? What do they expect of others who have been through this with them? What are their expectations of treatment providers or others with whom they have formed supportive relationships?

Clients also need to explore their beliefs and thoughts specific to the treatment process itself. What have they learned about treatment? Clients feel differently about treatment now that they have been in it for the duration of 10 modules. They may also view treatment differently and find that they have learned quite a bit about the purpose and nature of sex offender treatment. (With regards to this point, treatment providers can measure or estimate how likely clients will be to value treatment progress and maintain gains they have made.) Similarly, how have their perceptions about sex offending, as well as beliefs about their own maladaptive sexual behaviors, changed? What have they learned about the causes or precipitants of their own offending? Clients who had previously participated in other forms of treatment, or who had been influenced by others' interpretations of their behavior, entered treatment with set ideas about the cause of their sex offending. These beliefs probably changed as the result of their work in SOS. Treatment providers should help clients articulate these changes so that they can better conceptualize their progress, and so treatment providers can see just how much progress clients have (or have not) made in understanding their sexual offending within an SOS frame. Clients should also note changes in their beliefs about change. Initially, some clients may have expressed fears that they would never improve, while others were perhaps overconfident regarding their ability to never offend again. Hopefully they have developed a more balanced sense of what they are or are not capable of and reasonable expectations for maintaining behavioral change for the future.

A third component of this reflective process involves looking back at how their relationships and interpersonal interactions have changed. How do clients conceptualize boundaries? How have these boundaries changed during the course of treatment? This includes the ability to interpret and respect others' boundaries and to set and maintain their own boundaries with others. It may be helpful for clients to again review different types of boundaries for this discussion. They should also describe their experiences with healthy and unhealthy relationships, particularly noting how their relationship behaviors, persons with whom they are in relationships, or decisions about relationships have changed since the beginning of treatment. For clients with limited access to a diverse array of interpersonal interactions and relationships (i.e., clients who may be institutionalized), discussing how their perceptions and expectations of these relationships have changed, or how their relationships with staff members and peers have changed, would also be beneficial. Treatment providers can review useful strategies from Module 7 for building a healthy support system and for using effective problem-solving and conflict resolution strategies. Clients can identify any changes they have noted in their own problem-solving abilities that may be attributable to their participation in treatment.

Fourth, clients should discuss the process of developing skills— things like improving their self-monitoring abilities (so that they could identify dysregulated states and thus know when to use new strategies), learning new skills, practicing these skills, and looking for opportunities to reinforce new skills development. What challenges did they face during this process? What kinds of things prevented them from effectively using their skills? In what ways did they struggle with letting go of and replacing old patterns of maladaptive behavior? Clients may want to refer back to their discussions in Module 9 for a review of useful strategies and barriers to using new abilities. How did others encourage and support adaptive skills use, or in what ways did they perhaps reinforce maladaptive behavioral strategies?

Lastly, what strengths have clients developed or relied upon during the treatment process? In Modules 1 and 5, clients described strengths that could aid them in treatment. These may have been directly related to treatment, like motivation to change, knowledge of treatment concepts, or ability to self-monitor. Others may be more indirect but still helpful, such as consistent treatment attendance, willingness to participate in treatment discussions, or ability to understand new ideas and provide examples. How did their strengths change or develop, and what contributed to this change? For example, as clients felt more confident in treatment maybe they made more progress, or vice versa. Strengths related to new skills development might have improved other areas of their lives, such as relationships, occupational functioning, or self-esteem. (These ideas will be revisited later in the module, as clients discuss new strengths and how these will contribute to their continued success post-treatment.)

Looking Forward

One purpose of this module is to help clients transition to new settings or different treatment opportunities. With the completion of treatment, some clients will be released from institutional or residential care, while others may move on to a different form of supervision. Some who complete treatment will no longer be expected to attend sex offender treatment programming, whereas others will continue SOS with more refined or specific treatment goals. Given the many possibilities, it is important for clients to look ahead at what is needed for each of them individually. Clients may have difficulty imagining what they still need to do. Thinking about this in the context of dysregulation, refer them to their self-monitoring sheets and what they continually monitor on a day-to-day basis. How might they be able to translate these into future treatment goals or needs?

For example, clients who continue to self-monitor strong emotions, and who experience intense mood swings or high degrees of anger, sadness, anxiety, or loneliness, might want to look at treatment targeting these emotions (e.g., anger management, treatment for depression) or general emotion modulation. Clients who struggle with psychotic processes and delusional beliefs and who monitor these may benefit from continued medication management and treatment emphasizing illness management and recovery. Clients whose self-monitoring centers primarily on relationship behaviors and boundaries could solicit treatment emphasizing relationship functioning, communication and social skills, and problem-solving abilities. Clients who struggle with strong urges, or who continue to engage in varied maladaptive behaviors, may need continued focus on adaptive skills development.

Treatment providers should review with clients their long- and short-term goals. Clients established these goals in the first module of treatment, and they were reviewed throughout the treatment process, often at the end of each module. Goals were revisited and revised depending on the nature of the material presented in that particular module, and clients may have modified their goals several times prior to the end of treatment. What do their goals look like now? Looking ahead, what are their long-term goals for themselves and for treatment, and what short-term goals will aid them in achieving these targets?

STAGES OF CHANGE (SESSIONS 9–10)

In Modules 1 and 5, clients discussed the five stages of change (Prochaska & DiClemente, 1983; Prochaska et al., 1992). Here, they will review these stages again in relation to their current level of commitment (see Table 14.2). Many clients will say that they are in the "maintenance" stage simply because they are in the last module of SOS treatment. However, not everyone is truly in maintenance, and variations in their current stage of change reflect the complexity of these behaviors and the ongoing nature of change. Treatment providers should challenge clients to think of important differences between the action phase and the maintenance phase. Many clients will remain in the action phase for quite some time, as they are continuously monitoring important emotions, thoughts, interactions, and urges, and developing and practicing new self-regulatory strategies.

TABLE 14.2. Stages of Change (Sessions 9–10)

- Clients review each of the five stages of change
  - Where were they at in the beginning of treatment?
  - Where are they now?
  - How did their commitment change throughout the process?
  - Clients describe what it will take to maintain progress and commitment.

With regards to discussing these stages, clients will not only need to review where they are currently "at," but also how their level of commitment to change has varied. As was noted in Module 1, change is not a linear process. Though we always hope for clients to continually move forward in their efforts to improve and learn, this is not always the case. As clients experience frustrations and setbacks, they will inevitably move to stages reflecting less motivation and commitment. Clients will need to review their progression through the stages of change since the beginning of treatment. Below are some questions associated with each stage for clients to consider.

1. *Pre-recognition.* How did you deny or minimize your problem to others? How did you deny or minimize your problem to yourself? How did this denial impact your treatment progress? How did you overcome it? What got in your way of moving past this stage? What caused you to go back to this stage at any point during treatment?

2. *Recognition.* Which people, circumstances, issues, or decisions helped you realize that you had a problem? Did recognizing the problem change your view of yourself? Did it change how others view you? At the time, what did you think? What do you think now about having been in this stage?

3. *Planning.* What steps did you take as you prepared for treatment? What got in your way of fully committing to treatment? Were there parts of the plan that did not work? What parts did work? How did others help you make a treatment plan?

4. *Action.* What changes did you try to work on first? How did you expect your life to change as you made progress in treatment? Were you right? What actually did change? What helped keep you motivated as you made changes? How did others support you during this active phase of treatment and behavioral change? What was the most difficult thing about being involved in treatment?

5. *Maintenance.* What kinds of changes will you need to maintain? What steps will you need to take in order to do this? Who will help you do this? What kinds of challenges will you face as you try to maintain your treatment gains?

This discussion also provides clients with the opportunity to give one another validation, encouragement, and feedback, even if sometimes negative, regarding their progress in treatment. It can be helpful for them to reflect and "compare notes," so to speak. They can also give one another supportive reminders of things that may have caused fluctuations in their commitment and motivation in earlier modules of treatment. This will help those clients who experience an "out of sight, out of mind" approach to remembering their commitment throughout the lengthy duration of treatment.

COMMITTING TO ADAPTIVE SKILLS
(SESSIONS 11–15)

Clients who have made it this far in treatment obviously have evidenced some degree of commitment to treatment. They may not have always been committed in the same way—some clients commit to change their maladaptive behaviors, while others make a more superficial commitment to participate in treatment programming for some other gain (e.g., fulfilling placement or agency requirements, obtaining early release, or satisfying family members or others). Despite important differences between surface and deeper commitments, treatment providers should still acknowledge and foster clients' abilities and willingness to change. Even a superficial or begrudging commitment is an improvement over none at all, and it may be an early step toward becoming more involved in the change process. An overview of these sessions is described in Table 14.3.

TABLE 14.3. Committing to Adaptive Skills (Sessions 11–15)

- Making the commitment to positive life changes
  - Clients define commitment.
    o What are their own reasons for making a commitment?
  - Clients discuss what is involved in their commitment to treatment and how they or their lives have changed.
- Maintaining the commitment
  - Clients think ahead about how to maintain their commitment
    o What kind of changes will they need to maintain?
    o What challenges will they face?
    o What supports will clients need?
    o What will they do when their commitment starts to waver, or when they start to slip back into old habits?

Making the Commitment to Positive Life Changes

Changing one's behavior requires a strong commitment, especially in the face of long-held patterns of reinforcement and automatic responding. For many clients, the type and intensity of their commitment has changed since the time of their first offense, first arrest, or first involvement in sex offender treatment. To highlight such changes, clients should first think about what commitment means. Defining commitment may involve concepts like dedication, persistence, values, or change-supportive decisions. To facilitate such a discussion, clients should identify various commitments they have made over the course of their lives. How did they reach a decision regarding that commitment? What was involved? How did they accomplish it?

It is assumed that the clients still involved in SOS in Module 9 are in some way committed to their treatment. What does their commitment look like? In other words, what is involved in this commitment? How do they define this commitment in their own words? How do they see commitment in each other? For each client, commitment to change or to treatment will look a bit different. Different work and different sacrifices are involved for each person, and these can change at each step of their journey. Some ideas representing different definitions of commitment, or different reasons for commitment, are listed below for client discussion.

- "I want to change my behavior."
- "I have lost something important to me, and I see that I need to change."
- "In order to achieve my goals, I have to work in sex offender treatment."
- "I want to prove that I can do something about my behavior."
- "I want others to trust me again."
- "I believe I am capable of making myself a better person."
- "I have to work hard to make this happen."
- "I have a hard time thinking about what all I need to do, but I still do it anyway."
- "I have to get other people involved in my treatment to make this a success."
- "I have to go it on my own because no one else can help me."

Remember that as a part of this discussion, treatment providers will need to respond by using the six levels of validation. For clients who are more interpersonally dysregulated or who have difficulty with maintaining commitments involving others (e.g., people with antisocial personality disorder, significant egocentricity, or psychopathic features), treatment providers will want to use as much radical genuineness (i.e., Level 6 Validation) as is necessary to still provide them meaningful feedback. For example, some of these individuals may say: "I'm only still here because I have to be. I don't need this. It doesn't matter to me whether or not people think I've changed." A potential response from treatment providers could be: "I know, and I can sense that from you. It really doesn't seem like others' opinions are important. But I still think it's useful that you've stuck it out, and hopefully you were able to get something out of this experience." With other clients, the validation will be smoother and will come more easily. Helping clients understand the nature of their commitment can support and even encourage growth of their commitment in the future.

For clients, how has life changed since making a commitment to change their behavior? Have clients list ways that their lives have changed, hopefully for the better, as a result of their involvement in treatment. This can include feelings of accomplishment as they reach their goals; improved ability to regulate strong emotions, thoughts, interpersonal relationships, and urges; skills development; or other relevant areas of their lives. Understanding and verbalizing changes that result from their work in treatment helps clients see the value of maintaining their commitment to adaptive self-regulation. Hearing about others' improvements can also make subtle changes more salient. For example, many clients overlook the value of better attendance and participation in treatment, increased sincerity, or even improved ability to internally process feelings of guilt and shame to allow for better functioning on a day-to-day basis. From experiences with SOS in the pilot stages, the consensus has been that clients look too much at the "big picture" of treatment commitment and behavioral change, and in doing so sell themselves short on the smaller and more gradual changes that naturally occur in long-term treatment. These small changes are not irrelevant, as they build into larger, "big picture" changes and meanwhile offer meaning and hope in the clients' lives.

Maintaining the Commitment

As clients reach the end of SOS with Module 10, it does not necessarily mean that sex offender treatment is "finished." Since SOS emphasizes an individualized approach to client goals and progress, it is probable that each client is at a different point as the end of the 10-module program draws near. Some have made significant progress, while others have more yet to accomplish. Even those for whom the end of the treatment means discharge, transfer, or simply the completion of a necessary requirement will need to maintain their progress and commitment to behavioral change. For clients whose sex offender treatment must continue (whether through a return to SOS or some other companion treatment), they will need to maintain their commitment in the face of perhaps indefinite treatment participation. Thus, for all clients, working to maintain commitment is a valuable goal.

Clients will need to think ahead about what it means to maintain their commitment to change and what is involved in this process. Clients and treatment providers should have an open discussion of the following points:

1. "What kinds of changes will you need to maintain?" This question will prompt a helpful review of the changes clients have made. These will include those "big picture" changes that they most easily see, like engaging in healthier, nonoffending patterns of behavior, the less-recognizable but still significant changes like developing healthier relationships and establishing better boundaries with others, and subtle changes like increased sincerity, recognition of risk or need for treatment, and consistent willingness and commitment to change.

2. "What are challenges you will face in trying to stay committed?" Clients don't like to think of their hard work being easily undone, or that they may not be able to handle whatever comes their way in the future. Realistically, however, there will be challenges that may weaken their commitment or even negate some of their progress. In truth, clients have already faced some of these challenges during treatment, though they might not always be aware of them. Discussing factors like lack of support (or perceived lack of support), overconfidence in one's success, a sense of being overwhelmed by dysregulation or strong urges, negative reactions from other people, and other relevant challenges will help clients plan ahead for maintaining their commitment to change, or their commitment to continuing treatment.

3. "Are there supports you will need in order to maintain your progress?" Hopefully clients have established increased systems of support and developed healthier relationships with others during their time in treatment. They will need to retain these support systems and develop additional resources after the completion of treatment efforts.

Their support system may include obvious supports, such as therapists, case managers, or other mental health providers, family members, and friends. Other less obvious support systems may include occupational activities, educational efforts, religious affiliations, recreational activities, or volunteer associations. These supports will help clients create healthy and adaptive relationships, foster new opportunities for learning adaptive skills, and strengthen their commitment to positive behavioral change.

4. "What will you do when you feel your commitment wavering, or when you notice that you're starting to slip back into old habits (e.g., maladaptive regulatory strategies)?" Clients should plan ahead for the possibility that they will be less committed to change, or that they will have problems. Clients want to think that they will always do well—that once they have made progress, it will stay that way. However, we know that there will be realistic challenges that cause them to give in to their urges in harmful ways, to engage in maladaptive strategies, or to think that they don't need to change any further. They need to think about how this might "look" for them, and what they may do in the moment when this happens.

PROGRESS AND FUTURE TREATMENT (SESSIONS 16–20)

Here, clients will need to engage in a more in-depth discussion of their goals and progress (see Table 14.4). The development of goals is a fluid

---

TABLE 14.4. Progress and Future Treatment (Sessions 16–20)

- My treatment: Where I've been
    - Clients review their goals, progress, and changes in behavior
    - Clients rank their goals
    - How have others noticed changes in their behavior?
- My treatment: Where I'm going
    - Clients discuss whether or not they still need continuing treatment, or what they may still need to work on.
        o How did they meet their goals?
        o What are their other treatment needs?
        o What skills do they still need?
        o What are their supervision requirements?
    - Clients and treatment providers work together to figure out what is best for continuing care.

process in SOS, with treatment providers and clients working together collaboratively to refine and supplement clients' goals throughout the treatment process.

My Treatment: Where I've Been

What were clients' long- and short-term goals? How did those change? What things did they monitor each week in order to work toward those goals? How did their behaviors improve? What did others notice about them as they made progress in treatment? And what did they struggle with? Which goals or behaviors did not improve much? What were their major setbacks? Answering these questions for themselves will help them clarify how they have achieved (or not yet achieved) each of their goals in treatment. (A client handout for facilitating this discussion is provided in Form 14.1 at the end of the chapter.) Treatment providers will probably need to remind clients that sometimes they will not achieve all of their goals. Some goals may have been too far-fetched (e.g., the "perfection" goal), unhealthy (e.g., the "no urges ever again" goal, or the "no relationships with others" goal), or simply impossible (e.g., the "avoid women" or "avoid children" goal). Additionally, goals may change, and as new goals are identified, old goals become less relevant.

As clients review their goals and progress, have them rank each of their goals. Which were the most important—and how important were they—at the beginning of treatment? How do they rank now? Treatment providers should also have clients rate how much they have accomplished each of these goals on a 1–10 scale. How much would others say they have achieved their goals on this same scale? This is an opportunity for treatment providers and other clients to comment on these achievements. They may also need to talk about clients' expectations of how permanent these achievements are. For example, clients whose goal is to more effectively manage their sexual urges may think that they have finished this goal following a period of treatment success. However, we want them to recognize that this is a continuing and evolving process, and that reaching this goal of effective self-management does not mean that they can simply stop trying or ignore their urges in the future.

Another way of viewing progress is to ask clients what others have noticed about changes in their behaviors. This includes feedback that clients received from their treatment providers, peers in sex offender treatment group, others involved in their treatment (e.g., case managers, members of a treatment team), supervision agents, or friends and family members who remain in contact on a somewhat regular basis. Sometimes seeing themselves from another person's perspective or thinking back on what others have said can help clients see progress that they might have missed, or perhaps ground them in the reality of continued treatment needs. Behavioral change is something that can be fairly evident and observable, so it is easier to measure than more abstract changes, like emotional stability, attitude improvement, or increased sense of self-identity and self-worth.

My Treatment: Where I'm Going

Since many clients involved in SOS or any form of sex offender treatment are often there to satisfy court or agency requirements, thinking about continued treatment is a challenge. Such clients are hoping to be "done." But most clients will need continued treatment in some form, even if it is for other relevant but non-sex-offender issues, like substance abuse, relationship problems, or trauma. A discussion of whether or not they need treatment and how to recognize this need will help them frame their treatment future. Treatment providers can guide this discussion by using the following outline:

1. Treatment goals
   - "Did I reach all of my goals?"
   - "Are there some goals I still need to work on?"
   - "Do others have goals for me?"
   - "What are my own personal goals?"
   - "Do I feel like this is 'finished?' How will I know when it is?"
2. Other treatment needs
   - *Mental health needs.* This may include depression, anxiety, anger problems, psychosis, cognitive or learning deficits, or personality and relationship pathology.
   - *Continuing dysregulation.* While clients (and everyone else) will experience dysregulation throughout their lives in different situations and relationships, some clients may still struggle with intense and frequent dysregulated states.
   - *Traumatic experiences.* Once clients have the requisite skills and emotional and interpersonal stability, they may be prepared to begin working on their own traumatic experiences.
   - *Relationship problems.* Clients may need help reconnecting with family members and developing healthy relationships

once they are more stable and familiar with adaptive regulatory skills.

- *Substance use issues.* Many clients involved in sex offender treatment programming have also struggled with problematic substance use in the past. They may need continued treatment and support to address these behaviors.
- *Support* – As a group, sex offenders often lack support due to negative societal perceptions and legal restrictions on their activities, occupational choices, and movement. They may need to work on navigating these limitations and stigma while still achieving a balanced and healthy lifestyle.

3. Skills use
   - *Skills development.* "What skills do I still need to work on?"
   - *Skills practice.* "How can I continue practicing new skills? What are new situations that may require skills practice?"
   - *Skills coaching.* "Are people available to help me learn and use skills? How can I access these resources?"

4. Supervision requirements
   - "What is required of me now?"
   - "Do I still have to attend mandated treatment?"
   - "What do others expect of me?"
   - "What will happen if I fail to meet these requirements or expectations?"

Once clients have made a decision about the need for continued therapy, they will need to define what treatment is for and what works best for them. It may be helpful to think back to their targets and areas of improvement in SOS, including future coping skills, risk of future sex offending behaviors, relationships with others, and the ability to self-regulate. Be careful though—the assumption is that more treatment is better, but this is not true for all clients. The risk–needs–responsivity approach to sex offender treatment suggests that the most intensive and varied interventions are still the most effective for the highest risk offenders, while low-risk offenders may have fewer treatment needs than their higher risk counterparts. This may also mean that continuing treatment is less necessary for those at lower risk, or that future interventions may involve fewer areas of treatment focus.

Treatment providers should review available treatment options with clients. How to present these options and prepare clients for changes in their treatment, such as transitioning to relapse prevention, the good lives model, or sexual addiction treatment, are presented in further depth in Chapter 15 to guide this discussion.

CHALLENGES IN TREATMENT AND AFTERCARE (SESSIONS 21–23)

In this section, clients will consider aftercare issues, including potential risk, challenges and obstacles to maintaining progress, aftercare services, and working with supervision. For treatment providers, many of these issues are discussed in far greater detail and from the perspective of effective risk management in Chapter 15. In order to help with these discussions, treatment providers may also want to refer to Appendix A, a client aftercare packet. This section is described further in Table 14.5.

Life after Treatment

Clients often have an idealized view of life after treatment. They think they will be "cured"; that family members, friends, and society will eagerly welcome them home; and that they will never again have uncomfortable urges or problems with others. They think that after treatment, they will have "perfect" families, jobs, homes, and finances. They believe that no one will know about their history of sex offending, or that even if people do know, they will overlook it because they have done so well in treatment. Few clients believe all of these things; realistically, many clients do see potential challenges. But they will all have some areas in which they maintain an idealized view of life after treatment. Clients may thus underestimate the extent of the challenges they will face.

Clients will need to discuss potential obstacles and challenges, including stigma or negative perceptions by others, continued struggles

---

TABLE 14.5. Challenges in Treatment and Aftercare (Sessions 21–23)

- Life after treatment
  - What are posttreatment challenges?
  - What do they still need?
  - What parts of treatment were most helpful?
- Working with supervision
  - Clients discuss their emotional reactions to being under supervision.
  - What are the pros and cons of supervision?

with dysregulation and strong urges, self-doubt, overconfidence in treatment gains, problematic relationships, or lack of continued support. There are also practical issues for clients to consider. Do they know who to contact if they are in trouble? Do they have access to emergency mental health or other services? Do they have a list of strategies that they can carry with them in case of problems with self-regulation in the moment? This should be a fairly open-ended discussion, as clients will each have their own individualized issues to consider. Clients will be transitioning into different situations and environments dependent on their treatment progress and current circumstances, so treatment providers will want to facilitate this discussion in such a way so that each client can think about issues most relevant to him or her.

At the beginning of this module, clients reviewed initial and current expectations of themselves, peers, treatment providers, and supportive others involved in their treatment. They will now consider similar expectations of the future—what do they expect of themselves, the community (or others in their current setting), future treatment providers, supervisory agents like probation or parole officers, and support systems? Some clients have idealized views of these relationships, and their expectations will reflect this idealization. Others have overwhelmingly negative expectations regarding these relationships. For example, clients could believe that their family members will always be supportive and available, whereas they think that supervisory agents are simply going to harass and criticize them. Treatment providers can help them balance these expectations and think of potential obstacles and sources of support. Examples from treatment providers' own experiences with the clients can help illustrate these points (e.g., "I remember that when you started treatment you really didn't trust me. It got better over time. You may find that it's the same way with your case manager in the community.").

TABLE 14.6. Termination (Sessions 24–25)

- For the treatment providers
  - Treatment providers should take some time at the end to reinforce client progress, validate client anxieties, and say good-bye.
- For the clients
  - Clients in a group setting say good-bye to one another and reinforce their mutual support.

To further plan for continued care and life after treatment, clients should identify components of treatment that were helpful or success-ful, as well as those that were not. This may involve describing charac-teristics of treatment providers, support systems, or treatment discus-sions that they found useful and figuring out what modality of treatment, views of sexuality, or response to behavior that they think is most ben-eficial for them. These considerations allow them to make informed and experienced choices regarding future treatment approaches and modalities. Finally, clients will need to develop a list of their most useful adaptive strategies, including skills for prevention, distraction, and self-soothing strong emotions; skills for monitoring and changing problem-atic thoughts or beliefs; and skills for problem solving and communica-tion in interpersonal relationships.

Working with Supervision

Another reality for clients involved in sex offender treatment is that they are often supervised in the community or other settings. This may come from institutional or residential care or community supervision agents like probation and parole officers. Clients might have strong feelings about this supervision, even though many of them are already aware of these requirements and have had time to think about them prior to this stage of treatment. This is good, in that it is expected and not surprising, but it also contributes to reluctance, resentment, and negative anticipa-tion.

Clients have already discussed their emotional reactions to being involved in sex offender treatment, including both positive and negative feelings. They also discussed the pros and cons, or advantages and dis-advantages, of being in treatment. Now, we want clients to apply these principles to their feelings about supervision and risk management, and the pros and cons of being supervised in their current or other settings. In this discussion, we want to validate their emotions and perceptions, but also focus on ways that clients can overcome negative emotions and judgments in order to work more effectively with supervisory agents.

A useful skill for this is acceptance—supervision is their reality, and while they don't have to feel positively about it, they do have to abide by supervisory rules and requirements. To help with this acceptance, clients should think about how to use supervision as a support system. Many do not think of supervision in this way, and quite frequently supervi-sion agents themselves might not view themselves as a positive support for their sex offending clients. However, this is often a front-line source of information about how the client is doing and an available resource for the client. Therefore, they should expect supervision agents to help them maintain their progress, monitor their dysregulation and treatment needs, and provide needed resources in other settings.

TERMINATION (SESSIONS 24–25)

Much of this module has been for the purposes of terminating the therapy. The standard process of termination usually includes a review of the therapy experience, things that the client has learned, things that still need to be accomplished, and future plans for support and maintenance of treatment gains. The last part of termination is an opportunity for clients and their treatment providers to say goodbye, or to conclude their therapy sessions (see Table 14.6). This is an interesting process for individuals with a history of sexual offending. With SOS, the relationship between the client and the treatment provider is different than in other treatment modalities. The therapeutic relationship is a real relationship, even if it is not like other relationships in the clients' lives. It is a collaborative relationship, and one in which the treatment provider makes efforts to validate and engage the client in the change process. So even though the treatment provider doesn't agree with or condone the client's behavior, he or she does value the client, and the relationship is one of therapeutic support.

For the Treatment Providers

Treatment providers should reflect on the clients' successes, struggles, and progress through treatment, validating clients' anxieties and concerns as they move on. They should also feel free to comment on their own perceptions and struggles with the process as they feel able and comfortable. Depending on where clients are headed following their current treatment experience, some treatment providers may continue their contact with clients in either sex offender treatment or some other therapeutic capacity. This continued contact will impact the nature of these termination sessions.

For the Clients

Termination with a group also involves group members saying their farewells to each other. Some of them will be relieved, whereas others have formed supportive and reciprocal relationships with one another and will miss their peers. These sessions also allow group members to give each other final feedback and encouragement, and to make plans for shared support, if applicable and feasible.

In all, these concluding sessions reflect the clients' progress and the benefits of treatment. Summarizing their commitment to change, actual progress toward change, and newly learned self-management strategies will help prepare them for the transition into their improved lives.

FORM 14.1

Reviewing My Treatment Progress

My main treatment goals were:

1. _____

2. _____

3. _____

Things I monitored each week were:

_____   _____

_____   _____

_____   _____

_____   _____

How did my behaviors improve?

1. _____

2. _____

3. _____

Something others noticed about me as I made progress in treatment:

1. _____

2. _____

3. _____

I struggled most with:

1. _____

2. _____

3. _____

(cont.)

Reviewing My Treatment Progress *(page 2 of 2)*

Goals or behaviors that might not have improved much:

1. _____
2. _____
3. _____

Some of my setbacks were:

_____ _____

_____ _____

_____ _____

_____ _____

What do I still need to work on?

1. _____
2. _____
3. _____

CHAPTER 15

Family and Community Reintegration
Preparing the Client for Aftercare

When clients near the end of treatment with SOS, even if they have not yet completed all 10 modules of treatment, treatment providers, treatment teams, supervisors, and other risk management agents will need to address community reintegration and family reunification. Even if the current discharge plan does not include community release, contact with the community is a future reality for many clients in sex offender treatment. Helping clients reenter and reintegrate with the community is a complex and potentially volatile process, fraught with anxiety, judgment, anger, and shame. Additionally, many clients in sex offender treatment still maintain ties with family members and other supportive persons who want greater involvement in client recovery. Questions about potential risk, supervision requirements, the realities of community reintegration, and continuing treatment services are now more salient to clients and their treatment providers.

This chapter assists treatment providers with conceptualizing and examining these issues with their clients, treatment teams, and community supervision or risk management agents. The issues discussed here may also be relevant to agencies that frequently make release and placement decisions for clients who have successfully completed sex offender treatment. The primary goal of this chapter is to describe issues of family and community reintegration as well as risk and continued treatment planning. A supplementary goal is to help treatment providers individualize aftercare planning and guide clients through this process. Because many of these issues must be addressed at multiple points during the treatment process (e.g., in Module 7 during discussions of support and healthy relationships, in Module 8 regarding relationships and healing), we recommend that treatment providers read and review this chapter prior to initiating treatment with clients using SOS.

FAMILIES AND SUPPORT SYSTEMS

Clients present for treatment with a great variability in their available support and family relationships. Some have little social support or damaged what few social supports they did have by committing sexual offenses. There is a range of family contact—some are still supportive and involved, others have severed all ties, and some are only superficially involved in the client's life. Maintaining support systems like family, friends, clergy, employers, and others is often difficult when offenders are incarcerated, hospitalized, or placed in residential treatment as a result of their offending. Physical separation from their support systems, as well as accompanying changes in the client's life focus and day-to-day activities, can further widen the gap between the client and his or her support system. Supportive relationships are also challenged by fears about the client's behavior, uncertainties about what will happen postrelease, and the stigma that family members and friends may experience from continued contact with the offender.

So how do we maintain support for the client, or keep interested families involved in treatment efforts? A crucial point here is that we only want to explore these options when family members, friends, or others *want* to be involved. Though it may be painful for the clients, we are not in a position to force family members or others in the client's former support network to continue their support. That is a choice that they must make. But for those who do choose to remain involved, it can be difficult to identify ways of being supportive, integrate them into treatment, and involve them in aftercare planning.

If family members were victims, involving them in the treatment process is particularly difficult and will involve collaboration with other agencies or services to ensure continued safety for victims. In some cases, the client is prohibited from contact with victims. This ban should be respected, and it is understood that these persons will not be involved in the client's treatment. However, when family reunification is a viable goal and is supported by those involved in the care and treatment or the client and his or her family, family-based interventions and support may be needed. Treatments like multisystemic therapy (Henggeler, Schoenwal, Borduin, Rowland, & Cunningham, 1998), for example, integrate multiple areas of the client's life, including family, to look at systemic problems. Involving family members and supportive others as a system can create a healthier and more supportive system for all involved.

Systemic change (which does assume some problem within the family system at the outset, even if the problem is merely that something violent happened within the family) is one method of family intervention. Another involves the healing process. To reintegrate the client with his or her family, healing and relationship repair are necessary. In Module 8 clients discussed forgiveness and acceptance, learning that they may never truly find forgiveness for everything or undo the harm they caused to others, but that they can try to repair the damages caused by their behaviors. This includes damage to their families, such as loss of trust, sadness and disappointment, embarrassment and shame, feelings of regret or self-blame, anger, sense of violation or loss of safety in the home, or living with the doubt and judgment of others. There may be other practical damages, depending on the situation. Clients who offended against children, for example, may have family members who had worked with children prior to the offense, and who have since lost their jobs or experienced discomfort and mistrust due to their relationship with the client. Similarly, clients and their family members who live in small communities may find themselves isolated and less supported by others in the community. Thus, a simple acknowledgment and discussion of these damages in a therapeutic framework and efforts to make repairs are crucial steps in the healing process.

Family members and support systems are also important components of the client's aftercare plan. Teaching family members and supportive others how to help the client maintain success—including learning about the client's areas of dysregulation, self-monitoring practices, and newly learned adaptive strategies—can provide continuity of care once the client has left the immediate treatment environment. However, members of the client's support network are not expected to be solely responsible for monitoring and managing the client's dysregulation, as the point of SOS is *self*-monitoring and *self*-management. Still, helping supportive persons recognize potential problems and encourage or facilitate adaptive skills use reinforces the client's positive efforts to maintain treatment change and future self-management practices.

Those in the client's support system can also be positive role models for adaptive strategy development and practice. As noted in Module 9, there are times when important support persons have been models for both maladaptive and adaptive behaviors. But educating the client and these supportive persons more thoroughly regarding adaptive self-regulatory behaviors can facilitate the use of adaptive strategies. Family members or others who truly wish to support the client in his or her efforts to maintain treatment gains should continue to use adaptive strategies and demonstrate effective and healthy self-regulation. This may involve working with those persons to identify important differences between maladaptive and adaptive behaviors (either within the context of family sessions or family education groups), but such work can be informative for both clients and members of their primary support group. Persons in the support network can also provide opportunities for clients to engage in establishing healthy boundaries and practicing healthy relationship behaviors.

Finally, a difficult and somewhat controversial task of family members and supportive persons may be to monitor the client's risk, compliance with supervision requirements, or difficulties with maintaining adaptive behaviors. This is such a conflict: family members or others close to the client want to ensure safety and prevent future offending, but they don't want to police their loved one and report transgressions that may result in additional charges, incarceration or institutionalization, or added anxiety and stress for the client. It is perhaps easier if family members don't have to take on this role as well, but given that they have more contact with the client, greater knowledge and insight into his or her struggles and well-being, and the ability to monitor his or her behaviors in a more personal way, it makes sense that they will naturally assume some of this role. A way of managing this complex issue without causing damage to an already-fragile relationship or limiting the effectiveness of their support is for treatment providers to coach members of the support network in talking with the client about problems with self-monitoring and self-management, preferably before he or she reaches critical mass. Family members, supportive others, and clients are empowered to set their own boundaries with regards to monitoring and reporting the reemergence of maladaptive behaviors.

REALITIES OF COMMUNITY RELATIONSHIPS

Once clients are ready to reintegrate with the community, they will face many challenges. One such challenge is dealing with the reality of how others will react to them as sexual offenders. Here we will discuss these challenges and ways to prepare clients for such obstacles throughout SOS.

The most obvious barrier for clients is the stigma associated with being a sexual offender. Clients discussed societal perceptions in Module 1, so they are familiar with others' beliefs and expectations concerning individuals who have committed sexual crimes. They may feel strongly that this stigma is unfair, and that it interferes with their ability to form supportive relationships, to trust others, or to manage their cognitive, emotional, and interpersonal dysregulation. Others, however, may implicitly agree with these stigmatizing beliefs. For example, some clients may feel that they are bad people deserving of punishment. Having this self-image reinforced by negative treatment in the community will only further their isolation, resentment, loneliness, and lack of healthy, supportive relationships.

Clients can also suffer dual stigmas from co-occurring serious mental illness or intellectual and developmental disabilities, thus complicating the development of positive community relationships. Additional stigmas associated with their sexual offending include the stigma of being an ex-convict, a hospital patient, having to report to supervision agents, and so on. Therefore, being a sex offender is sometimes only the starting point for judgment, negative perceptions, and shame that clients experience in the community. While we don't necessarily want clients to focus on the negative aspects of their posttreatment future, it is important for them to at least have some awareness of these factors so that they can mentally, emotionally, and socially prepare in advance of being placed in a community setting.

Community registration and notification requirements are an additional challenge. Most jurisdictions in the United States and Canada currently have registration, notification, and residency requirements for those who have been convicted of sexual offenses. These typically require offenders to notify law enforcement agencies of their residence in the community, to check in periodically, and to restrict their residence and movement to areas of the community where they have limited access to children or other potential victims. There are also community notification practices requiring public dissemination of information about the offender, which may include the person's name, address, crime, or other important personal details. Though these laws were enacted to increase a sense of community safety, understandably they also increase difficulties clients face with stigma and judgment from community members.

Research describing the effectiveness of such legislation is limited, though primarily negative. For example, few people make routine use of such registration and community notification lists to take precautions against sexual violence in their communities (e.g., Anderson, 2008; Anderson & Sample, 2008), and in many instances strict residency restrictions have led to homelessness, failure to register, or excessive burden on the part of family members and friends who would be willing to support an offender in their homes. Recent research examining the impact of residency restrictions and community registration and notification practices suggests that these policies may in fact place offenders at greater risk, through increasing their sense of isolation and loneliness, increasing anxiety and shame, limiting available social supports, and prohibiting skillful work, recreational, religious, or other opportunities that may actually be adaptive strategies or protective factors (e.g., Levenson & Cotter, 2005).

With regards to the impact of these registration requirements and effects of stigma, treatment providers will need to emphasize adaptive strategies to help with shame, anxiety, fear, anger, resentment, and other risky emotional states; strategies to aid with acceptance, responsibility, problem solving, and healthy expectations of others; and strategies to improve relationship functioning, boundaries, conflict resolution, and self-esteem and assertiveness. As clients learn these strategies, they can think ahead about how to apply them in real-world situations, like the community. In Modules 9 and 10 clients should revisit these strategies in the context of coping ahead and building supportive relationships with others.

A third challenge for clients will be their involvement with supervisory agents. Some leave treatment still facing a term of probation or parole. Those in forensic mental health systems may have a similar monitoring system in place. Others may be beholden to more restrictive supervision requirements than these, through day programs, residential care facilities, or other semisupervised, structured living arrangements. At a minimum, many clients will still be required to report their whereabouts and activities to law enforcement agents as part of sex offender registration procedures. Few clients will leave treatment unsupervised, with the exception of some deemed "low risk." Even so, treatment providers should anticipate a need for clients to interact with supervision agents in the community and include preparation for this in the aftercare plan. (Relevant points for aftercare planning are outlined further in Appendix A.) An important component of aftercare planning is knowing what is expected in terms of frequency of contact, types of information clients will need to share, specific restrictions, behavioral requirements (e.g., drug testing, call-in reporting), or participation in monitoring programs (e.g., electronic monitoring, GPS tracking). Advance awareness and preplanning will help clients address their emotions concerning, doubts about, and reactions to supervision in the community.

Additionally, clients may have to consider their relationships with supervision agents. For some, the relationship is supportive and helpful. We are always pleased to meet members of probation and parole services and often find that they show compassion and concern for the well-being of their clients, despite the somewhat adversarial perception of their relationship. However, this is not always the case, and clients will determine the strength of these supportive relationships through their own actions. Being secretive, oppositional, or demonstrating unhealthy boundaries can cause damage to these relationships. Being open about their commitment to treatment, their struggles, and their needs and anxieties can help solidify or strengthen these relationships. Therefore, clients will need to view supervision through several lenses: What does supervision mean to the community? The client? The victim? Other potential victims? The supervision agent? Those involved in continuing treatment? This encourages clients to appreciate the various roles and responsibilities of supervision agents, and also prepares them for coping with supervision requirements and being effectively involved in their own supervision.

A fourth challenge is the potential lack of adaptive, healthy, and supportive relationships. Limited access to supportive relationship is related to many factors. Stigma can limit the development of new relationships or the continuation of old relationships. Client family members, for example, may not want to face others' judgments or hostility when they knowingly welcome back a family member who engaged in problematic sexual behavior. Those who learn of a client's sex offending history may be nervous about engaging in a new friendship, offering an employment opportunity, or considering a romantic partnership. Lack of social support also results from factors related to the offender's lifestyle, such as limited employment or residential opportunities, lengthy periods of incarceration or institutionalization (isolating him or her from community supports), or learned dependence on institutional and supervisory agents. Other characteristics common in a sex offender population may be similarly limiting, such as mental illness, poor social skills, intimacy deficits, illicit substance use, impulsivity, or continued problems with healthy boundaries. And finally, we have to face the reality that not all individuals in a client's life are healthy and supportive. They may come from abusive backgrounds or maintain contact with friends and family members who are sources of interpersonal dysregulation and negative reinforcement and modeling. These are pertinent issues for discussion in Module 9, when clients describe persons who represent adaptive and maladaptive coping.

With SOS, treatment providers can facilitate building and maintaining healthy boundaries (Module 7) and repairing supportive relationships that were damaged by the client's sexual behavior (Module 8). Treatment providers will need to help clients balance the difficulties of establishing and maintaining adaptive and supportive relationships with the benefits of having such relationships. Helping clients recognize differences between healthy and unhealthy relationships, healthy boundaries with others, and strategies for managing relationship conflict or discord, can help them manage these challenges. In terms of interpersonal dysregulation, clients can use their adaptive interpersonal strategies to help them cope with isolation, unhealthy relationships, or conflict in their relationships.

Another challenge, though certainly not the last they will face during the process of community reintegration, is what they and others expect. They will face anxiety, suspicion, fear, guilt, and intense doubt. These emotions and experiences come from themselves and others in the community. This will be dysregulating, and they will need to think about skills that will help cope ahead and in the moment. Also, clients will have to deal with the "perfection" myth, that they will be perfect after completing treatment and will no longer be at risk of committing sexual offenses or engaging in any maladaptive behaviors. It is fairly common throughout treatment for clients to indicate that their goal is to "never do it again," or that the outcome of treatment is to be "cured." A goal of SOS is to help clients monitor and manage their urges and maladaptive behaviors, so that we never truly expect clients to be finished. And while many clients do desist from offending, for higher risk offenders, their ability to desist is the result of careful practice and considerable effort. Even so, they do not reach "perfection." Treatment providers will need to carefully watch for this perfection myth in the development of an aftercare plan. Including occupational and educational opportunities, family support, other available supports, and continued struggles with dysregulation and intense behavioral urges will help clients adopt a more balanced view of community reintegration.

FACING VICTIMS

In Module 8 clients discussed acceptance and forgiveness. These discussions addressed their own feelings of guilt and shame, experiences of victims, and self-criticism and self-judgment. While it was noted that clients may never have the opportunity to speak with their victims, or to resolve their emotions within the context of victim relationships, they were encouraged to repair damage that they had caused to the community and others. And while we want clients to accept the reality that they may never see their victims again, or that victim contact is inadvisable, there are situations in which they do have continued contact with victims, primarily (though not exclusively) during the family reunification and community reintegration process.

People often return to the same or similar environment from which they came following incarceration, hospitalization, or residential treatment. Under these circumstances, they are likely to happen upon prior victims or the friends and family members of those victims. Clients' expectations regarding these encounters may vary widely. Some will want complete avoidance, hoping not to see victims at all or planning to ignore victims and their family members. They will expect hostility, anger, resentment, or fear. Others may desire such contact for the purpose of making amends, apologizing, or seeking forgiveness. They may also expect anger, resentment, or blame, but they will also harbor the belief that their apology will initiate acceptance and forgiveness. Of greater concern are those who expect that their meetings with victims will be meaningless and detached. They may be surprised to find that victims have emotional reactions to seeing the perpetrator in their environment again, and they may not understand the depth and intensity of victims' emotional experiences. Such clients may feel entitled to move on with their lives without "interference" from victims, and they may generally have a limited ability to appreciate the impact of their behaviors on others.

Regardless of how they view their victims or what they expect from them, treatment providers and clients must generate ideas as to how to respond to such encounters. Depending on supervision requirements, there may be specific sanctions or rules about contact with victims, and these should be strictly followed. Clients may need education about these rules and the consequences for violating such rules. When there are no set restrictions, clients need to consider how the victim may feel, and the potential impact of such contact, whether incidental or more extensive, on the victim. Clients should consider the potential for victims' shock, fear, anger, shame, or other possible emotions, and should think about what the victim may want. Ultimately, clients will need to cope with victim encounters in a skillful and effective way. Helpful strategies for doing this include recognizing their own and others' boundaries, examining their reasons for wanting to seek out or speak with victims, and practicing or at least identifying skills ahead of time.

In the discussions of victimization in Modules 2 and 8, treatment providers may also find it useful to discuss victim impact research with clients. Sexual assault and abuse have individualized effects on victims. Offenders have usually been taught that victims are permanently and irrevocably damaged by sexual victimization, and that these crimes leave the person scarred and incapable of functioning normally. It is true that many victims carry negative effects of their victimization for much of their lives, but believing that it has permanently ruined them is likely an exaggeration for most victims. Most empirical research suggests a more moderate impact—the long-term effects of sexual victimization vary greatly depending on characteristics of the victim and situational factors idiosyncratic to their abuse experiences. Offenders may never be fully able to predict the impact of their sexual behaviors on their victims. Simply because one victim "handled it well" (as some clients have been known to say) does not mean that the next one will. Clients must learn to balance their understanding of the negative effects of sexual abuse with resilience factors that may allow their victims (and themselves, if they have a history of adverse childhood experiences) to survive and lead productive lives.

RISK MANAGEMENT: TREATMENT PROGRESS AND CONTINUED RISK

One of the first questions that treatment providers are asked about their clients is "How is he or she doing?" The answer will facilitate decisions regarding effective risk management for that particular client. In SOS, this means assessing how well the client understands his or her dysregulation, how this dysregulation relates to maladaptive behaviors (including those that are not sexual in nature), whether or not the client is able to effectively self-monitor these and other relevant states, how committed the client is to change, and how the client is doing with regards to building new, adaptive regulatory skills and practicing them in the moment. An in-depth understanding of these factors helps treatment providers answer questions regarding the client's progress, needed supports, and continued risk.

More specifically, however, treatment providers will need to describe progress in the context of dynamic risk factors identified through empirical research that predicts future sexual offending in known sexual offenders. Problems with self-regulation have been consistently identified as predictive of sexual recidivism, but there are many types of self-regulatory problems or deficits that contribute to this finding (Hanson & Morton-Bourgon, 2004). As noted in Chapter 2, a number of well-studied dynamic risk factors can be conceptualized in the context of dysregulation. For example, negative affect, anger, and loneliness are forms of emotional dysregulation predictive of increased risk (Hanson & Harris, 1998; Hanson et al., 2007; Hanson & Morton-Bourgon, 2004). (For a review of these factors, we refer readers to pp. 20–24 of this book.) Thus, treatment providers can continually assess a client's developing self-regulatory abilities and continued struggles with dysregulation as measures of dynamic risk.

In general, measures of dynamic risk for sexual recidivism heavily emphasize treatment participation and progress. Therefore, in addition to assessing client progress with regards to specific forms of dysregulation and self-regulatory deficits, treatment providers will also need to consider how willing, engaged, and committed clients have been to treatment over time. The risk assessment literature notes that common stereotypes associated with treatment progress, such as the belief that denial predicts risk, or that clients who deny or minimize offenses cannot make meaningful progress in treatment, are in fact not predictive of sexual risk. This finding is important since SOS holds the belief that clients may remain willing and committed to self-monitor important sources of dysregulation and to develop new skills, even if they struggle with openly and publicly acknowledging all aspects of their offending behaviors. However, individuals who show no recognition of the wrongness of their behaviors, or who deny any wrongdoing whatsoever, have not always made good progress in treatment and may still be at risk. They may deny or minimize because they lack insight (a risk factor). Also, remember that many clients who acknowledge their offenses still present with significant risk of sexual harm to others.

CHALLENGES WITH CONTINUING TREATMENT

Once clients have completed the activities, discussions, and adaptive skills practice associated with SOS, they will have other options for continuing treatment needs. Some clients can continue their work in SOS, revisiting their motivation and commitment to change, and then establishing newer, perhaps more complex, treatment goals related to their maladaptive sexual behaviors. This course is especially appropriate when clients primarily focused on low-level goals, like attending and participating in treatment, or learning about healthy relationships and boundaries. Such clients may now be prepared to target other, more difficult goals related to their dysregulation and history of serious and pervasive sexual offending. Thus, if available, high-risk clients or those with complex treatment needs who have made a successful first pass through SOS could benefit from an additional round of treatment using this same approach. A repeat course would focus more specifically on behavioral chain analysis of continued maladaptive behaviors, more in-depth discussion of areas of dysregulation, and daily self-monitoring and skills practice.

For lower risk clients, those who have met many of their sex offender treatment goals, and those with complex needs related to other behavioral concerns (e.g., substance abuse, trauma, continued mental health needs), moving into other realms of treatment may further improve their lives and facilitate positive change. Transitioning into treatments that emphasize adaptive skills building and self-regulation, like DBT (Linehan, 1993), may be helpful for successful SOS clients who continue to struggle with emotion or mood regulation and relationship instability. Principles of illness management and recovery (Mueser et al., 2002; Substance Abuse and Mental Health Services Administration, 2010), a treatment emphasizing education and recovery planning, help those with prominent posttreatment mental health issues and medication compliance needs. Also, for clients with histories of trauma, cognitive-behavioral-based interventions are available to assist them with the emotional, cognitive, and interpersonal sequelae associated with those experiences. Not all clients will need specific mental health or relationship therapies following their course of sex offender treatment, nor will they always need to wait until treatment has been completed in order to accomplish these goals. These are considerations for clients who need extra support or continued therapy beyond their immediate need for sex offender treatment programming.

As clients transition from residential care or institutional settings into less restrictive or community placements, they will need case management services. This may be particularly true for clients with serious and persistent mental illness, intellectual or developmental disabilities, lengthy periods of institutionalization that have kept them segregated from community life, or high-risk offenders with many supervision needs. Through case management and other associated services (e.g., vocational rehabilitation), clients can continue self-monitoring and utilizing skills learned in SOS, and learn new skills to help them manage their lives in the community. Services designed to help clients maintain stability posttreatment, including employment, residency, and social support services; involvement with supervisory agents; and participation in treatment activities can be as stabilizing and supportive in some cases as treatment itself. It also provides a needed "check-in" service for many clients, who may continue to struggle with expressing their needs, soliciting help from the environment, fostering social support systems, and effectively managing stress.

Transitioning into other residential placements or community settings may result in a change in available treatment programming. Understandably, not all treatment providers or agencies offer the same types of sex offender treatment. A variety of treatment modalities and approaches are available, depending on the resources in the client's area. When clients move to another agency or into a community setting and are still in need of follow-up treatment services, it is necessary to evaluate available treatments and the client's amenability to each alternative. For clients who have done well with SOS, it is also important to help them translate that progress into another approach. To facilitate this transition, we return to several of the common forms of sex offender treatment methods introduced in Chapter 1 and how SOS clients would best transition into such approaches.

Cognitive-Behavioral Therapy

CBT views sex offending behaviors as the result of problematic or dysfunctional belief systems that support offending behaviors. Such cognitions are viewed as "wrong," and therapy is meant to change them. SOS, on the other hand, characterizes the antecedents of maladaptive sexual behavior as dysregulation with corresponding deficits in adaptive regulatory strategies. Clients in SOS have been taught that having dysregulated thoughts is sometimes "normal," though the intensity, expectations, and inability to cope with such thoughts have the potential to lead to maladaptive behavior.

These two approaches share an understanding of the role of reinforcement in the development of sexual interests, urges, and ultimately behavior. However, SOS purports to reinforce new skill sets and eventually replace more maladaptive behaviors with more adaptive ones, while CBT approaches aim to make the maladaptive behaviors less reinforcing and aversive instead.

Many CBT programs also contain elements related to social skills training and the development of problem-solving abilities. This emphasis provides important crossover with SOS, as clients can continue their focus on the development of healthy relationships, healthy boundaries, and learning valuable interpersonal skills. Some programs additionally address the issue of intimacy deficits and early developmental experiences characterized by trauma and maltreatment. These shared components may help ease the transition from one treatment approach to the other.

Relapse Prevention

Relapse prevention strives to educate clients about the deviancy of their thoughts, decisions, and difficulties with sexual urges, with an ultimate goal of helping them avoid situational risks and change thought patterns that are supportive of offending. In SOS, the goal is to identify some of these same factors, though as sources of dysregulation, and to teach specific skills to help clients tolerate, accept, or change these states. Reporting urges in SOS is viewed as a positive step toward effective self-monitoring—doing the same in relapse prevention may be labeled a "lapse" leading to potential relapse. Bridging this gulf between treatment theory, goals, and terminology will help clients maintain their success and be aware of differing treatment expectations.

Another important difference is in the approach and conceptualization of the client. Many relapse prevention programs have traditionally been fairly confrontational, with a goal of "breaking down" client defenses and eliciting an acknowledgment of responsibility. Full offense disclosure is a key element of the treatment. This is vastly different from the way SOS deals with disclosure, denial, and minimization, as well as how SOS treatment providers approach and conceptualize clients and their progress. Treatment providers should be fairly straightforward about these differences, as some clients may actually lose ground if they are unprepared for how they may be treated once they enter a different treatment modality.

Both approaches are similar though in that they intend to identify relevant precursors of offending and help clients develop a plan for dealing with them. Clients transitioning into relapse prevention can already demonstrate a reasonable understanding of these precursors, albeit within the context of dysregulation and self-regulatory deficits, and can communicate these with an intention of "coping ahead" and developing skills to address them in the moment.

Good Lives Model

SOS and the good lives model share a positive psychology view of sex offending behavior: clients are viewed as people capable of change through highlighting and fostering positive life goals. However, SOS accomplishes this end through identifying self-regulatory deficits and enhancing adaptive skills use in several domains. Therefore, clients who have already participated in SOS may struggle with a treatment that does not focus on self-monitoring dysregulation and reinforcing newly learned skills.

The basic approach, however, may be attractive to those who have participated in SOS, in that clients are viewed in a positive way, and that their strengths and capabilities are valued. Client–therapist interactions may also be similar, as highly confrontational and blaming methods are discouraged in both SOS and the Good Lives model. A crucial point, however, is that there have been concerns regarding the dissention between the good lives model and the RNR model, and SOS does emphasize the principles of risk, needs, and responsivity. So while both approaches endorse a positive and adaptational approach to improving clients' lives, they accomplish this in dissimilar ways and may differentially measure risk and progress in treatment.

Sexual Addiction Therapy/Sexual Abusers Anonymous

With sexual addition therapy, the emphasis is on abstinence (rather than harm reduction); avoidance of situations, thoughts, or urges consistent with sex offending behaviors; the idea that sexual offending is an out-of-control disease: and the view that some sexual urges or behaviors are considered to be treatment failure. It thus goes without saying that these etiological, conceptual, and philosophical elements are vastly divergent from those of SOS. Clients who intend to pursue such treatments will face significant challenges in making such a transition. The SOS philosophy that sexual urges, continued sexual relationships, and experiences of dysregulation are normative human experiences may be problematic in such a different treatment modality. There are those, however, who will find a different approach helpful after a limited course of treatment with SOS. Those who struggled with accepting and tolerating continued urges, for example, may find that this type of treatment gives them comfort; they may want to be free of such experiences. This largely depends on client preferences, their own views of sex offending behaviors, and their goals at the time of treatment.

CONCLUDING THOUGHTS

Treatment providers and clients both will be faced with many challenges as they move toward the completion of SOS and the client's transition into new settings. Taking steps toward family and community reintegration and making important decisions regarding continued treatment goals and approaches are all part of this process. Thinking about risk and risk management will involve collaboration between clients, treatment providers, and other agents throughout the course of treatment. Treatment providers can help clients work through these issues by understanding available options and resources, reviewing potential challenges, and highlighting client progress, risk issues, and continued needs.

APPENDICES

Client Aftercare Packet

Clients and treatment providers should think about the "end" of treatment, even as early as Module 1. Anticipating the completion of treatment will cue clients to develop a plan and know what they need as Module 10 nears. Whether clients go into the community or other residential placements, treatment providers can prepare them for aftercare services. In this appendix, we have listed materials and information that treatment providers should collect and give to clients to ease their transition and ensure continuity of care. Many of these materials are individualized to the client, and although we have provided references here for finding generic forms within the text, treatment providers and clients should develop a plan unique to each client's needs.

TREATMENT

- Copies of self-monitoring sheets (refer to sample self-monitoring sheets in Table 6.9)
- List of client's common forms of dysregulation
- List of adaptive skills (refer to pp. 276–280 of Chapter 13)
- List of maladaptive skills (refer to Form 14.1)
- Personal goals and strengths
- Signs or symptoms of worsening mental illness

RISK MANAGEMENT

- Name and contact information of supervisory agents (e.g., probation and parole officers, forensic management agents)
- Name and contact information of case manager
- Basic plan for coping in the community or another placement
- Plan for dealing with harassment and stigma
- Information for securing a job, residence, and continued treatment services (for sex offender treatment, mental illness, etc.)
- Jurisdictional and federal sex offender registration and notification requirements, and information about where the client needs to go to do this
- Any special restrictions, like prohibitions on alcohol use, victim contact, affiliation with other offenders, or certain job types

(cont.)

SUPPORT

- Information for health care and insurance coverage
- Medication refills
- Emergency information
- Supportive people who are models of adaptive skills use
- Benefits paperwork, if eligible for state or federal assistance
- Contact information for local support and service agencies (e.g., day programs, community assistance programs, residential and food support agencies)
- Vocational rehabilitation services
- Educational opportunities
- Spiritual or religious support groups
- Contact information of anticipated treatment providers
- Contact information of current treatment providers (if appropriate)
- A quick reference list or programmed cell phone list of immediate contacts

Additional Client Handouts

FORM B1

My Treatment Progress

My goals for this group are:

1. _____

2. _____

3. _____

Things I have learned in this group during Module _____:

About dysregulation: _____

_____

_____

_____

About my self-monitoring practice: _____

_____

_____

_____

About how my dysregulation affects my sexual behavior: _____

_____

_____

_____

(cont.)

About adaptive skills: _____

_____

_____

_____

Other things I have learned in this module: _____

_____

_____

How's my treatment progress?

1. How have my behaviors improved?

2. How am I meeting my goals?

3. What do I still need to learn?

How Do I Feel about Being in Sex Offender Treatment?

Everyone reacts differently when they think about being in treatment, whether they have been in treatment for a while or just a short time. Think about your own emotional reaction to being in this group. Circle the emotions below that best describe how you feel RIGHT NOW about being in a sex offender group.

Angry	Ashamed
Disappointed	Enthusiastic
Afraid	Hopeless
Resentful	Suspicious
Hostile	Nervous
Desperate	Safe
Curious	Confused
Relieved	Annoyed
Disinterested	Excited
Hopeful	Frustrated
Sad	Betrayed

References

Abracen, J., Looman, J., & Anderson, D. (2000). Alcohol and drug abuse in sexual and nonsexual violent offenders. *Sexual Abuse: A Journal of Research and Treatment, 12*(4), 263–274.

Ahlmeyer, S., Kleinsasser, D., Stoner, J., & Retzlaff, P. (2003). Psychopathology of incarcerated sex offenders. *Journal of Personality Disorders, 17*(4), 306–318.

American Psychiatric Association. (2000). *Diagnostic and statistical manual of mental disorders* (4th ed., text rev.). Washington, DC: Author.

Anderson, A. L. (2008). *Understanding the passage and use of sex offender laws: Assumptions vs. reality.* Atlanta: Association for the Treatment of Sexual Abusers.

Anderson, A. L., & Sample, L. L. (2008). Public awareness and action resulting from sex offender community notification laws. *Criminal Justice Policy Review, 19*(4), 371–396.

Andrews, D. A., Bonta, J., & Hoge, R. D. (1990). Classification for effective rehabilitation. *Criminal Justice and Behavior, 17*(1), 19–52.

Anestis, M. D., Selby, E. A., & Joiner, T. E. (2007). The role of urgency in maladaptive behaviors. *Behaviour Research and Therapy, 45*(12), 3018–3029.

Babchishin, K. M., Hanson, R. K., & Helmus, L. (2011). *The RRASOR, Static-99R, and Static-2002R all add incrementally to the prediction of recidivism among sex offenders* (User Report 2011-02). Ottawa, ON: Public Safety Canada.

Baumeister, R. F., Catanese, K. R., & Wallace, H. M. (2002). Conquest by force: A narcissistic reactance theory of rape and sexual coercion. *Review of General Psychology, 6*(1), 92–135.

Baumeister, R. F., & Vohs, K. D. (Eds.). (2004). *Handbook of self-regulation: Research, theory, and applications.* New York: Guilford Press.

Baumeister, R. F., & Vohs, K. D. (Eds.). (2010). *Handbook of self-regulation: Research, theory, and applications* (2nd ed.). New York: Guilford Press.

Beck, A. T., Rush, A. J., Shaw, B. F., & Emery, G. (1979). *Cognitive therapy of depression.* New York: Guilford Press.

333

Becker, J. V. (1988). The effects of child sexual abuse on adolescent sex offenders. In G. E. Wyatt & G. J. Powell (Eds.), *Lasting effects of child sexual abuse* (pp. 193–207). Newbury Park, CA: Sage.

Becker, J. V., & Stinson, J. D. (2011). Extending rehabilitative principles to violent sex offenders. In J. Dvoskin, J. L. Skeem, R. W. Novaco, & K. S. Douglas (Eds.), *Using social science to reduce violent offending* (pp. 223–243). New York: Oxford University Press.

Becker, J. V., Stinson, J. D., Tromp, S., & Messer, G. (2003). Characteristics of individuals petitioned for civil commitment. *International Journal of Offender Therapy and Comparative Criminology, 47*(2), 185–195.

Beech, A., & Fordham, A. S. (1997). Therapeutic climate of sexual offender treatment programs. *Sexual Abuse: A Journal of Research and Treatment, 9*(3), 219–237.

Beers, S. R., & DeBellis, M. D. (2002). Neuropsychological function in children with maltreatment-related posttraumatic stress disorder. *American Journal of Psychiatry, 159,* 483–486.

Bellack, A. S., Mueser, K. T., Gingerich, S., & Agresta, J. (2004). *Social skills training for schizophrenia: A step-by-step guide* (2nd ed.). New York: Guilford Press.

Blaske, D. M., Borduin, C. M., Henggeler, S. W., & Mann, B. J. (1989). Individual, family, and peer characteristics of adolescent sex offenders and assaultive offenders. *Developmental Psychology, 25*(5), 846–855.

Bloomquist, M. L. (2005). *Skills training for children with behavior problems: A parent and practitioner guidebook* (rev. ed.). New York: Guilford Press.

Blumenthal, S., Gudjonsson, G., & Burns, J. (1999). Cognitive distortions and blame attribution in sex offenders against adults and children. *Child Abuse and Neglect, 23*(2), 129–143.

Boer, D. P., Hart, S. D., Kropp, P. R., & Webster, C. D. (1997). *Manual for the Sexual Violence Risk–20: Professional guidelines for assessing risk of sexual violence.* Vancouver: British Columbia Institute Against Family Violence.

Bonta, J., & Andrews, D. A. (2007). *Risk–need–responsivity model for offender assessment and rehabilitation* (User Report 2007-06). Ottawa, ON: Public Safety Canada.

Bouffard, L. A. (2010). Exploring the utility of entitlement in understanding sexual aggression. *Journal of Criminal Justice, 38*(5), 870–879.

Bremner, J. D., Elzinga, B., Schmahl, C., & Vermetten, E. (2007). Structural and functional plasticity of the human brain in posttraumatic stress disorder. *Progress in Brain Research, 167,* 171–186.

Briere, J. (1995). *Trauma Symptom Inventory.* Odessa, FL: Psychological Assessment Resources.

Briere, J. (2001). *Detailed Assessment of Posttraumatic Symptoms (DAPS).* Odessa, FL: Psychological Assessment Resources.

Briggs, F., & Hawkins, R. M. F. (1996). A comparison of the childhood experiences of convicted male child molesters and men who were sexually abused in childhood and claimed to be non-offenders. *Child Abuse and Neglect, 20*(3), 221–233.

Briken, P., & Kafka, M. P. (2007). Pharmacological treatments for paraphilic patients and sex offenders. *Current Opinions in Psychiatry, 20,* 609–613.

Bumby, K. M. (1996). Assessing the cognitive distortions of child molesters and rapists: Development and validation of the MOLEST and RAPE scales. *Sexual Abuse: A Journal of Research and Treatment, 8*(1), 37–54.

Bushman, B. J., Bonacci, A. M., van Dijk, M., & Baumeister, R. F. (2003). Narcissism, sexual refusal, and aggression: Testing a narcissistic reactance model of sexual coercion. *Journal of Personality and Social Psychology 84*(5), 1027–1040.

Calkins, S. D. (2004). Early attachment processes and the development of emotional self-regulation. In R. F. Baumeister & K. D. Vohs (Eds.), *Handbook of self-regulation: Research, theory, and applications* (pp. 324–339). New York: Guilford Press.

Caputo, A. A., Frick, P. J., & Brodsky, S. L. (1999). Family violence and juvenile sex offending: The potential mediating role of psychopathic traits and negative attitudes toward women. *Criminal Justice and Behavior, 26,* 338–356.

Carnes, P. (1983). *Out of the shadows: Understanding sexual addiction.* Center City, MN: Hazelden.

Carr, E. G., Dunlap, G., Horner, R. H., Koegel, R. L., Turnbull, A. P., Wailor, W., et al. (2002). Positive behavior support: Evolution of an applied science. *Journal of Positive Behavior Interventions, 4*(1), 4–16.

Check, J. V., & Malamuth, N. M. (1983). Sex role stereotyping and reactions to depictions of stranger versus acquaintance rape. *Journal of Personality and Social Psychology, 45*(2), 344–356.

Cicchetti, D., Ganiban, J., & Barnett, D. (1991). Contributions from the study of high-risk populations to understanding the development of emotion regulation. In J. Garber & K. A. Dodge (Eds.), *The development of emotion regulation and dysregulation* (pp. 15–48). Cambridge, UK: Cambridge University Press.

Cole, P. M., Martin, S. E., & Dennis, T. A. (2004). Emotion regulation as a scientific construct: Methodological challenges and directions for child development research. *Child Development, 75*(2), 317–333.

Cortoni, F., & Marshall, W. L. (2001). Sex as a coping strategy and its relationship to juvenile sexual history and intimacy in sexual offenders. *Sexual Abuse: A Journal of Research and Treatment, 13*(1), 27–43.

Crossmaker, M. (1991). Behind locked doors—Institutional sexual abuse. *Sexuality and Disability, 9*(3), 201–219.

Davidson, R. J., Putnam, K. M., & Larson, C. L. (2000). Dysfunction in the neural circuitry of emotion regulation: A possible prelude to violence. *Science, 289,* 591–594.

Davison, S., & Taylor, P. J. (2001). Psychological distress and severity of personality disorder symptomatology in prisoners convicted of violent and sexual offenses. *Psychology, Crime, and Law, 7,* 263–274.

DiClemente, R. J., Hansen, W. B., & Ponton, L. E. (Eds.). (1996). *Handbook of adolescent health risk behavior.* New York: Plenum Press.

Dimeff, L. A. (2008). DBT validation principles and strategies. Retrieved from *http://behavioraltech.org/ol/details_validation.cfm.*

Dimeff, L. A., & Koerner, K. (Eds.). (2007). *DBT in clinical practice: Applications across disorders and settings.* New York: Guilford Press.

DonGiovanni, V. J., & Travia, T. (2007). *Sex offender treatment: A Pennsylvania civil commitment program.* Paper presented at the conference of the National Association of State Mental Health Program Directors, Forensic Division, San Antonio, TX.

Dvoskin, J., Skeem, J. L., Novaco, R. W., & Douglas, K. S. (Eds.). (2011). *Using social science to reduce violent offending.* New York: Oxford University Press.

Eisenberg, N., Fabes, R. A., Carlo, G., & Karbon, M. (1992). Emotional responsivity to others: Behavioral correlates and socialization antecedents. *New Directions for Child Development, 55,* 57–73.

Eisenberg, N., Fabes, R. A., Murphy, B., Karbon, M., Smith, M., & Maszk, P. (1996). The relations of children's dispositional empathy-related responding to their emotionality, regulation, and social functioning. *Developmental Psychology, 32*(2), 195–209.

Eisenberg, N., Smith, C. L., Sadovsky, A., & Spinrad, T. L. (2004). Effortful control: Relations with emotion regulation, adjustment, and socialization in childhood. In R. F. Baumeister & K. D. Vohs (Eds.), *Handbook of self-regulation: Research, theory, and applications* (pp. 259–282). New York: Guilford Press.

Epperson, D. L., Kaul, J. D., & Hesselton, D. (2005). *Minnesota Sex Offender Screening Tool, Revised (MnSOST-R): Development, performance, and recommended risk level cut scores.* St. Paul: Minnesota Department of Corrections.

Fehrenbach, P. A., Smith, W., Monastersky, C., & Deisher, R. W. (1986). Adolescent sexual offenders: Offender and offense characteristics. *American Journal of Orthopsychiatry, 56*(2), 225–233.

Firth, H., Balogh, R., Berney, T., Bretherton, K., Graham, S., & Whibley, S. (2001). Psychopathology of sexual abuse in young people with intellectual disability. *Journal of Intellectual Disability Research, 45*(3), 244–252.

Garland, R. J., & Dougher, M. J. (1992). Motivational intervention in the treatment of sex offenders. In W. R. Miller & S. Rollnick, *Motivational interviewing: Preparing people to change addictive behavior* (pp. 303–313). New York: Guilford Press.

Giltay, E. J., & Gooren, L. J. G. (2009). Potential side effects of androgen deprivation treatment in sex offenders. *Journal of the American Academy of Psychiatry and the Law, 37*(1), 53–58.

Glaser, B. (2011). Paternalism and the Good Lives Model of sex offender rehabilitation. *Sexual Abuse: A Journal of Research and Treatment, 23*(3), 329–345.

Gold, S. N., & Heffner, C. L. (1998). Sexual addiction: Many conceptions, minimal data. *Clinical Psychology Review, 18*(3), 367–381.

Goodyear-Brown, P., Fitzgerald, M. M., & Cohen, J. (2012). Trauma-focused cognitive-behavioral therapy. In P. Goodyear-Brown (Ed.), *Handbook of child sexual abuse: Identification, assessment, and treatment* (pp. 199–228). Hoboken, NJ: Wiley.

Graham, K. R. (1996). The childhood victimization of sex offenders: An underestimated issue. *International Journal of Offender Therapy and Comparative Criminology, 40*(3), 192–203.

Granic, I., & Patterson, G. R. (2006). Toward a comprehensive model of antisocial development: A dynamic systems approach. *Psychological Review, 113*(1), 101–131.

Guerino, P., & Beck, A. J. (2011). *Sexual victimization reported by adult correctional authorities, 2007–2008*. Washington, DC: U.S. Department of Justice.

Guidry, L. L., & Saleh, F. M. (2004). Clinical considerations of paraphilic sex offenders with comorbid psychiatric conditions. *Sexual Addiction and Compulsivity, 11*, 21–34.

Haapasalo, J., & Kankkonen, M. (1997). Self-reported childhood abuse among sex and violent offenders. *Archives of Sexual Behavior, 26*(4), 421–431.

Hanh, T. N. (2010). *You are here: Discovering the magic of the present moment*. Boston: Shambhala.

Hall, G. C. N., & Hirschman, R. (1991). Toward a theory of sexual aggression: A quadripartite model. *Journal of Consulting and Clinical Psychology, 59*, 62–669.

Hall, G. C. N., & Hirschman, R. (1992). Sexual aggression against children: A conceptual perspective of etiology. *Criminal Justice and Behavior, 19*, 8–23.

Hanish, L. D., Eisenberg, N., Fabes, F. A., Spinrad, R. L., Ryan, P., & Schmidt, S. (2004). The expression and regulation of negative emotions: Risk factors for young children's peer victimization. *Development and Psychopathology, 16*, 335–353.

Hanson, R. K. (1997). *The development of a brief actuarial risk scale for sexual offense recidivism* (User Report 97-04). Ottawa, ON: Department of the Solicitor General of Canada.

Hanson, R. K., Bourgon, G., Helmus, L., & Hodgson, S. (2009a). *A meta-analysis of the effectiveness of treatment for sexual offenders: Risk, need, and responsivity* (User Report 2009–01). Ottawa, ON: Public Safety Canada.

Hanson, R. K., Bourgon, G., Helmus, L., & Hodgson, S. (2009b). The principles of effective correctional treatment also apply to sexual offenders: A metaanalysis. *Criminal Justice and Behavior, 36*(9), 865–891.

Hanson, R. K., Gizzarelli, R., & Scott, H. (1994). The attitudes of incest offenders: Sexual entitlement and acceptance of sex with children. *Criminal Justice and Behavior, 21*(2), 187–202.

Hanson, R. K., & Harris, A. J. R. (1998). *Dynamic predictors of sexual recidivism*

(User Report 1998-1). Ottawa, ON: Department of the Solicitor General of Canada.

Hanson, R. K., Harris, A. J. R., Scott, T. L., & Helmus, L. (2007). *Assessing the risk of sexual offenders on community supervision: The Dynamic Supervision Project* (User Report 2007-05). Ottawa, ON: Public Safety Canada.

Hanson, R. K., & Morton-Bourgon, K. E. (2004). *Predictors of sexual recidivism: An updated meta-analysis* (User Report 2004-02). Ottawa, ON: Public Safety and Emergency Preparedness Canada.

Hanson, R. K., & Morton-Bourgon, K. E. (2005). The characteristics of persistent sexual offenders: A meta-analysis of recidivism studies. *Journal of Consulting and Clinical Psychology, 73*(6), 1154–1163.

Hanson, R. K., & Thornton, D. (2000). Improving risk assessments for sex offenders: A comparison of three actuarial scales. *Law and Human Behavior, 24*(1), 119–136.

Hanson, R. K., & Thornton, D. (2003). *Notes on the development of Static-2002.* (User Report 2003-01). Ottawa, ON: Department of the Solicitor General of Canada.

Happel, R. M., & Auffrey, J. J. (1995). Sex offender assessment: Interrupting the dance of denial. *American Journal of Forensic Psychology, 13*, 5–22.

Hare, R. D. (1991). *The Hare Psychopathy Checklist, Revised.* Toronto, ON: Multi-Health Systems.

Hare, R. D. (1999). *Without conscience: The disturbing world of the psychopaths among us.* New York: Guilford Press.

Harkins, L., & Beech, A. R. (2007). A review of the factors that can influence the effectiveness of sexual offender treatment: Risk, need, responsivity, and process issues. *Aggression and Violent Behavior, 12*(6), 615–627.

Hart, S. D., & Hare, R. D. (1997). Psychopathy: Assessment and association with criminal conduct. In D. M. Stoff, J. Breiling, & J. D. Maser (Eds.), *Handbook of antisocial behavior* (pp. 22–35). Hoboken, NJ: Wiley.

Hazlett, E. A., New, A. S., Newmark, R., Haznedar, M. M., Lo, J. N., Speiser, L. J., et al. (2005). Reduced anterior and posterior cingulated gray matter in borderline personality disorder. *Biological Psychiatry, 58*(8), 614–623.

Helmus, L., Thornton, D., Hanson, R. K., & Babchishin, K. M. (2011). *Assessing the risk of older sex offenders: Developing the Static-99R and Static-2002R* (User Report 2011-01). Ottawa, ON: Public Safety Canada.

Hendriks, J., & Bijleveld, C. C. J. H. (2004). Juvenile sexual delinquents: Contrasting child abusers with peer abusers. *Criminal Behavior and Mental Health, 14*(4), 238–250.

Henggeler, S. W., Schoenwald, S. K., Borduin, C. M., Rowland, M. D., & Cunningham, P. B. (1998). *Multisystemic treatment of antisocial behavior in children and adolescents.* New York: Guilford Press.

Herman, P. D., & Polivy, J. (2004). The self-regulation of eating: Theoretical and practical problems. In R. F. Baumeister & K. D. Vohs (Eds.), *Handbook of self-regulation* (pp. 492–508). New York: Guilford Press.

Hill, S. Y., Wang, S., Kostelnik, B., Carter, H., Holmes, B., McDermott, M., et al.

(2009). Disruption of orbitofrontal cortex laterality in offspring from multiplex alcohol dependence families. *Biological Psychiatry, 65*(2), 129–136.

Hirschi, T. (2004). Self-control and crime. In R. F. Baumeister & K. D. Vohs (Eds.), *Handbook of self-regulation* (pp. 537–552). New York: Guilford Press.

Hull, J. G., & Slone, L. B. (2004). Alcohol and self-regulation. In R. F. Baumeister & K. D. Vohs (Eds.), *Handbook of self-regulation* (pp. 466–491). New York: Guilford Press.

Izard, C. E. (1991). *The psychology of emotions.* New York: Plenum Press.

Izard, C. E., & Kobak, R. R. (1991). Emotions system functioning and emotion regulation. In J. Garber & K. A. Dodge (Eds.), *The development of emotion regulation and dysregulation* (pp. 303–321). Cambridge, UK: Cambridge University Press.

Jacques-Tiura, A. J., Abbey, A., Parkhill, M. R., & Zawacki, T. (2007). Why do some men misperceive women's intentions more frequently than others do?: An application of the confluence model. *Personality and Social Psychology Bulletin, 33*(11), 1467–1480.

Johnson, L., & Ward, T. (1996). Social cognition and sexual offending: A theoretical framework. *Sexual Abuse: A Journal of Research and Treatment, 8*(1), 55–80.

Jones, E. E., & Harris, V. A. (1967). The attribution of attitudes. *Journal of Experimental Social Psychology, 3,* 1–24.

Jonson-Reid, J., & Way, I. (2001). Adolescent sexual offenders: Incidence of childhood maltreatment, serious emotional disturbance, and prior offenses. *American Journal of Orthopsychiatry, 71*(1), 120–130.

Kafka, M. P., & Hennen, J. (2002). A DSM-IV Axis I co-morbidity study of males with paraphilias and paraphilia-related disorders. *Sexual Abuse: A Journal of Research and Treatment, 14*(4), 349–366.

Kobayashi, J., Sales, B. D., Becker, J. V., Figueredo, A. J., & Kaplan, M. S. (1995). Perceived parental deviance, parent–child bonding, child abuse, and child sexual aggression. *Sexual Abuse: A Journal of Research and Treatment, 7*(1), 25–44.

La Greca, A. M., Prinstein, M. J., & Fetter, M. D. (2001). Adolescent peer crowd affiliation: Linkages with health-risk behaviors and close friendships. *Journal of Pediatric Psychology, 26*(3), 131–143.

Lambrick, F., & Glaser, W. (2004). Sex offenders with an intellectual disability. *Sexual Abuse: A Journal of Research and Treatment, 16*(4), 381–392.

Langevin, R., & Lang, R. A. (1990). Substance abuse among sex offenders. *Annals of Sex Research, 3*(4), 397–424.

Langevin, R., Langevin, M., Curnoe, S., & Bain, J. (2006). Generational substance abuse among male sexual offenders and paraphilics. *Victims and Offenders, 1*(4), 395–409.

Langevin, R., Wright, P., & Handy, L. (1989). Characteristics of sex offenders who were sexually victimized as children. *Annals of Sex Research, 2*(3), 227–253.

Laws, D. R. (Ed.). (1989). *Relapse prevention with sex offenders.* New York: Guilford Press.

Laws, D. R., Hudson, S. M., & Ward, T. (2000). *Remaking relapse prevention with sex offenders: A sourcebook.* Thousand Oaks, CA: Sage.

Leary, M. R. (2004). The sociometer, self-esteem, and the regulation of interpersonal behavior. In R. F. Baumeister & K. D. Vohs (Eds.), *Handbook of self-regulation: Research, theory, and applications* (pp. 373–391). New York: Guilford Press.

Leue, A., Borchard, B., & Hoyer, J. (2004). Mental disorders in a forensic sample of sexual offenders. *European Psychiatry, 19*(3), 123–130.

Levenson, J. S. (2011). "But I didn't do it!": Ethical treatment of sex offenders in denial. *Sexual Abuse: A Journal of Research and Treatment, 23*(3), 346–364.

Levenson, J. S., & Cotter, L. P. (2005). The impact of sex offender residence restrictions: 1000 feet from danger or one step from absurd? *International Journal of Offender Therapy and Comparative Criminology, 49*(2), 168–178.

Lindsay, W. R. (2002). Research and literature on sex offenders with intellectual and developmental disabilities. *Journal of Intellectual Disability Research, 46*(Suppl. 1), 74–85.

Linehan, M. M. (1993). *Cognitive-behavioral treatment of borderline personality disorder.* New York: Guilford Press.

Linz, D. G., Donnerstein, E., & Penrod, S. (1988). Effects of long-term exposure to violent and sexually degrading depictions of women. *Journal of Personality and Social Psychology, 55,* 758–768.

Lochman, J. E. (1987). Self and peer perceptions and attributional biases of aggressive and nonaggressive boys in dyadic interactions. *Journal of Consulting and Clinical Psychology, 55,* 404–410.

Lösel, F., & Schmucker, M. (2005). The effectiveness of treatment for sexual offenders: A comprehensive meta-analysis. *Journal of Experimental Criminology, 1*(1), 117–146.

Luborsky, L., Auerbach, A. H., Chandler, M., Cohen, J., & Bachrach, H. M. (1971). Factors influencing the outcome of psychotherapy: A review of quantitative research. *Psychological Bulletin, 75*(3), 145–185.

Malamuth, N. M., & Check, J. V. P. (1981). The effects of mass media exposure on acceptance of violence against women: A field experiment. *Journal of Research in Personality, 15,* 436–446.

Malamuth, N. M., & Check, J. V. P. (1985). The effects of aggressive pornography on beliefs in rape myths: Individual differences. *Journal of Research in Personality, 19,* 299–320.

Malatesta-Magai, C. (1991). Development of emotion expression during infancy: General course and patterns of individual difference. In J. Garber & K. A. Dodge (Eds.), *The development of emotion regulation and dysregulation* (pp. 49–68). Cambridge, UK: Cambridge University Press.

Maletzky, B. M. (1991). The use of medroxyprogesterone acetate to assist in the treatment of sexual offenders. *Annals of Sex Research, 4,* 117–129.

Maletzky, B. M., Tolan, A., & McFarland, B. (2006). The Oregon Depo-Provera

Program: A five-year follow-up. *Sexual Abuse: A Journal of Research and Treatment, 18*, 303–316.

Mann, R. E. (2000). Managing resistance and rebellion in relapse prevention intervention. In R. D. Laws, S. M. Hudson, & T. Ward (Eds.), *Remaking relapse prevention with sex offenders: A sourcebook* (pp. 187–200). Thousand Oaks, CA: Sage.

Mann, R. E., Webster, S. D., Schofield, C., & Marshall, W. L. (2004). Approach versus avoidance goals in relapse prevention with sexual offenders. *Sexual Abuse: A Journal of Research and Treatment, 16*(1), 65–75.

Marques, J. K., Wiederanders, M., Day, D. M., Nelson, C., & Van Ommeren, A. (2005). Effects of a relapse prevention program on sexual recidivism: Final results from California's Sex Offender Treatment and Evaluation Project (SOTEP). *Sexual Abuse: A Journal of Research and Treatment, 17*(1), 79–107.

Marshall, W. L. (1989). Intimacy, loneliness, and sexual offenders. *Behaviour Research and Therapy, 27*(5), 491–504.

Marshall, W. L. (1993). The role of attachments, intimacy, and loneliness in the etiology and maintenance of sex offending. *Sexual and Marital Therapy, 8*(2), 109–121.

Marshall, W. L. (2005). Therapist style in sexual offender treatment: Influence on indices of change. *Sexual Abuse: A Journal of Research and Treatment, 17*(2), 109–116.

Marshall, W. L., Anderson, D., & Champagne, F. (1997). Self-esteem and its relationship to sex offending. *Psychology, Crime, and Law, 3*(3), 161–186.

Marshall, W. L., Anderson, D., & Fernandez, Y. (1999). *Cognitive behavioural treatment of sexual offenders.* New York: Wiley.

Marshall, W. L., Jones, R., Ward, T., Johnston, P., & Barbaree, H. E. (1991). Treatment outcome with sex offenders. *Clinical Psychology Review, 11*(4), 465–485.

Marshall, W. L., & Moulden, H. (2001). Hostility toward women and victim empathy in rapists. *Sexual Abuse: A Journal of Research and Treatment, 13*(4), 249–255.

Marshall, W. L., Thornton, D., Marshall, L. E., Fernandez, Y. M., & Mann, R. (2001). Treatment of sexual offenders who are in categorical denial: A pilot project. *Sexual Abuse: A Journal of Research and Treatment, 13*(3), 205–215.

Marshall, W. L., Ward, T., Mann, R. E., Moulden, H., Fernandez, Y. M., Serran, G., et al. (2005). Working positively with sexual offenders: Maximizing the effectiveness of treatment. *Journal of Interpersonal Violence, 20*(9), 1096–1114.

Masters, W. H., & Johnson, V. E. (1966). The sexual response cycle. In *Human sexual response* (pp. 3–8). Boston: Little, Brown, & Company.

Maughan, A., & Cicchetti, D. (2002). Impact of child maltreatment and interadult violence on children's emotion regulation abilities and socioemotional adjustment. *Child Development, 73*(5), 1525–1542.

McCabe, L. A., Cunningham, M., & Brooks-Gunn, J. (2004). The development of self-regulation in young children: Individual characteristics and environmental contexts. In R. F. Baumeister & K. D. Vohs (Eds.), *Handbook of self-regulation: Research, theory, and applications* (pp. 340–356). New York: Guilford Press.

McConaghy, N., Blaszczynski, A., & Kidson, W. (1988). Treatment of sex offenders with imaginal desensitization and/or medroxyprogesterone. *Acta Psychiatrica Scandinavica, 77,* 199–206.

McGrath, R. J. (2005). *Treatment Intervention and Progress Scale for Sexual Abusers with Intellectual Disabilities: Scoring manual.* Middlebury, VT: McGrath Psychological Services.

McGrath, R. J., & Cumming, G. F. (2003). *Sex Offender Treatment Needs and Progress Scale manual.* Middlebury, VT: McGrath Psychological Services.

McGrath, R. J., Cumming, G. F., Burchard, B. L., Zeoli, S., & Ellerby, L. (2010). *Current practices and emerging trends in sexual abuser management: The Safer Society 2009 North American Survey.* Brandon, VT: Safer Society Press.

McGrath, R. J., Hoke, S. E., & Vojtisek, J. E. (1998). Cognitive-behavioral treatment of sex offenders: A treatment comparison and long-term follow-up study. *Criminal Justice and Behavior, 25*(2), 203–225.

McGuire, R. J., Carlisle, J. M., & Young, B. G. (1964). Sexual deviations as conditioned behavior: A hypothesis. *Behaviour Research and Therapy, 2*(2–4), 185–190.

Messer, S. B., & Wampold, B. E. (2002). Let's face facts: Common factors are more potent than specific therapy ingredients. *Clinical Psychology: Science and Practice, 9*(1), 21–25.

Mihailides, S., Devilly, G. J., & Ward, T. (2004). Implicit cognitive distortions and sexual offending. *Sexual Abuse: A Journal of Research and Treatment, 16*(4), 333–350.

Miller, W. R., & Rollnick, S. (1992). *Motivational interviewing: Preparing people to change addictive behavior.* New York: Guilford Press.

Miller, W. R., & Rollnick, S. (2002). *Motivational interviewing* (2nd ed.): *Preparing people to change.* New York: Guilford Press.

Miller, W. R., & Rollnick, S. (2013). *Motivational interviewing* (3rd ed.). New York: Guilford Press.

Millon, T., & Davis, R. D. (1996). *Disorders of personality: DSM-IV and beyond* (2nd ed.). New York: Wiley.

Millon, T., Simonsen, E., Birket-Smith, M., & Davis, R. D. (Eds.). (1998). *Psychopathy: Antisocial, criminal, and violent behavior.* New York: Guilford Press.

Mills, J. F., Anderson, D., & Kroner, D. G. (2004). The antisocial attitudes and associates of sex offenders. *Criminal Behavior and Mental Health, 14*(2), 134–145.

Miner, M. H., Marques, J. K., Day, D. M., & Nelson, C. (1990). Impact of relapse prevention in treating sex offenders: Preliminary findings. *Sexual Abuse: A Journal of Research and Treatment, 3*(2), 165–185.

Miner, M. H., & Munns, R. (2005). Isolation and normlessness: Attitudinal comparisons of adolescent sex offenders, juvenile offenders, and nondelinquents. *International Journal of Offender Therapy and Comparative Criminology, 49*(5), 491–504.

Minzenberg, M. J., Fan, J., New, A. S., Tang, C. Y., & Siever, L. J. (2007). Fronto-limbic dysfunctiong in response to facial emotion in borderline personality disorder: An event-related fMRI study. *Psychiatry Research: Neuroimaging, 155*(3), 231–243.

Minzenberg, M. J., Fan, J., New, A. S., Tang, C. Y., & Siever, L. J. (2008). Fronto-limbic structural changes in borderline personality disorder. *Journal of Psychiatric Research, 42*(9), 727–733.

Moffitt, T. E. (1993). Adolescence-limited and life-course persistent antisocial behavior: A developmental taxonomy. *Psychological Review, 100*(4), 674–701.

Mueser, K. T., Corrigan, P. W., Hilton, D. W., Tanzman, B., Schaub, A., Gingerich, S., et al. (2002). Illness management and recovery: A review of the research. *Psychiatric Services, 53*, 1272–1284.

Nezu, C. M., Nezu, A. M., Dudek, J. A., Peacock, M. A., & Stoll, J. G. (2005). Social problem-solving correlates of sexual deviancy and aggression among adult child molesters. *Journal of Sexual Aggression, 11*(1), 27–36.

Patrick, C. J. (Ed.). (2007). *Handbook of psychopathy.* New York: Guilford Press.

Peugh, J., & Belenko, S. (2001). Examining the substance use patterns and treatment needs of incarcerated sex offenders. *Sexual Abuse: A Journal of Research and Treatment, 13*(3), 179–195.

Pithers, W. D., Marques, J. K., Gibat, C. C., & Marlatt, G. A. (1983). Relapse prevention with sexual agressiveness: A self-control model of treatment and maintenance of change. In J. G. Greer & I. R. Stuart (Eds.), *The sexual aggressor* (pp. 124–239). New York: Van Nostrand Reinhold.

Porter, S., Campbell, M. A., Woodworth, M., & Birt, A. R. (2001). A new psychological conceptualization of the sexual psychopath. In F. Columbus (Ed.), *Advances in psychology research* (Vol. 7, pp. 21–36). Huntington, NY: Nova Science.

Pritchard, C., & Bagley, C. (2001). Suicide and murder in child murderers and child sexual abusers. *Journal of Forensic Psychiatry, 12*(2), 269–286.

Pritchard, C., & King, E. (2005). Differential suicide rates in typologies of child sex offenders in a 6-year consecutive cohort of male suicides. *Archives of Suicide Research, 9*(1), 35–43.

Prochaska, J. O., & DiClemente, C. C. (1983). Stages and processes of self-change of smoking: Toward an integrative model of change. *Journal of Consulting and Clinical Psychology, 51*(3), 390–395.

Prochaska, J. O., DiClemente, C. C., & Norcross, J. C. (1992). In search of how people change: Applications to addictive behaviors. *American Psychologist, 47*(9), 1102–1114.

Quinsey, V. L., Harris, G. T., Rice, M. E., & Cormier, C. A. (1998). *Violent offenders: Appraising and managing risk.* Washington, DC: American Psychological Association.

Quinsey, V. L., Harris, G. T., Rice, M. E., & Lalumiere, M. L. (1993). Assessing treatment efficacy in outcome studies of sex offenders. *Journal of Interpersonal Violence, 8*(4), 512–523.

Quinsey, V. L., Khanna, A., & Malcolm, P. B. (1998). A retrospective evaluation of the regional treatment centre sex offender treatment program. *Journal of Interpersonal Violence, 13*(5), 621–644.

Raver, C. C. (2004). Placing emotional self-regulation in sociocultural and socio-economic contexts. *Child Development, 75,* 346–353.

Rice, M. E., & Harris, G. T. (2003). *What we know and don't know about treating adult sex dangerous offenders: Law, justice, and therapy* (pp. 101–118). Washington, DC: American Psychological Association.

Rice, M. E., Quinsey, V. L., & Harris, G. T. (1991). Sexual recidivism among child sexual offenders released from a maximum security psychiatric institution. *Journal of Consulting and Clinical Psychology, 59,* 381–386.

Rogers, R., & Dickey, R. (1991). Denial and minimization among sex offenders. *Sexual Abuse: A Journal of Research and Treatment, 4*(1), 49–63.

Ross, L. (1977). The intuitive psychologist and his shortcomings: Distortions in the attribution process. In L. Berkowitz (Ed.), *Advances in experimental social psychology* (Vol. 10, pp. 173–220). New York: Academic Press.

Rothbart, M. K., Ziaie, H., & O'Boyle, C. G. (1992). Self-regulation and emotion in infancy. *New Directions for Child Development, 55,* 7–23.

Ryan, R. M., Kuhl, J., & Deci, E. L. (1997). Nature and autonomy: An organizational view of social and neurobiological aspects of self-regulation in behavior and development. *Development and Psychopathology, 9,* 701–728.

Sarason, I. G., Johnson, J. H., & Siegel, J. M. (1978). Assessing the impact of the Life Experiences Survey. *Journal of Consulting and Clinical Psychology, 46,* 932–946.

Scaramella, L. V., & Leve, L. D. (2004). Clarifying parent–child reciprocities during early childhood: The early childhood coercion model. *Clinical Child and Family Psychology Review, 7*(2), 89–107.

Segal, Z. V., & Marshall, W. L. (1985). Heterosexual social skills in a population of rapists and child molesters. *Journal of Consulting and Clinical Psychology, 53*(1), 55–63.

Seghorn, T. K., Prentky, R. A., & Boucher, R. J. (1987). Childhood sexual abuse in the lives of sexually aggressive offenders. *Journal of the American Academy of Child and Adolescent Psychiatry, 26*(2), 262–267.

Seidman, B. T., Marshall, W. L., Hudson, S. M., & Robertson, P. J. (1994). An examination of intimacy and loneliness in sex offenders. *Journal of Interpersonal Violence, 9*(4), 518–534.

Serran, G., Fernandez, Y., Marshall, W. L., & Mann, R. E. (2003). Process issues in treatment: Application to sex offender programs. *Professional Psychology: Research and Practice, 34*(4), 368–374.

Shapiro, S. L., & Carlson, L. E. (2009). *The art and science of mindfulness: Integrating mindfulness into psychology and the helping professions.* Washington, DC: American Psychological Association.

Shaw, D. S., Owens, E. B., Giovannelli, J., & Winslow, E. B. (2001). Infant and toddler pathways leading to early externalizing disorders. *Journal of the American Academy of Child and Adolescent Psychiatry, 40*(1), 36–43.

Siegle, G. J. (2007). Brain mechanisms of borderline personality disorder at the intersection of cognition, emotion, and the clinic. *American Journal of Psychiatry, 164*(12), 1776–1779.

Smallbone, S. W., & Milne, L. (2000). Associations between trait anger and aggression used in the commission of sexual offenses. *International Journal of Offender Therapy and Comparative Criminology, 44*, 606–617.

Smallbone, S., & Wortley, R. K. (2004). Criminal diversity and paraphilic interests among adult males convicted of sexual offenses against children. *International Journal of Offender Therapy and Comparative Criminology, 48*(2), 175–188.

Smith, A. D., & Taylor, P. J. (1999). Serious sex offending against women by men with schizophrenia: Relationship of illness and psychotic symptoms to offending. *British Journal of Psychiatry, 174*, 233–237.

Stinson, J. D., & Becker, J. V. (2010, October). *Safe Offender Strategies: Pilot data and outcomes from a new manualized treatment approach.* Poster presentation at the meeting of the Association for the Treatment of Sexual Abusers, Phoenix, AZ.

Stinson, J. D., & Becker, J. V. (2011). Sexual offenders with serious mental illness: Prevention, risk, and clinical concerns. *International Journal of Law and Psychiatry, 34*(3), 239–245.

Stinson, J. D., Becker, J. V., & Sales, B. D. (2008). Self-regulation and the etiology of sexual deviance: Evaluating causal theory. *Violence and Victims, 23*(1), 35–52.

Stinson, J. D., & Gonsalves, V. (2011, November). *Suicide and self-harm behaviors in a psychiatric sex offender sample.* Poster presentation at the meeting of the Association for the Treatment of Sexual Abusers, Toronto, Ontario, Canada.

Stinson, J. D., Robbins, S. B., & Crow, W. C. (2011). Self-regulatory deficits as predictors of sexual, aggressive, and self-harm behaviors in a psychiatric sex offender population. *Criminal Justice and Behavior, 38*(9), 885–895.

Stinson, J. D., Sales, B. D., & Becker, J. V. (2008). *Sex offending: Causal theories to inform research, prevention, and treatment.* Washington, DC: American Psychological Association.

Substance Abuse and Mental Health Services Administration. (2010). *Illness management and recovery evidence-based practices kit* (Publication SMA09-4463). Retrieved from *http://store.samhsa.gov/product/SMA09–4463.*

Tomkins, S. S. (1962). *Affect imagery consciousness: Vol. I. The positive affects.* London: Tavistock.

Tomkins, S. S. (1963). *Affect imagery consciousness: Vol. II. The negative affects.* London: Tavistock.

Tomkins, S. S. (1991). *Affect imagery consciousness: Vol. III. The negative affects: Anger and fear.* New York: Springer.

Veneziano, C., Veneziano, L., & LeGrand, S. (2000). The relationship between adolescent sex offender behaviors and victim characteristics with prior victimization. *Journal of Interpersonal Violence, 15*(4), 363–374.

Vess, J., Murphy, C., & Arkowitz, S. (2004). Clinical and demographic differences between sexually violent predators and other commitment types in a state forensic hospital. *Journal of Forensic Psychiatry and Psychology, 15*(4), 669–681.

Vohs, K. D., & Ciarocco, N. J. (2004). Interpersonal functioning requires self-regulation. In R. F. Baumeister & K. D. Vohs (Eds.), *Handbook of self-regulation: Research, theory, and applications* (pp. 392–407). New York: Guilford Press.

Walters, G. D. (1995). The Psychological Inventory of Criminal Thinking Styles, Part I: Reliability and preliminary validity. *Criminal Justice and Behavior, 22*(3), 307–325.

Walters, G. D. (2002). The Psychological Inventory of Criminal Thinking Styles (PICTS): A review and meta-analysis. *Assessment, 9*(3), 278–291.

Ward, T. (2000). Sexual offenders' cognitive distortions as implicit theories. *Aggression and Violent Behavior, 5*(5), 491–507.

Ward, T., & Brown, M. (2004). The Good Lives Model and conceptual issues in offender rehabilitation. *Psychology, Crime, and Law, 10*(3), 243–257.

Ward, T., Fon, C., Hudson, S. M., & McCormack, J. (1998). A descriptive model of dysfunctional cognitions in child molesters. *Journal of Interpersonal Violence, 13*(1), 129–155.

Ward, T., & Gannon, T. A. (2006). Rehabilitation, etiology, and self-regulation: The comprehensive Good Lives Model of treatment for sexual offenders. *Aggression and Violent Behavior, 11*(1), 77–94.

Ward, T., Hudson, S. M., Johnston, L., & Marshall, W. L. (1997). Cognitive distortions in sex offenders: An integrative review. *Clinical Psychology Review, 17*(5), 479–507.

Ward, T., Hudson, S. M., & Keenan, T. (1998). A self-regulation model of the sexual offense process. *Sexual Abuse: A Journal of Research and Treatment, 10*(2), 141–157.

Ward, T., & Keenan, T. (1999). Child molesters' implicit theories. *Journal of Interpersonal Violence, 14*(8), 821–838.

Ward, T., & Mann, R. E. (2004). Good lives and the rehabilitation of offenders: A positive approach to sex offender treatment. In P. A. Linley & S. Joseph (Eds.), *Positive psychology in practice* (pp. 598–616). Hoboken, NJ: Wiley.

Ward, T., Mann, R. E., & Gannon, T. A. (2007). The Good Lives Model of offender rehabilitation: Clinical implications. *Aggression and Violent Behavior, 12*(1), 87–107.

Ward, T., & Siegert, R. J. (2002). Toward a comprehensive theory of child sexual abuse: A theory knitting perspective. *Psychology, Crime, and Law, 8*, 319–351.

Ward, T., & Stewart, C. A. (2003a). Good lives and the rehabilitation of sexual offenders. In T. Ward, D. R. Laws, & S. M. Hudson (Eds.), *Sexual deviance: Issues and controversies* (pp. 21–44). Thousand Oaks, CA: Sage.

Ward, T., & Stewart, C. A. (2003b). The treatment of sex offenders: Risk management and good lives. *Professional Psychology: Research and Practice, 34,* 353–360.

Weinrott, M. R., & Saylor, M. (1991). Self-report of crimes committed by sex offenders. *Journal of Interpersonal Violence, 6*(3), 286–300.

Whiteside, S. P., & Lynum, D. R. (2001). The five-factor model and impulsivity: Using a structural model of personality to understand impulsivity. *Personality and Individual Differences, 30*(4), 669–689.

Worling, J. R. (1995). Sexual abuse histories of adolescent male sex offenders: Differences on the basis of the age and gender of their victims. *Journal of Abnormal Psychology, 104*(4), 610–613.

Yates, P. M., Prescott, D., & Ward, T. (2010). *Applying the Good Lives and Self-Regulation Models to sex offender treatment: A practical guide for clinicians.* Brandon, VT: Safer Society Press.

Yochelson, S., & Samenow, S. E. (1976). *The criminal personality: Vol. 1. A profile for change.* New York: Jason Aronson.

Zgourides, G., Monto, M., & Harris, R. (1997). Correlates of adolescent male sexual offense: Prior adult sexual contact, sexual attitudes, and use of sexually explicit materials. *International Journal of Offender Therapy and Comparative Criminology, 41*(3), 272–283.

Index